MOSBY'S
COMPREHENSIVE REVIEW
of RADIOGRAPHY
THE COMPLETE STUDY GUIDE AND CAREER PLANNER

Sixth Edition

MOSBY'S COMPREHENSIVE REVIEW
of RADIOGRAPHY

THE COMPLETE STUDY GUIDE AND CAREER PLANNER

Sixth Edition

WILLIAM J. CALLAWAY, MA, RT(R)

Director, Associate Degree Radiography Program
Academic Services Division
Lincoln Land Community College
Springfield, Illinois

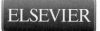

ELSEVIER
MOSBY

3251 Riverport Lane
St. Louis, Missouri 63043

MOSBY'S COMPREHENSIVE REVIEW OF RADIOGRAPHY:
THE COMPLETE STUDY GUIDE AND CAREER PLANNER

ISBN: 978-0-323-08078-1

Notices

Knowledge and best practice in this field are constantly changing. As new research and experience
broaden our understanding, changes in research methods, professional practices, or medical treatment
may become necessary.

Practitioners and researchers must always rely on their own experience and knowledge in evaluating
and using any information, methods, compounds, or experiments described herein. In using such
information or methods they should be mindful of their own safety and the safety of others, including
parties for whom they have a professional responsibility.

With respect to any drug or pharmaceutical products identified, readers are advised to check the
most current information provided (i) on procedures featured or (ii) by the manufacturer of each
product to be administered, to verify the recommended dose or formula, the method and duration of
administration, and contraindications. It is the responsibility of practitioners, relying on their own
experience and knowledge of their patients, to make diagnoses, to determine dosages and the best
treatment for each individual patient, and to take all appropriate safety precautions.

To the fullest extent of the law, neither the Publisher nor the authors, contributors, or editors, assume
any liability for any injury and/or damage to persons or property as a matter of products liability,
negligence or otherwise, or from any use or operation of any methods, products, instructions, or ideas
contained in the material herein.

Library of Congress Cataloging-in-Publication Data

Callaway, William J. (William Joseph), 1951-
  Mosby's comprehensive review of radiography : the complete study guide and career planner / William J.
Callaway. – 6th ed.
    p. ; cm.
  Comprehensive review of radiography
  Radiography
  Includes bibliographical references and index.
  ISBN 978-0-323-08078-1 (pbk. : alk. paper)
  I. Title. II. Title: Comprehensive review of radiography. III. Title: Radiography.
  [DNLM: 1. Technology, Radiologic–Examination Questions. 2. Radiography–Examination Questions.
3. Vocational Guidance–Examination Questions. WN 18.2]
  616.07′572076–dc23

                                                          2011048775

Content Strategy Director: Jeanne Olson
Associate Content Development Specialist: Amy Whittier
Publishing Services Managers: Julie Eddy and Hemamalini Rajendrababu
Project Managers: Janine Waters and Srikumar Narayanan
Designer: Ashley Eberts

Printed in the United States of America

Last digit is the print number: 9 8 7 6 5 4 3 2 1

William J. Callaway, MA, RT(R), has been involved in radiography education for more than 30 years. He has directed both collegiate associate degree and hospital-sponsored programs, as well as taught the subjects covered in this text. He is coauthor of *Introduction to Radiologic Technology,* also published by Elsevier, and has had writings published in state and national radiologic technology journals. He has also coauthored a quality customer service guide for radiology.

Mr. Callaway has an extensive background in staff development and has served as a management and quality service consultant for health care institutions all over the United States.

He is widely known for his *Key Points Presentations* for students, educators, and practicing technologists at international, national, state, and local radiologic technology meetings. He has given more than 500 of his *Key Points Presentations,* which include "A Fresh Perspective on Patient Care," "I'd Rather Die Than Give a Presentation," "Practical Physics for the Radiographer (and You Thought Physics Had to Be Boring!)," "Preparing for the Certification Exam", and "Finding and Keeping Your Dream Job."

To our family's next generation, our grandchildren:
Alex, Kailin, Mariah, Jacob, Mikella, Makenna,
Troy, Madalyn, and those yet to arrive

Angie Anderson, MA, RT (R) (CT), (QM)
Director, Radiography Program
Prince George's Community College
Largo, Maryland

Alberto Bello, MEd, RT(R), (CV)
Program Director, Radiologic
　Technology
Danville Area Community College
Danville, Illinois

Karen Callaway, MA, SPHR
Vice-President, Human Resources
　in the Healthcare Industry
H.D. Smith
Springfield, Illinois

Dianne Castor, RSRT(R)
Retired Radiologic Science Program
　Director
Retired College of Coastal Georgia
Brunswick, Georgia

Andrea Cornuelle, MS, RT(R)
Professor, Radiologic Technology
Northern Kentucky University
Highland Heights, Kentucky

Kenneth W. Delbow, RT(R)
Course Supervisor, Diagnostic
　Imaging Apprentice (Phase II)

United States Air Force Academy
Colorado Springs, Colorado

Sherry Floerchinger, MA, RT(N) (QM)
Program Director, Radiography
　Department
Dixie State College of Utah
Saint George, Utah

Joe Garza, MS, RT(R)
Professor, Radiologic Science
Lone Star College-Montgomery
Conroe, Texas

Eugene Hasson, MS RT(R)
Program Director, Medical Imaging
Charles Drew University of
　Medicine and Science
Los Angeles, California

Carol Howard, MHSc, RT(R)(MR)
Program Director, Radiography
　Department
Randolph Community College
Asheboro, North Carolina

Terra Lage, BSRS, RT(R)
Instructor
Allen College
Waterloo, Iowa

Tricia Leggett, DHEd, RT(R) (QM)
Program Director, Radiologic
　Technology
Associate Professor
Zane State College
Zanesville, Ohio

Mary Ellen Newton, MSM, RT(R)(M)
Program Director, School of
　Radiography
Saint Francis School of
　Resurrection, Resurrection
　Healthcare
Evanston, Illinois

Theresa Roberts, MHS, RT(R) (MR)
Program Director, Radiology
Keiser University
Melbourne, Florida

Robert Slothus, MS, RT(R)
Associate Professor
Pennsylvania College of Technology
Williamsport, Pennsylvania

Nathan Stallings, MS, BT(R)
Department Chair, Radiologic
　Technology
Tyler Junior College
Tyler Texas

CONTENT AND ORGANIZATION

Mosby's Comprehensive Review of Radiography is designed for students as a study guide throughout their radiography education and as a review book as they prepare to take the Registry examination.

Part One begins right where students need to begin: guiding them through an assessment of their study skills and time management, both critical to success in the radiography program and reviewing. The complete topic outline of the radiography exam administered by the American Registry of Radiologic Technologists (ARRT) is provided to help students visualize the breadth of information they need to master. Tips on answering multiple-choice questions ensure that students will be able to manage the styles of questions they will encounter on the ARRT exam.

The highlight of Part One is a comprehensive review, in outline form, of the five major content areas covered on the ARRT exam in radiography. Each content review is followed by a set of 100 questions related specifically to that topic. After students have reviewed all five subject areas, they are ready to take the three 200-question challenge tests in Chapter 7. All of the questions are written in formats used by the ARRT. Answers and rationales for the review questions and challenge tests are provided in Appendix A.

To prepare students to master the material and be fully prepared for the Registry exam, the Evolve website that accompanies the text provides hundreds of additional questions taken right from the Registry exam content outline and written in formats used by the ARRT.

Unlike other review books, *Mosby's Comprehensive Review of Radiography* also serves students as a career planner. Part Two, Career Planning, provides students the opportunity to inventory their interests and set goals for professional development. It gives suggestions for satisfying professional continuing education requirements. Valuable information and resources on radiologic specialties and academic degrees are presented to further assist students with career planning. Part Two also offers examples of real resumes and cover letters, as well as important information and tips on interviewing. To further ease the transition into the healthcare workplace, this part describes employer expectations in detail. No other book provides all of this valuable information to help students make the transition to their careers as practicing radiographers.

NEW CONTENT AND FEATURES

This new edition is written to the latest radiography exam content specifications used by the ARRT effective January 1, 2012, making this the most up-to-date review book

available. Coverage of digital imaging, included in previous editions, has been expanded to reflect its importance on the certification exam. Of particular significance is the inclusion of numerous images from the Online Digital Imaging Academy (ODIA) to greatly enhance the coverage of digital imaging. Used with permission of the ARRT, these images have been used extensively to educate practicing radiographers. This is the first text that makes them available to radiography students.

One of the most popular features of this study guide is the material available on the Evolve website. Those questions can be accessed anywhere the student has Internet access, whether at home or in the palm of their hand. These questions are designed to simulate the computer-based exam administered by the ARRT. In tutorial mode, students may answer hundreds of multiple-choice questions for each ARRT content area. Rationales and study tips provide immediate feedback, and questions can be bookmarked for later reference. In test mode a virtually unlimited number of randomly generated, 200-question multiple-choice exams are available.

These resources make this the premier radiography review book and study guide, all in one product.

HOW TO USE THIS BOOK

This study guide is particularly effective for use throughout the radiography program. The content outline may be referenced as a supplement to most courses in the radiography curriculum. The study questions are excellent aids to learning in all of the subject areas.

As a review book, this text provides a logical, well-thought-out approach to preparing for the Registry exam. The content outline, so effective throughout the educational program, is particularly appreciated at review time. All content that may be tested is presented in a format that is easy to use and understand. Because I teach these subjects, my approach to the reader is the same as if class were being held each time the book is opened.

Care has been taken to create questions that cover the primary information taught in radiography programs and are therefore relevant to the ARRT exam. This philosophy, coupled with the outline form, helps students make optimal use of study time. Explanations of answers are written in the same style I use in my own classes. This student-friendly approach will be appreciated for its direct communication to the users of this text. Students who have difficulty understanding an answer are advised to return to the study guide for additional review. This text should not be viewed as a substitute for a textbook or coursework that comprehensively covers a subject area.

A final note on the use of this guide: Variation in the details of test content occurs across certification exams. Therefore, inclusion of specific information in this guide does not guarantee that it will be tested, and the exclusion of certain information is not meant to suggest its absence from the exam. The ARRT does not review, evaluate, or endorse publications. Permission to reproduce ARRT copyrighted materials within this publication should not be construed as an endorsement of the publication by the ARRT.

ACKNOWLEDGMENTS

Elsevier once again assembled a great team to bring this project to fruition. Special acknowledgment goes to Jeanne Olson for her leadership and enthusiastic support of this text. Amy Whittier provided expert editing, as well as guiding manuscript development throughout this entire project. Jan Waters moved the project towards completion by providing copyedited chapters in a timely and workable manner. Given the talents of the entire Elsevier staff, any errors or omissions from this book are solely mine.

I extend my thanks to the hundreds of educators and thousands of students who have used this text and given it their overwhelming support. Their positive comments and suggestions have been incorporated and make it better than ever. I express my sincere appreciation to the reviewers for going over this text line by line and question by question.

Very special recognition goes to my family, for their love and support of my professional endeavors, from speaking to writing. Thanks to my wife, Karen; our children Amy, Adam, Cara, David, and Kim; and our grandchildren Alex, Kailin, Mariah, Jacob, Mikella, Makenna, Troy, and Madalyn.

William J. Callaway

CONTENTS

PART I

Review and Study Guide

Preparation for Review

The future belongs to those who believe in the beauty of their dreams.

WELCOME TO YOUR STUDY GUIDE AND CAREER PLANNER!

Congratulations on acquiring the most complete study guide available to prepare for radiography classes throughout the educational program and to master the radiography certification examination. This student-friendly guide, coupled with your commitment to excellence and management of study time, will take you on a journey culminating in the achievement of your goals.

By reviewing the major subject areas contained in Part One, "Review and Study Guide," of this book, answering and studying the exam questions in the text and the online resource, and understanding the skills involved in various areas of radiography, you will be well on the way to achieving the goal of excelling in class and passing the radiography examination.

Passing the courses and the examination is only one of several steps in building your new career, however. As you look toward graduation, you are probably contemplating your transition into the work environment or considering further education. In addition to preparing you thoroughly for the exam, this book helps you develop your career goals. In Part Two, "Career Planning," you will have an opportunity to describe the events that have been rewarding and motivating during your education. This activity will enable you to set goals for establishing your practice of medical radiography and to plan for either immediate employment or continued education.

The most important tools used during the transition into the workforce are the resume and the interview, which are covered in Chapters 9 and 10 to prepare you thoroughly for marketing yourself in today's ever-changing health care environment. So that you may be fully aware of your role as an entry-level radiographer, Chapter 11 is dedicated to helping you anticipate on-the-job expectations for your first postgraduate position. The competitive, and at times chaotic, nature of health care delivery requires that you understand these expectations well as you prepare your first resume or have your first interview. This information is presented to ease your transition from student to entry-level radiographer.

Because the American Registry of Radiologic Technologists (ARRT) requires proof of continuing education for recertification, this important topic is included in Chapter 8, "Career Paths." Chapter 8 also addresses advanced-level examinations, academic degrees, and many options available to you as you plan your professional career.

If you are using this text as a program-long study guide, you will want to become familiar with Chapters 2 through 6 quickly. These chapters may be used as a supplement to the text you have for each course in your program. They are effective for a quick overview of subject matter and a review before a quiz or test. Whether using this guide throughout the program or as a Registry review, be sure to take time with the rest of Chapter 1. A key to success in your classes and the radiography exam is prioritizing and managing your time. Investing time now in Chapter 1 will pay big dividends as your review process moves along in an organized fashion.

PRIORITIZING SUBJECTS AND SCHEDULING STUDY TIME

DETERMINING THE LENGTH OF REVIEW

As you begin the task of planning your review for the ARRT examination, take a few moments to think about how you want to go about the review process. It is never too early to begin studying for the exam. Because you may take the exam immediately after graduation, you will probably want to begin your review very soon. If you are also using this text as a study guide throughout your radiography program, you are already becoming familiar with the topics and use of the book. Most radiography educators recommend that students begin a well-thought-out review approximately 6 months before taking the exam. Not all students require that much time to prepare adequately; students who are better able to retain the material they have already learned may complete their review more quickly.

Another factor that can greatly influence how far in advance you should begin studying is the amount of time you have available. In all likelihood, you are beginning to review while still taking other courses in your educational program. Those courses must be given a high priority as you begin budgeting your time. It does little good to review for the certification examination only to find that you are hopelessly behind in another required course. In addition, you may have employment obligations that take up a considerable amount of time or family commitments that must not be allowed to falter while you prepare for the exam. Be aware, however, that exam preparation takes a lot of time and that your success depends on it.

Begin reviewing at least 6 months before the exam. If you need to begin reviewing earlier, based on the exercises that follow, then do so. If you finish your review before 6 months is up, you can either stop reviewing or go back over the material in less detail one more time. If you wait to begin reviewing only 3 or 4 months before the exam, you may have insufficient time to go over the material thoroughly and as a result may need to postpone your exam date.

Before you begin budgeting your review time, consider the suggestions and encouragement provided by your instructors, who probably have several years' experience in working with students about to prepare for the exam. Their wisdom and advice should be taken seriously. If you follow the routine they suggest and the guidelines contained in this review book, you should be more than adequately prepared to pass the exam. Remember, however, that managing the quality and quantity of your review time is ultimately up to you. Now that you have successfully reached this point in your educational program, you should use your energy, time, and skills wisely during these final months of preparation. Just as with running a race, finish strong!

PLANNING THE REVIEW PROCESS

If one advances confidently in the direction of their dreams and endeavors to lead a life which they have imagined, they will meet with a success unexpected in common hours.

Henry David Thoreau

It is now time to turn your attention to the review process and begin to set priorities. Look through the chapters containing the review material if you have not already done so. In the following space provided, make a list of the subject areas in which you feel particularly strong or weak. By listing the subject areas in this way, you will be able to prioritize the material you need to cover. Second-year radiography students preparing for the exam commonly make the mistake of reviewing the easiest material first. This is the opposite of what you should do.

Weaker Subjects

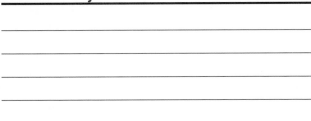

Stronger Subjects

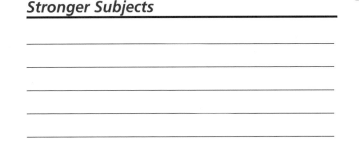

Look again at the entries you made. Transfer these subjects to the spaces that follow, ranking the weakest subjects first. Then progress, in order, to the subjects in which you are strongest.

Priority of Study Topics, Weaker to Stronger

I need to study the following subjects in this order:

1.

2.

3.

4.

5.

6.

7.

8.

9.

10.

11.

_____

12.

_____

The rationale for studying more difficult content first is twofold: (1) The more difficult material will require more time, which you will have in greater supply at the beginning of the 6-month period than at the end; (2) if you have had serious difficulty with some of the subject areas and you study those first, you will have additional time to seek explanation from your instructors and to read the material again. Save for last the subjects with which you are the most comfortable. These will require the least amount of study, and if your time becomes limited, reviewing them quickly will not be as detrimental.

The time you spend now on planning a study calendar and prioritizing your study needs will pay great dividends as you begin the review process. Such planning should allow you to proceed more efficiently and dedicate more time to studying. If you are not filling in a calendar or prioritizing your study needs as you read this chapter, take the time right now to select a day and time within the next 5 days when you will reread Chapter 1 and follow the directions for time management and prioritizing.

_____ I have completed my planner calendar and prioritized my subject areas for study.
_____ I will complete my planner calendar and prioritize my subject areas for study on _____ (day), _____ (date) at _____ am/pm.

Now that you have established your priorities or made an appointment with yourself to plan your calendar, you have set your first goal for reviewing and passing the certification examination. Even more important, you have taken the initial step toward your first radiography job or continued education. Be sure to congratulate yourself on accomplishing this task, and then finish reading this chapter.

Although some may scoff at your calendar planning and the amount of time you choose to spend reviewing, others may feel that you are not spending enough time preparing. If you are receiving conflicting advice, you may become confused by all of the suggestions, hints, and guidelines. You should refer to the suggestions made by your instructors and the suggestions contained in this study guide.

SCHEDULING YOUR STUDY TIME

Go through the process of planning your study time and evaluating your commitments so that you may set goals for reviewing all of the material. Browse through Chapters 2 through 6 and briefly refresh your memory about the topics. Are there large amounts of information that you can't recall? Is information there that you have never seen before? Does most of it look familiar, and is it easy to recall?

Try answering a few of the exam questions after each section, and sample some of the questions from the comprehensive exams in Chapter 7. Were you able to answer the questions easily? Do you feel confident about your answers, or were they educated guesses? How many did you get correct compared with the number you missed? Are there specific subject areas in which you feel particularly strong or weak? Will you need to spend more time studying one area than another? You have to answer all of these questions as you attempt to budget your review time. Pause now to consider each of them carefully.

If you are already using some form of daily, weekly, or monthly calendar to plan your study time, you simply need to decide where within your study schedule to include your review. If you have not been using a calendar to budget your time, this is a great time to start. You don't have to buy an expensive time planner. Most students use a calendar with squares large enough to write in times and planned activities. Others plan their time using the software in their particular brand of smartphone, tablet, or other mobile device. Figure 1-1 is an example of a simple calendar being used to budget time for current classes and for review.

The importance of writing study time on a calendar cannot be overemphasized. You are much more likely to adhere to a study schedule if you have thought it through, written it down, and posted it where you see it daily. It is highly recommended that once you plan your review time, you make a copy of your calendar and give it to your instructor. Educators can be powerful motivators by occasionally reminding a student of a written commitment to review. Filling in a calendar in this way is also a form of establishing a written contract with yourself. In so doing, you recognize that only _you_ are ultimately responsible for covering the review material. If the college or hospital you are attending provides you access to a study skills department, meet with one of the professionals there, share your ideas for time and study management, and gain even more support for attaining your goals.

When you are setting up a review calendar, being regular and consistent is important. Set aside specific time to review on a regular basis. Don't save review for times when you have nothing else to do. State your commitment in such terms as the following: "I will review physics every Thursday evening for the next 8 weeks for approximately 2 hours each time." This contract with yourself describes the activity, the time commitment, and the subject involved. Avoid such entries as "I will study physics four times this month." There is little commitment to that statement, and the goal it sets forth is not likely to be accomplished.

Sunday	Monday	Tuesday	Wednesday	Thursday	Friday	Saturday
				1 10:00 *Advanced Positioning* 1:00 *Pathology Class*	2 7:30 *Clinical Education* 7:00 *Review: Radiation Biol*	3 *No Study Day*
4 7:00 *Review: Radiation Biol*	5 7:30 *Clinical Education*	6 10:00 *Advanced Positioning* 1:00 *Pathology Class*	7 7:30 *Clinical Education*	8 10:00 *Advanced Positioning* 1:00 *Pathology Class*	9 7:30 *Clinical Education* 7:00 *Review: Physics*	10 *No Study Day*
11 7:00 *Review: Physics*	12 7:30 *Clinical Education*	13 10:00 *Advanced Positioning* 1:00 *Pathology Class*	14 7:30 *Clinical Education*	15 10:00 *Advanced Positioning* 1:00 *Pathology Class*	16 7:30 *Clinical Education* 7:00 *Review: Quality Control*	17 *No Study Day*
18 7:00 *Review: Quality Control*	19 7:30 *Clinical Education*	20 10:00 *Advanced Positioning* 1:00 *Pathology Class*	21 7:30 *Clinical Education*	22 10:00 *Advanced Positioning* 1:00 *Pathology Class*	23 7:30 *Clinical Education* 7:00 *Review: Image Intensifier*	24 *No Study Day*
25 7:00 *Review: Image Intensifier*	26 7:30 *Clinical Education*	27 10:00 *Advanced Positioning* 1:00 *Pathology Class*	28 7:30 *Clinical Education*	29 10:00 *Advanced Positioning* 1:00 *Pathology Class*	30 7:30 *Clinical Education* 7:00 *Review: Skull Anatomy*	

FIGURE 1-1 Calendar for scheduling study time.

As an adult learner, you have probably developed an awareness of your strengths and weaknesses relative to time management and commitment to studies. Whatever your self-appraisal, the fact that you are using this book suggests that you are a successful student with the capability to manage your time effectively. You should now spend some time applying your scheduling and time management skills to the planning of your review.

If you are allotting at least 6 months to prepare for the exam, you should have plenty of time to cover all of the material and take and review the exams in this book. If you do all of the expected regular studies and review, you should have little difficulty on the exam. I hope that by the time you take the exam, you will regard it as just another quiz.

STUDY HABITS

Study habits mirror the individuality of each student. Some students prefer to study alone. They may read small sections of a chapter at a time, pausing to reflect on the content and taking additional notes if necessary, or they may recite the material aloud. Others choose to read over a section or an entire chapter many times, reviewing the

material to facilitate their recall. Some students find it helpful to study in groups, taking turns quizzing one another and answering practice questions.

By now, you probably have formed your own set of effective study habits. In using this book to prepare for the exam, you should consider every suggestion that may improve your method of study. However, do not greatly alter study habits that have already proved successful. Also, keep in mind that as you review for the exam, you should not be learning new material. By definition, a *review* should be a revisiting of material that you have already learned and learned well. In addition, your review should be as comprehensive as possible, including all of the topics.

Before discussing study habits, let's address concerns that many second-year students have after talking with others who have recently taken the exam. You may have been told to give little attention to certain subject areas because they did not appear on the exam. You may hear that the exam was particularly easy and that you should not worry about it. You may also be surprised to hear such comments as "There was almost no positioning on the exam" or "It was *all* physics!" The radiography examination adheres to content specifications that are included in this chapter. In most cases, when test takers think one category had significantly more questions than another category, this is a reflection of their command of the category's content or of their preparation, or lack thereof, for the exam. Although individuals who are providing you with feedback about the exam may have good intentions, the reliability of their memory of the exam items is questionable. Besides, because of the size of the item bank for the exam, the questions vary each time the examination is administered. Even if the individuals with whom you are speaking accurately recall the exam content, you will not be taking the same exam. Each radiography examination is different from the preceding exam.

Most importantly, you should be aware that passing along test question content is a violation of the ARRT Standards of Ethics. It is best to avoid such conversations from both preparation and ethical standpoints. Finally, by choosing to ignore advice from even the most well-intentioned person who has recently taken the exam and instead following the study routine that you are planning under the guidance of your instructors and this book, you will guarantee that you are the one controlling the exam outcome and can be assured that you are undertaking the best preparation for the exam.

A few reminders about study habits or study conditions are in order. Remember to choose your most difficult subjects to study first. You have already listed these in the previous section. When you study, be sure you have set aside time when you can be quiet with no interruptions. Some people study better with soft music in the background, whereas others prefer silence. Other types of music and television simply interfere with concentration. Although you should be comfortable while studying, you should not be too comfortable. Remaining upright is particularly important.

Take regular but infrequent breaks. Be sure that lighting is adequate and the room temperature is controllable and comfortable. Arrange the study conditions so that you can focus all of your attention on what you are doing. Regardless of the study method used, quiet concentration is of utmost importance. You may wish to reinforce your learning by reciting the material aloud—a practice requiring a study setting that is isolated and free from distractions. In addition, study at the time of day when your mind is most alert. Some students prefer to study early in the morning, whereas others have found that they study better later in the afternoon or early evening. Cramming late at night or into the early hours of the morning is ineffective for most individuals. Besides, if review is a priority, you will want to assign it an important place in your schedule.

EXAMINATION SPECIFICATIONS

Although the exam specifications for the ARRT radiography examination (Table 1-1) do not divulge specific questions, they do give the reader the outline from which the exam is constructed. In addition, the approximate number of questions in each category is listed to allow you

KEY REVIEW POINTS
Reviewing

- Begin at least 6 months before test day.
- Perform an inventory of strengths and weaknesses by topic.
- Commit your study schedule to a calendar.
- Base review on ARRT exam specifications; avoid coaching from previous test-takers.
- Use study habits that have proven successful in the past.
- Study difficult subjects first.
- Study with no interruptions.
- Be comfortable during study but not too comfortable.
- Review during the time of day when you are most alert.

TABLE 1-1	Specifications for the ARRT Radiography Examination	
Content Category	**Percent of Test**	**Number of Questions**
A. Radiation Protection	22.5	45
B. Equipment Operation and Quality Control	11.0	22
C. Image Acquisition and Evaluation	22.5	45
D. Imaging Procedures	29.0	58
E. Patient Care and Education	15.0	30
Total	*100*	*200*

From American Registry of Radiologic Technologists www.arrt.org, 2010.

to see the relative importance placed on the different subject areas.

You may wonder why these particular categories were selected for the exam and are weighted in this way. The ARRT periodically performs an extensive study called a *task analysis*. The resulting task inventory (see Chapter 11) for radiographers lists all of the specific skills normally performed by an entry-level radiographer.

The skills in the task inventory should coincide with the terminal competencies of all approved educational programs. From this task inventory, the categories for the exam are constructed, and the relative importance of each is weighted. The review of the major categories on the exam is covered in the next five chapters.

ANALYSIS OF CATEGORY COMPONENTS

An approximate number of questions for each of the major subject areas is shown in the detailed list that follows.* The percentages of subcategory content within the major areas are general guidelines and may vary to a certain extent with each exam administration.

---

*Adapted from American Registry of Radiologic Technologists: *Content specifications for the examination in radiography,* St Paul, MN, 2010, ARRT.

A. Radiation Protection (45 questions)

I. Biological Aspects of Radiation (10)
  A. Radiosensitivity
    1. Dose-response relationships
    2. Relative tissue radiosensitivities (e.g., LET, RBE)
    3. Cell survival and recovery (LD_{50})
    4. Oxygen effect
  B. Somatic Effects
    1. Short-term versus long-term effects
    2. Acute versus chronic effects
    3. Carcinogenesis
    4. Organ and tissue response (e.g., eye, thyroid, breast, bone marrow, skin, gonadal)
  C. Acute Radiation Syndromes
    1. CNS
    2. Hematopoietic
    3. GI
  D. Embryonic and Fetal Risks
  E. Genetic Impact
    1. Genetic significant dose
    2. Goals of gonadal shielding
  F. Photon Interactions with Matter
    1. Compton effect
    2. Photoelectric absorption
    3. Coherent (classical) scatter
    4. Attenuation by various tissues
      a. thickness of body part (density)
      b. type of tissue (atomic number)
II. Minimizing Patient Exposure (15)
  A. Exposure Factors
    1. kVp
    2. mAs
  B. Shielding
    1. Rationale for use
    2. Types
    3. Placement
  C. Beam Restriction
    1. Purpose of primary beam restriction
    2. Types (e.g., collimators)
  D. Filtration
    1. Effect on skin and organ exposure
    2. Effect on average beam energy
    3. NCRP recommendations (NCRP #102, minimum filtration in useful beam)
  E. Exposure Reduction
    1. Patient positioning
    2. Automatic exposure control (AEC)
    3. Patient communication
    4. Digital imaging
    5. Pediatric dose reduction
    6. ALARA
  F. Image Receptors (e.g., types, relative speed, digital versus film)
  G. Grids
  H. Fluoroscopy
    1. Pulsed
    2. Exposure factors
    3. Grids
    4. Positioning
    5. Fluoroscopy time
III. Personnel Protection (11)
  A. Sources of Radiation Exposure
    1. Primary x-ray beam
    2. Secondary radiation
      a. scatter
      b. leakage
    3. Patient as source
  B. Basic Methods of Protection
    1. Time
    2. Distance
    3. Shielding
  C. Protective Devices
    1. Types
    2. Attenuation properties
    3. Minimum lead equivalent (NCRP #102)
  D. Special Considerations
    1. Portable (mobile) units
    2. Fluoroscopy
      a. protective drapes
      b. protective Bucky slot cover
      c. cumulative timer
    3. Guidelines for fluoroscopy and portable units (NCRP #102, CFR-21)
      a. fluoroscopy exposure rates
      b. exposure switch guidelines
IV. Radiation Exposure and Monitoring (9)
  A. Units of Measurement*
    1. Absorbed dose
    2. Dose equivalent
    3. Exposure
  B. Dosimeters
    1. Types
    2. Proper use
  C. NCRP Recommendations for Personnel Monitoring (NCRP #116)
    1. Occupational exposure
    2. Public exposure
    3. Embryo/fetus exposure
    4. ALARA and dose equivalent limits
    5. Evaluation and maintenance of personnel dosimetry records
  D. Medical Exposure of Patients (NCRP #160)
    1. Typical effective dose per exam
    2. Comparison of typical doses by modality

---

*Conventional units are generally used. However, questions referenced to specific reports (e.g., NCRP) use SI units to be consistent with such reports.

B. Equipment Operation and Quality Control (22 questions)

I. Principles of Radiation Physics (9)
  A. X-Ray Production
    1. Source of free electrons (e.g., thermionic emission)
    2. Acceleration of electrons
    3. Focusing of electrons
    4. Deceleration of electrons
  B. Target Interactions
    1. Bremsstrahlung
    2. Characteristic
  C. X-Ray Beam
    1. Frequency and wavelength
    2. Beam characteristics
      a. quality
      b. quantity
      c. primary versus remnant (exit)
    3. Inverse square law
    4. Fundamental properties (e.g., travel in straight lines, ionize matter)
II. Imaging Equipment (9)
  A. Components of Radiographic Unit (Fixed or Mobile)
    1. Operating console
    2. X-ray tube construction
      a. electron sources
      b. target materials
      c. induction motor
    3. Automatic exposure control (AEC)
      a. radiation detectors
      b. back-up timer
      c. density adjustment (e.g., +1 or −1)
    4. Manual exposure controls
    5. Beam restriction devices
  B. X-Ray Generator, Transformers, and Rectification System
    1. Basic principles
    2. Phase, pulse, and frequency
  C. Components of Fluoroscopic Unit (Fixed or Mobile)
    1. Image intensifier
    2. Viewing systems
    3. Recording systems
    4. Automatic brightness control (ABC)
  D. Components of Digital Imaging (CR and DR)
    1. PSP - Photostimulable phosphor
    2. Flat panel detectors—direct and indirect
    3. Start up and shut down
    4. CR plate erasure
    5. Equipment cleanliness (imaging plates, CR plates)
  E. Types of Units
    1. Dedicated chest unit
    2. Tomography unit
  F. Accessories
    1. Stationary grids
    2. Bucky assembly
    3. Image receptors

III. Quality Control of Imaging Equipment and Accessories (4)
  A. Beam Restriction
    1. Light field to radiation field alignment
    2. Central ray alignment
  B. Recognition and Reporting of Malfunctions
  C. Digital Imaging Receptor Systems
    1. Artifacts (e.g., nonuniformity, erasure)
    2. Maintenance (e.g., detector fog)
    3. Display monitor quality assurance
  D. Shielding Accessories (e.g., lead apron and glove testing)

C. Image Acquisition and Evaluation (45 questions)

I. Selection of Technical Factors (20)
  A. Factors Affecting Radiographic Quality (Table 1-2). (Refer to Attachment C to clarify terms that may occur on the exam.)
  B. Technique Charts
    1. Preprogrammed techniques—anatomically programmed radiography (APR)
    2. Caliper measurement
    3. Fixed versus variable kVp
    4. Special considerations
      a. casts
      b. anatomic and pathologic factors
      c. pediatrics
      d. contrast media
  C. Automatic Exposure Control (AEC)
    1. Effects of changing exposure factors on radiographic quality
    2. Detector selection
    3. Anatomic alignment
    4. Density control (+1 or −1)
  D. Digital Imaging Characteristics
    1. Spatial resolution
      a. sampling frequency
      b. detector element size (DEL)
      c. receptor size and matrix size
    2. Image signal (exposure related)
      a. quantum mottle (noise)
      b. signal to noise ratio (SNR) or contrast to noise ratio (CNR)
II. Image Processing and Quality Assurance (12)
  A. Image Identification
    1. Methods (e.g., photographic, radiographic, electronic)
    2. Legal considerations (e.g., patient data, examination data)
  B. Film Screen Processing
    1. Film storage
    2. Components*

---

*Specific chemicals in the processing solutions are not covered (e.g., glutaraldehyde).

TABLE 1-2	Factors Affecting Radiographic Quality			
	1. Density/Brightness	**2. Contrast/Gray Scale**	**3. Recorded Detail/ Spatial Resolution**	**4. Distortion**
a. MAs	X			
b. kVp	X	X		
c. OID		X (air gap)	X	X
d. SID	X		X	X
e. Focal spot size			X	
f. Grids*	X	X		
g. Filtration	X	X		
h. Film-screen	X		X	
i. Beam restriction	X	X		
j. Motion			X	
k. Anode heel effect	X			
l. Patient factors (size, pathology)	X	X	X	X
m. Angle (tube, part, or receptor)			X	X

From American Registry of Radiologic Technologists: *Content specifications for the examination in radiography*, January 2010.
Note: X indicates topics covered on the exam.
*Includes conversion factors for grids.

    a. developer
    b. fixer
  3. Maintenance/malfunction
    a. start up and shut down procedure
    b. possible causes of malfunction (e.g., improper temperature, contamination, replenishment, water flow)
 C. Digital Imaging Processing
  1. Electronic collimation (masking)
  2. Gray-scale rendition (look-up table [LUT], histogram)
  3. Edge enhancement/noise suppression
  4. Contrast enhancement
  5. System malfunctions (e.g., ghost image, banding, erasure, dead pixels, readout problems)
  6. CR reader components
 D. Image Display
  1. Viewing conditions (i.e., luminance, ambient lighting)
  2. Spatial resolution
  3. Contrast resolution/dynamic range
  4. DICOM grayscale function
  5. Window level and width function
 E. Digital Image Display Informatics
  1. PACS
  2. HIS
  3. RIS (modality work list)
  4. Networking (e.g., HL7, DICOM)
  5. Workflow (e.g., inappropriate documentation, lost images, mismatched images, corrupt data)
III. Criteria for Image Evaluation (13)
 A. Brightness/Density (e.g., mAs, distance)
 B. Contrast/Gray Scale (e.g., kVp, filtration, grids)

 C. Recorded Detail (e.g., motion, poor film-screen contact)
 D. Distortion (e.g., magnification, OID, SID)
 E. Demonstration of Anatomical Structures (e.g., positioning, tube–part–image receptor alignment)
 F. Identification Markers (e.g., anatomical, patient, date)
 G. Patient Considerations (e.g., pathological conditions)
 H. Image Artifacts (e.g., film handling, static, pressure, grid lines, Moiré effect or aliasing)
 I. Fog (e.g., age, chemical, radiation, temperature, safelight)
 J. Noise
 K. Acceptable Range of Exposure
 L. Exposure Indicator Determination
 M. Gross Exposure Error (e.g., mottle, light or dark, low contrast)

D. Imaging Procedures (58 questions)

This section addresses imaging procedures for the anatomic regions listed (I through VII). Questions cover the following topics:

1. Positioning (e.g., topographic landmarks, body positions, path of central ray, immobilization devices)
2. Anatomy (e.g., physiology, basic pathology, and related medical terminology)
3. Technical factors (e.g., adjustments for body habitus, trauma, pathology, breathing techniques).

I. Thorax (10)
 A. Chest
 B. Ribs

C. Sternum

D. Soft Tissue Neck

II. Abdomen and GI Studies (8)

A. Abdomen

B. Esophagus

C. Swallowing Dysfunction Study

D. Upper GI Series, Single or Double Contrast

E. Small Bowel Series

F. Barium Enema, Single or Double Contrast

G. Surgical Cholangiography

H. ERCP

III. Urological Studies (3)

A. Cystography

B. Cystourethrography

C. Intravenous Urography

D. Retrograde Pyelography

IV. Spine and Pelvis (10)

A. Cervical Spine

B. Thoracic Spine

C. Scoliosis Series

D. Lumbar Spine

E. Sacrum and Coccyx

F. Sacroiliac Joints

G. Pelvis and Hip

V. Head (5)

A. Skull

B. Facial Bones

C. Mandible

D. Zygomatic Arch

E. Temporomandibular Joints

F. Nasal Bones

G. Orbits

H. Paranasal Sinuses

VI. Extremities (20)

A. Toes

B. Foot

C. Calcaneus (Os Calcis)

D. Ankle

E. Tibia, Fibula

F. Knee

G. Patella

H. Femur

I. Fingers

J. Hand

K. Wrist

L. Forearm

M. Elbow

N. Humerus

O. Shoulder

P. Scapula

Q. Clavicle

R. Acromioclavicular Joints

S. Bone Survey

T. Long Bone Measurement

U. Bone Age

V. Soft Tissue/Foreign Bodies

VII. Other (2)

A. Arthrography

B. Myelography

E. Patient Care and Education (30 questions)

I. Ethical and Legal Aspects (4)

A. Patient's Rights

1. Informed consent (e.g., written, oral, implied)

2. Confidentiality (HIPAA)

3. Additional rights (e.g., Patient's Bill of Rights)

a. privacy

b. extent of care (e.g., DNR)

c. access to information

d. living will; health care proxy

e. research participation

B. Legal Issues

1. Examination documentation (e.g., patient history, clinical diagnosis)

2. Common terminology (e.g., battery, negligence, malpractice)

3. Legal doctrines (e.g., respondeat superior, res ipsa loquitur)

4. Restraints versus immobilization

C. ARRT Standards of Ethics

II. Interpersonal Communication (5)

A. Modes of Communication

1. Verbal/written

2. Nonverbal (e.g., eye contact, touching)

B. Challenges in Communication

1. Patient characteristics

2. Explanation of medical terms

3. Strategies to improve understanding

4. Cultural diversity

C. Patient Education

1. Explanation of current procedure

2. Response to inquiries about other imaging modalities (e.g., CT, MRI, mammography, sonography, nuclear medicine, bone densitometry regarding dose differences, types of radiation, and patient preps)

III. Infection Control (5)

A. Terminology and Basic Concepts

1. Asepsis

a. medical

b. surgical

c. sterile technique

2. Pathogens

a. fomites, vehicles, vectors

b. nosocomial infections

B. Cycle of Infection

1. Pathogen

2. Source or reservoir of infection

3. Susceptible host

4. Method of transmission

a. contact (direct, indirect)

b. droplet

c. airborne/suspended
d. common vehicle
e. vector borne

C. Standard Precautions
1. Handwashing
2. Gloves, gowns
3. Masks
4. Medical asepsis (e.g., equipment disinfection)

D. Additional or Transmission-Based Precautions
1. Airborne (e.g., respiratory protection, negative ventilation)
2. Droplet (e.g., particulate mask, restricted patient placement)
3. Contact (e.g., gloves, gown, restricted patient placement)

E. Disposal of Contaminated Materials
1. Linens
2. Needles
3. Patient supplies (e.g., tubes, emesis basin)

IV. Physical Assistance and Transfer (4)
A. Patient Transfer and Movement
1. Body mechanics (balance, alignment, movement)
2. Patient transfer

B. Assisting Patients with Medical Equipment
1. Infusion catheters and pumps
2. Oxygen delivery systems
3. Other (e.g., nasogastric tubes, urinary catheters, tracheostomy tubes)

C. Routine Monitoring
1. Equipment (e.g., stethoscope, sphygmomanometer)
2. Vital signs (e.g., blood pressure, pulse, respiration)
3. Physical signs and symptoms (e.g., motor control, severity of injury)
4. Documentation

V. Medical Emergencies (5)
A. Allergic Reactions (e.g., contrast media, latex)
B. Cardiac or Respiratory Arrest (e.g., CPR)
C. Physical Injury or Trauma
D. Other Medical Disorders (e.g., seizures, diabetic reactions)

VI. Pharmacology (3)
A. Patient History
1. Medication reconciliation (current medications)
2. Premedications
3. Contraindications
4. Scheduling and sequencing examinations

B. Complications/Reactions
1. Local effects (e.g., extravasation/infiltration, phlebitis)
2. Systemic effects
a. mild
b. moderate
c. severe
3. Emergency medications
4. Radiographer's response and documentation

VII. Contrast Media (4)
A. Types and Properties (e.g., iodinated, water soluble, barium, ionic versus non-ionic)
B. Appropriateness of Contrast Media to Examination
1. Patient condition (e.g., perforated bowel)
2. Patient age and weight
3. Laboratory values (e.g., BUN creatinine, GFR)
C. Patient Education
1. Verify informed consent
2. Instructions regarding preparation, diet, and medications
3. Preexamination and postexamination instructions (e.g., discharge instructions)
D. Venipuncture
1. Venous anatomy
2. Supplies
3. Procedural technique
E. Administration
1. Routes (e.g., intravenous, oral)
2. Supplies (e.g., enema kits, needles)

EXAMINATION PROCEDURE

APPLICATION PROCESS

At the appropriate point in your educational program, your program director will provide you with a booklet published by the ARRT to apply to take the radiography certification examination. Read everything in the handbook! You should pay close attention to the ARRT Rules and Regulations and the Standards of Ethics and Code of Ethics. Although your program director may highlight and discuss certain portions of the booklet, you are responsible for understanding everything it contains. This may be the most important exam you will have taken so far in your career, so be sure to read the materials provided.

After you read the entire booklet, it is important to fill out the application, providing all of the information requested. Be sure to print legibly and to fill in all information and dates accurately. Pay close attention to the photo requirements. You can submit the application up to 3 months before your anticipated graduation date.

After you have signed the application and your program director has signed it, insert the document along with a check or money order for the application fee into the envelope provided in the handbook. It is important that you mail the envelope yourself. Do not include it in a large envelope with applications from other members of your class, and do not trust anyone else to mail the application for you. Be sure to send your application as certified mail and to request a return receipt. Although this costs slightly more than regular mail, you will receive verification that your application has been delivered.

Several weeks after receipt of your application, the ARRT will send you examination information and test center admission instructions. When you receive the admission information, you should immediately check it to verify the examination window dates, the examination to be taken, and the personal identification on the form. If any of this information is incorrect or has changed, or if you fail to receive this mailing after an appropriate period of time, it is your responsibility to contact the ARRT office immediately at (651) 687-0048. Carefully read the process for making an appointment with the test center. Once you have received these documents, put them in a safe place until the day of the exam.

You must have completed all of the educational requirements of your program to take the ARRT examination; this may be particularly significant if your program requires you to make up missed time after graduation. If you need to make up missed time, you will have to fulfill this requirement before taking the exam. If your program awards a degree as a condition of program completion, you must also satisfy all general education coursework requirements before being eligible to take the exam. Effective January 1, 2015, you will need to provide proof that you have earned a minimum of an associate degree in order to apply to take the Registry exam. Near your date of graduation, your program director will receive a form on which to verify your status, and he or she will sign the form and return it to the ARRT or use the online verification process to verify that you have completed the educational program and are eligible to take the exam. This includes verification that you have completed all required clinical and didactic competencies.

One of the most informative websites that you as an imaging professional should commit to memory is www.arrt.org.

MATERIALS NEEDED FOR THE EXAMINATION

You should take very few items with you to the exam center. No papers, books, calculators, purses, cell phones, or food or drink of any kind may be taken into the testing room. The items that you should bring include your admission ticket, all required photos, and identification materials required by the ARRT. If you wish to use a calculator during the examination, it will be provided by the test center.

Environmental conditions of the testing center can vary. The exam room may be warmer or cooler than you would prefer. If being too cool is a concern for you, consider taking a sweater into the exam room. A good way to prepare for a less-than-ideal situation is to study and take practice examinations under different conditions. By doing so, you will be able to adapt more easily to the variations in temperature and to the room

arrangements that you may face when you take the ARRT examination.

Careful reading of ARRT materials will ensure that you have everything you need for the examination. Addressing these issues well ahead of time will free your mind for the more important task—passing the examination.

EXAMINATION RESULTS

On completion of the test, you will receive your preliminary exam result on-screen. The result will include a preliminary scaled score and pass/fail status. Remember that a scaled score of at least 75 is required to pass the exam. This on-screen indication of your score still does not provide evidence of certification, and you may not yet use the credentials "R.T.(R)" following your name.

Certification becomes official when you receive your ARRT-approved scores and credentials in the mail. Be watching for the large envelope from the ARRT to arrive. You may also wish to visit the "check registration status" link at www.arrt.org (click on "Employers and Regulators") to verify whether or not your name has been added to the list of credentialed radiographers.

TEST-TAKING SKILLS

Do not fear the winds of adversity. Remember, a kite rises against the wind rather than with it.

PHYSICALLY AND MENTALLY PREPARING FOR THE EXAMINATION DAY

Although most of your preparation for the exam centers on reviewing your coursework, the physical and mental preparation must be taken into account as well. The question of how long before the exam date you discontinue your review has no definite answer. It is an individual decision based on how lengthy and thorough a review you have done and how comfortable you are with the material. Consulting your instructors or study skills professionals to clarify your specific needs will prove helpful in answering this question. A brief discussion of the points involved may assist you in deciding how long to study.

If you are the type of student who conducts a well-thought-out, carefully planned review of all of the material, as suggested in this chapter, it is reasonable to expect that studying will taper off within 2 to 3 weeks before the examination. If you use this review book effectively and cover all of the content areas over a period of at least 6 months, you should be well prepared for the examination and can draw your review to a close several weeks before the exam.

If you have not allowed yourself sufficient time to review and are attempting to compress your studying into a few weeks, you may wish to keep on reviewing until a date closer to the exam. Be aware that anxiety, which will tend to increase as the exam approaches, may interfere with learning and recalling even the most basic information as you continue to review. Also, if you have not learned the material over a period of time, there is little that you can learn in the last few weeks. Trying to cram for the examination is futile. If you have waited too long to begin studying, limit your review to the key points in all the major subject areas.

As you prepare mentally for the day of the test, realize that apprehension about the exam may surface in unexpected ways. It is not unusual for students to report having strange dreams about the exam. The content of these dreams may involve driving for hours but never reaching the test center or starting the exam, falling asleep, and waking up with only 5 minutes left and nearly 200 questions to answer. This is a normal response to your anticipation of a major event. It may also serve as a motivator to continue reviewing and preparing for the exam. You may wish to share your dream experiences with other students in your class. You will come to realize that most of them are having this response and that it is perfectly normal.

Another important aspect of preparation for the exam involves your physical readiness, which means having gathered all the materials you will need for the test and having prepared your body physically to take an exam of this type. Having the appropriate materials ready well in advance of the test has been discussed previously. Don't wait until the day before or the day of the exam to get your paperwork in order. Allowing several days to accomplish these tasks will ensure that you are prepared for any emergency that arises.

In preparing your body to take the exam, the basic rule of thumb is to treat exam day much as you would any other day. This phase of your preparation should begin the evening before the test. Intake of alcohol or large amounts of food should be avoided. You should get approximately the same amount of sleep as usual, waking at your usual time.

On the day of the exam, depending on the time of your appointment, use the time before the test to enhance your mental and physical readiness. Start the day by eating a substantial and healthy breakfast. Although you should do this every day, it is particularly important on test day. As the hour of the exam nears, you may feel less like eating. A light snack is a good idea, but avoid high-sugar snacks so that you do not experience a blood sugar drop as you go in to take the exam.

If you have an exercise regimen that you follow daily, follow it on the test day as well. Exercise helps relieve stress and anxiety for many people. You will probably find that trips to the rest room increase in number on the test day. This is a normal physiologic response to the stress associated with the anticipation of a major event.

Is such physical preparation really necessary? Why should you be attentive to this aspect of test taking? With all of the time and effort expended during your 2 years of education in medical radiography and during the review process, you want to be certain that fatigue and physical stress do not impede your ability to take the examination.

Your instructors probably gave you a series of review examinations in the last few months of the program, and you will have used the computer exams that accompany this text. These will have helped you to assess your strengths and weaknesses in the various subject areas. Another reason for these practice exams was to help you become accustomed to sitting for 3 or 4 hours while taking an examination. It is important not to let the physical aspect of test taking hamper your ability to pass the exam.

The writing of this book is grounded in more than 30 years of experience preparing students to take the ARRT examination. Attention to the details in this section will help relieve your anxiety about the exam and allow you to focus on the more important aspects of reviewing and taking the exam.

STRATEGIES FOR TAKING THE EXAMINATION

Everyone has a preferred system for taking a lengthy, mostly multiple choice format examination. If you have a method that has worked well in the past, continue to use it. If you seem to lose focus when taking such a test, however, consider the following suggestions for structuring your approach to this exam.

Just getting started may be difficult for some individuals and cause them to experience discomfort. Many graduates have reported that they were uneasy when beginning the test. This is usually the result of the apprehension and stress surrounding this important event. Such an initial response should not be viewed as abnormal, and you can be assured that several of your peers are feeling that same discomfort. If this occurs, close your eyes, breathe deeply several times, and start again. Unless you have severe exam anxiety or failed to review and prepare carefully ahead of time, you will be ready to begin answering the questions.

There are 200 test items on the exam, plus approximately 20 additional unscored pilot questions. You will have 3½ hours to answer all of the questions. Additional time is allotted to complete a tutorial before beginning the exam and a survey after the exam. Be sure to take the tutorial at the start and provide feedback to the ARRT at the end of the exam. Questions are asked randomly, not by category. A test item includes the *stem,* or question, and the set of possible answers. The stem will ask a question; only one of the possible answers will be correct.

The other choices are called *distracters*. Distracters are choices designed to make you think they are the correct answer. They usually consist of the most common incorrect responses. Each question has only one correct answer.

The people who construct the exam attempt to include only items for which there is a broad consensus regarding the correct response. Questions about specific departmental routines and information drawn from only one textbook are not used. Information that is proprietary in nature (i.e., specific to a manufacturer or supplier) is avoided. Several sources are consulted when questions for the exam are screened, and only the information common to several sources is used. The ARRT does not officially endorse any textbooks for screening or writing test items, so you may be assured that you will not be penalized on the exam because you did not use a certain textbook as a student.

As you begin taking the exam, read each question carefully. Accurate reading is one of the most important skills needed to pass the exam. Comprehension of what is being asked is crucial. Do not attempt to read more into the question than is printed. Do not assume that it is a "trick" question. The exam questions are carefully written and well constructed. There should be nothing on the test that you have not seen before in your studies and during your review. Be careful not to read the question the way you want it to be asked. Take the question at face value.

Questions on the ARRT examination are not all A-B-C-D multiple choice questions. Questions may be asked using one of several different formats. A valuable resource at www.arrt.org is the *Test Item Development for Radiologic Technology* manual that describes the various question formats you may encounter on the exam. Examples from that manual follow.*

In general, following are the question formats used, and not used, on the ARRT examination:

Used on ARRT Exams	Not Used on ARRT Exams
Direct question - multiple choice	True-false
Incomplete statement	Matching
Exhibits (e.g., radiographs, tables, illustrations, graphs)	Comparison
	Combined response
Hot spots or videos	Short answer and essay
Multi-select items	Other (fill-in-the-blank, true-false, none of the above, all of the above)
Sorted list items	
Combined response	

*© 2011, The American Registry of Radiologic Technologists

We will concentrate on the question formats you *may* encounter. Each of the following examples is © 2003 The American Registry of Radiologic Technologists.

The most commonly used format is called the *direct question*. Here you are asked a question and are provided with either three or four choices, as follows:

Which of the following refers to the degree of blackening seen on a radiograph?

A. Radiographic intensity
B. Radiographic contrast
C. Radiographic sharpness
D. Radiographic density

The *incomplete statement* format simply gives a statement to complete, as follows:

The degree of blackening seen on a radiograph is referred to as radiographic:

A. Intensity
B. Contrast
C. Sharpness
D. Density

A third form of test question is the *negatively worded* item. This item sometimes causes problems for students when the question is read too quickly. This item measures your knowledge of exceptions to the data you have learned. This type of question is used sparingly on the exam. Following is an example of a negatively worded question:

Which of the following will *not* result in grid cutoff?

A. An off-center tube
B. A tube that is perpendicular to the lead strips
C. Improper SID being used with a focused grid
D. Grid motion being started before exposure is made

The fourth format, one you will definitely encounter, is called an *exhibit question*. It is a question or series of questions referring to a diagram, a radiograph, a table, a chart, or a drawing. On the ARRT examination, 10% or more of the questions use an image or illustration of some kind. Numerous questions can be asked about exhibits, including using the computer mouse to click on a spot or region of the exhibit to identify a piece of information. Examples of exhibits that may be used are:

- Videos
- Medical images
- Anatomical illustrations
- Positioning photographs or diagrams
- Drawings or photographs of equipment and instrumentation
- Models of scientific principles or processes (e.g., x-rays interacting with a molecule, dose-response curves)
- Tables or graphs with technical factors, technique charts, equipment specifications, results of QC tests

A fifth question format may present a list of four to eight options that you are required to place in a correct sequence. This is done by using the computer mouse to drag and drop the answers into a table in their proper order.

Be aware that the Registry is always researching other question formats and may insert them into your exam as pilot questions being tested for future use.

Regardless of the test item format used, after you read the question and all of the choices, the first answer you choose usually is correct. Be careful not to begin second-guessing your choice of an answer. Do not watch for patterns of answers. For example, resist choosing A just because you haven't used it in a while, and do not be surprised if a certain answer choice is used for several consecutive questions. Also, all types of question formats may involve clinical scenarios.

There is no guessing penalty on the exam, so if you have no idea what the answer is, guess. However, have a strategy even when guessing. Do not choose an answer with terms that are unfamiliar to you. Students sometimes reason that such a choice must be the answer because they have never heard of it before. Most often, this is not the case. Make an educated guess by ruling out answers you are sure are wrong. Then choose from among the items containing familiar terminology.

Becoming familiar with the types of items that may be used will help you anticipate what the exam will be like and will assist you in studying and preparing. A variety of question types are used in this book. Most of these types of questions are commonly used on exams. The certification examination is nothing to fear if you review and prepare properly. Be sure to consider the suggestions and strategies presented here and those identified by your instructors. If you have practiced and studied and prepared your strategy, the exam will be just another quiz.

KEY REVIEW POINTS
The Certification Exam

- Questions on the exam are not confined to A-B-C-D multiple choice questions; other types of questions may be used.
- Carefully read and safely file *all* materials regarding the exam provided to you by your instructor and the ARRT.
- Taper off reviewing as the test day nears.
- Apprehension about the exam is normal; share your experiences with others.
- Assemble materials needed for test day well ahead of time; drive to the test center a few days before to be certain of its location.
- Maintain usual diet and exercise for test day; avoid large intake of food or alcohol.
- Be aware of test item formats used by the Registry: direct question, incomplete statement, negatively worded, combined response, and exhibit.
- Read all test questions and answer choices carefully.

YOU'RE ON YOUR WAY!

Using this first chapter as a planner, you are now ready to work toward one of the crowning achievements of your educational career. Do all that is expected, and use your time and talents wisely. Do not allow external distractions to send you off course. It is time to plan and work for what is yet to come—passing the radiography examination and moving on to the next phase of your career. You have numerous human and material resources available to assist you, one of which you are reading. Use them all and go for it!

Success is a journey, not a destination.

Review of Radiation Protection

To be a winner, all you need to give is all you have.

BASIC RADIATION PROTECTION TERMINOLOGY

Ionizing radiation radiation that possesses the ability to remove electrons from atoms by a process called *ionization*

Somatic effects effects of radiation on the body being irradiated

Genetic effects effects of radiation on the genetic code of a germ cell; affects next generation

Natural background radiation radiation contained in the unpolluted environment

Artificially produced radiation also called *man-made radiation* (e.g., medical x-rays)

Primary radiation radiation exiting the x-ray tube

Exit radiation (remnant radiation; image-producing radiation) x-rays that emerge from the patient and strike the image receptor

Attenuation absorption and scatter (loss of intensity) of the x-ray beam as it passes through the patient

Heterogeneous beam x-ray beam that contains photons of many different energies

Photoelectric effect absorption of x-ray photons in the atoms of the body

Compton effect scatter of x-ray photons from the atoms of the body

Roentgen (R) traditional unit of in-air exposure

Coulombs per kilogram (C/kg) SI unit of in-air exposure

Rad traditional unit of absorbed dose

Gray SI unit of absorbed dose

Rem traditional unit of equivalent dose and effective dose

Sievert SI unit of equivalent dose and effective dose

Curie traditional unit of activity

Becquerel SI unit of activity

National Academy of Sciences/ National Research Council Committee on the Biological Effects of Ionizing Radiation (NAS/NRC-BEIR) organization that studies biological effects of ionizing radiation and publishes resulting data

International Commission on Radiological Protection (ICRP) organization that publishes international radiation protection guidelines

National Council on Radiation Protection and Measurements (NCRP) organization that publishes radiation protection guidelines for the United States

Nuclear Regulatory Commission (NRC) organization that enforces radiation protection standards at the federal level related to use of radioactive material

NCRP Report #102 makes recommendations on equipment design and protection regarding lead shielding and fluoroscopic and mobile exposure rates

NCRP Report #116 makes recommendations pertaining to risk-benefit analysis of radiation exposure; states that somatic and genetic effects should be kept to a minimum when radiation is used for diagnostic imaging; defines annual exposure limits

NCRP Report #160 addresses radiation exposure from all sources to people living in the United States

Effective dose limit upper boundary dose that can be absorbed, either in a single exposure or annually, with a negligible risk of somatic or genetic damage to the individual; effective dose implies whole-body radiation exposure

Cumulative effective dose (CED) lifetime occupational exposure must not exceed the radiographer's age multiplied by 1 rem

Equivalent dose equal to the absorbed dose multiplied by the radiation weighting factor; formerly known as *dose equivalent*

Equivalent dose limit upper boundary dose that can be absorbed, either in a single exposure or annually, with a negligible risk of a deterministic effect

As low as reasonably achievable (ALARA) concept of radiologic practice that encourages radiation users to adopt measures that keep the dose to the patient and themselves at minimal levels

Dose-response curves graphs that illustrate the relationship between radiation dose and the response of the organism to exposure; may be linear or nonlinear, threshold or nonthreshold

Probabilistic effects randomly occurring effects of radiation; the probability of such effects is proportional to the dose (increased dose equals increased probability, not severity, of effects)

Deterministic effects effects of radiation that become more severe at high levels of radiation exposure and do not occur below a certain threshold dose

Genetically significant dose (GSD) average annual gonadal dose of radiation to individuals of childbearing age; addresses the relationship of gonadal doses to individuals versus an entire population and the overall effects

Linear energy transfer (LET) amount of energy deposited by radiation per unit length of tissue

Relative biologic effectiveness (RBE) ability to produce biological damage; varies with the LET

Direct effect effect that occurs when radiation directly strikes DNA in the cellular nucleus

Indirect effect effect that occurs when radiation strikes the water molecules in the cytoplasm of the cell

Radiolysis of water effect that occurs as radiation energy is deposited in the water of the cell; the result of radiolysis is an ion pair in the cell: a positively charged water molecule (HOH^+) and a free electron

Mutation erroneous information passed to subsequent generations via cell division

Law of Bergonié and Tribondeau cells are most sensitive to radiation when they are immature, undifferentiated, and rapidly dividing

Early somatic effects of radiation hematopoietic syndrome; gastrointestinal (GI) syndrome; central nervous system syndrome

Late somatic effects of radiation carcinogenesis; cataractogenesis; embryologic effects; thyroid dysfunction; life span shortening

Cardinal principles of radiation protection distance, time, shielding

Distance best protection against radiation exposure

Personnel monitoring devices optically stimulated luminescence (OSL) badge, film badge, thermoluminescent dosimeter (TLD)

Mean marrow dose average dose of radiation to the bone marrow

---

BASIC PRINCIPLES OF RADIATION PROTECTION

RESPONSIBILITY FOR RADIATION PROTECTION

A. Radiographer is primarily responsible for protecting the patient from unnecessary exposure
   1. Best accomplished by avoiding repeat exposures
   2. Should use smallest amount of radiation that produces a diagnostic radiograph
B. Radiologist and referring physician assume shared responsibility for radiation safety of the patient
   1. Best accomplished by consultation
   2. Should not order unnecessary examinations
C. Safe use of radiation in diagnostic imaging to determine the extent of disease or injury should outweigh the risk involved from the exposure

IONIZING RADIATION

A. X-radiation exposure involves a transfer of energy through photon-tissue interactions
   1. Possesses the ability to remove electrons from atoms by a process called *ionization*
   2. Results of ionization in human cells
      a. Unstable atoms
      b. Free electrons
      c. Production of low-energy x-rays
      d. Formation of new molecules harmful to the cell
      e. Cell damage may be exhibited as abnormal function or loss of function
B. General types of radiation damage
   1. *Somatic:* Damage to the exposed individual
   2. *Genetic:* Damage to the genetic code of the germ cell contained in the DNA; may be passed to the next generation
C. Sources of ionizing radiation (per NCRP Report #160)

1. This report addresses the dose, from all sources, to the population of the United States
2. All data represent annual effective dose per person
3. Total annual background radiation dose is 6.25 mSv (double compared with early 1980s)
4. Natural background radiation
   a. Contributes 3.11 mSv
   b. 50% of total radiation dose
   c. Largest sources of natural background radiation are radon (largest source) and thoron (2.28 mSv)
   d. Other sources of natural background radiation are terrestrial, internal, and space, which contribute 0.83 mSv
5. Medical background radiation
   a. Contributes 3.0 mSv (these data assume that medical doses would be spread equally across the entire population)
   b. 48% of total radiation dose
   c. Increase in total exposure is primarily attributed to increased use of CT
   d. CT effective dose is 1.47 mSv
   e. CT accounts for 24% of total radiation exposure
   f. CT and nuclear medicine account for 75% of medical radiation exposure
   g. CT and nuclear medicine account for 36% of total radiation exposure
   h. Conventional radiography and fluoroscopy contribute 0.33 mSv; typical doses per procedure:

Average Effective Dose	
Chest	0.1 mSv
Cervical spine	0.2 mSv
Thoracic spine	1.0 mSv
Lumbar spine	1.5 mSv
Upper GI	6.0 mSv
Abdomen (KUB)	0.7 mSv
Pelvis and hip	0.7 mSv
Extremities	negligible—0.005-0.008 mSv

i. Nuclear medicine procedures contribute 0.77 mSv

j. Interventional fluoroscopy contributes 0.43 mSv

6. Other human-made background radiation
   a. Remaining 2% of effective dose
   b. Sources—occupational exposure, various consumer products, and other sources

📱 KEY REVIEW POINTS
Ionizing Radiation

- Ionizing radiation is able to remove electrons from atoms; the process is called *ionization*
- Ionization may cause unstable atoms, free electrons, or formation of new molecules harmful to the cell
- Two types of cell damage may occur: somatic (damage to the cell itself) or genetic (damage to the cell's genetic code)
- Natural background radiation is present in the environment
- The greatest source of natural background exposure to humans is radon
- Human-produced radiation is created by human activities or inventions
- CT accounts for the largest increase in total dose and medical dose to the population
- Total radiation dose to the U.S. population has doubled since the 1980s

PHOTON-TISSUE INTERACTIONS

A. *Primary radiation:* Radiation exiting the x-ray tube

B. *Exit radiation (image-producing radiation):* X-rays that emerge from the patient and strike the image receptor; composed of primary and scattered photons

C. *Attenuation:* Absorption and scatter (loss of intensity) of the x-ray beam as it passes through the patient

D. *Heterogeneous beam:* X-ray beam that contains photons of many different energies

E. Most common photon-tissue interactions in diagnostic radiography are photoelectric and Compton interactions
   1. Photoelectric interaction (Figure 2-1)
      a. Photon absorption interaction
      b. Incoming x-ray photon strikes a *K*-shell electron
      c. Energy of x-ray photon is transferred to electron
      d. Electron is ejected from the *K*-shell and is now called a *photoelectron*
      e. X-ray photon has deposited all of its energy and ceases to exist
      f. Photon has been completely absorbed
      g. Photoelectron may ionize or excite other atoms until it has deposited all of its energy
      h. Hole in *K*-shell is filled by electrons from outer shells, releasing energy that creates low-energy characteristic photons that are locally absorbed

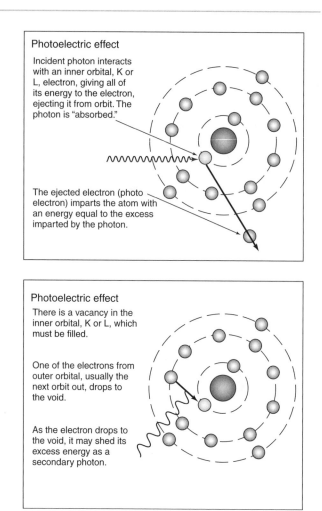

FIGURE 2-1 The photoelectric effect is responsible for total absorption of the incoming x-ray photon.

      i. Photoelectric interaction results in increased dose to the patient
      j. Photoelectric interaction produces contrast in the radiograph because of the differential absorption of the incoming x-ray photons in the tissues
   2. Compton interaction (Figure 2-2)
      a. Also called *Compton scattering* or modified scattering
      b. Incoming x-ray photon strikes a loosely bound, outer-shell electron
      c. Photon transfers part of its energy to the electron
      d. Electron is removed from orbit as a scattered electron, referred to as a *recoil electron*
      e. Ejected electrons may ionize other atoms or recombine with an ion needing an electron
      f. Photon scatters in another direction with less energy than before because of its encounter with the electron
      g. Scattered photon may interact with other electrons, causing more ionization, additional scattering events, or photoelectric absorption, or it may exit the patient

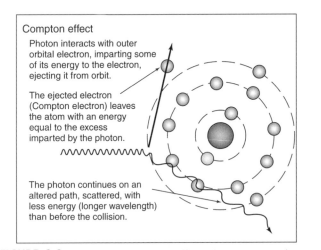

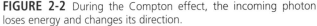

FIGURE 2-2 During the Compton effect, the incoming photon loses energy and changes its direction.

h. Scattered photons emerging from the patient travel in very divergent paths in random directions

i. Scattered photons may also be present in the room and expose the radiographer or radiologist

3. Coherent scatter (also known as *classic* or *Thompson's scatter*)

   a. Produced by low-energy x-ray photons
   b. Atomic electrons are not removed but vibrate because of the deposition of energy from the photon
   c. As the electrons vibrate, they emit energy equal to that of the original photon
   d. This energy travels in a path slightly different from the path of the original photon
   e. Ionization has not occurred, although the photon has scattered
   f. Does not affect image less than 70 kVp
   g. May have negligible effect on fog greater than 70 kVp

4. Pair production

   a. Does not occur in radiography
   b. Produced at photon energies greater than 1.02 million electron volts
   c. Involves an interaction between the incoming photon and the atomic nucleus

5. Photodisintegration—does not occur in diagnostic radiography

UNITS OF RADIATION MEASUREMENT

A. Traditional units used are roentgen, rad, rem, and curie
B. International System (SI) of units used are coulomb/kilogram, gray, sievert, and becquerel
   1. Adopted by International Commission on Radiation Units and Measurements (ICRU) in 1989
   2. Not yet in widespread use in the United States

C. Radiation exposure in air
   1. Measurement of positive and negative particles created when radiation ionizes the atoms in air (x-rays and gamma rays only, up to 3 million electron volts, in-air measurements only)
   2. This is the unit used to measure the output of an x-ray machine; it is also the amount of radiation that may be expected to strike an object placed near the source of radiation
   3. Traditional unit is the roentgen (R); 1 R equals 2.58×10^{-4} coulombs of positive and negative charges produced per kilogram of air
   4. SI unit is the coulomb/kilogram (C/kg)
   5. $1\ R = 2.58 \times 10^{-4}$ C/kg
   6. $1\ C/kg = \frac{1}{2.58} \times 10^{-4}$ C R

D. Unit of absorbed dose
   1. Amount of energy absorbed by the object
   2. Absorption of energy may result in biological damage
   3. As the atomic number of the object increases, so does the absorbed dose
   4. Traditional unit is the rad (radiation absorbed dose)—1 rad is 100 ergs of energy deposited per gram of tissue
   5. SI unit is the gray
      a. 1 gray = 1 joule of energy deposited per kilogram of tissue
      b. 1 gray = 100 rads
      c. 1 rad = $\frac{1}{100}$ gray

E. Unit of equivalent dose
   1. Used to take into account the different biological effects caused by different types of radiation
   2. A radiation weighting factor (W_R) is used to modify the absorbed dose amount to account for the greater damage inflicted by some forms of ionizing radiation (rad $\times W_R$ = equivalent dose [rem])
      a. W_R takes into account linear energy transfer (LET), which is the amount of energy transferred by ionizing radiation per unit length of tissue traveled

b. LET varies for different types of radiation
c. High-ionization radiations such as alpha particles and neutrons have high LET (cause more biological damage)
d. Lower ionization radiations such as x-rays and gamma rays have lower LET (cause less biological damage)
e. W_R for x-rays and gamma rays = 1
f. 100 rads of x-rays = 100 rem
g. W_R for neutrons = 20
h. 100 rads of neutrons = 2000 rem (a higher dose equivalency)
3. Traditional unit is the rem—1 rem = $\frac{1}{100}$ sievert

F. SI unit is the sievert—1 sievert = 100 rem

G. Radioactivity
1. Used to measure the quantity of radioactive material (is *not* used to measure the radiation emitted but rather the number of atoms decaying per second)
2. Used primarily in nuclear medicine
3. Traditional unit is the curie—1 curie = 3.7×10^{10} becquerels
4. SI unit is the becquerel

📱 KEY REVIEW POINTS
Units of Radiation Measurement

Traditional Units of Measurement
- Roentgen—unit of in-air exposure
- Rad—unit of absorbed dose
- Rem—unit of equivalent dose
- Curie—unit of activity

International System (SI) Units of Measurement
- Coulombs per kilogram—unit of in-air exposure
- Gray—unit of absorbed dose
- Sievert—unit of equivalent dose
- Becquerel—unit of activity

ANNUAL DOSE LIMITS

A. Agencies involved in dose-response evaluations
1. International Commission on Radiological Protection (ICRP)
   a. Conducts research and provides recommendations on radiation protection to the worldwide community based on fundamental scientific principles
   b. Has no legal power
   c. Most countries base radiation protection legislation on ICRP recommendations
2. National Council on Radiation Protection and Measurements (NCRP)
   a. Formulates and publishes scientifically researched recommendations on radiation protection and measurements in the United States

3. Nuclear Regulatory Commission (NRC)
   a. Enforces radiation protection standards relating to radioactive material at the federal level

B. Effective dose limit
1. Upper boundary dose that can be absorbed, either in a single exposure or annually, with a negligible risk of somatic or genetic damage to the individual
2. *As low as reasonably achievable* (ALARA)
   a. Concept of radiologic practice that encourages radiation users to adopt measures that keep the dose to the patient and themselves at minimal levels

C. Dose-response relationships
1. Linear-nonthreshold relationship (Figure 2-3)
   a. Indicates that no level of radiation can be considered completely safe
   b. A response occurs at every dose
   c. The degree of response to exposure is directly proportional to the amount of radiation received
2. Linear-threshold relationship (Figure 2-4)
   a. Indicates that at lower doses of radiation exposure (to the left of the line intersecting the *x*-axis), no response is expected
   b. When the threshold dose is exceeded, the response is directly proportional to the dose received
   c. As an example, cataractogenesis does not occur at low levels of radiation exposure; there is a threshold dose below which cataractogenesis does not occur
3. Nonlinear-threshold relationship (Figure 2-5)
   a. Indicates that at lower doses of radiation exposure (to the left of the curve intersecting the *x*-axis), no response is expected

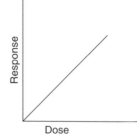

FIGURE 2-3 Linear-nonthreshold relationship.

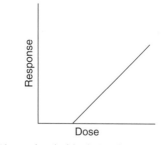

FIGURE 2-4 Linear-threshold relationship.

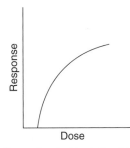

FIGURE 2-5 Nonlinear-threshold relationship.

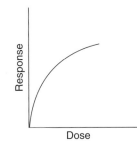

FIGURE 2-6 Nonlinear-nonthreshold relationship.

   b. When the threshold dose is exceeded, the response is not directly proportional to the dose received and is increasingly effective per unit dose
 4. Nonlinear-nonthreshold relationship (Figure 2-6)
   a. Indicates that no level of radiation can be considered completely safe
   b. A response occurs at every dose
   c. The degree of the response is not directly proportional to the dose received
   d. The effect is large even with a small increase in dose
 5. *Probabilistic effects:* Randomly occurring effects of radiation; the probability of such effects is proportional to the dose (increased dose equals increased probability, not severity, of effects)
 6. *Deterministic effects:* Effects that become more severe at high levels of radiation exposure and do not occur below a certain threshold dose
D. NCRP Report #116
 1. Recommends balance between the risk and benefit of using radiation for diagnostic imaging
 2. Recommends that somatic and genetic effects be kept to a minimum when using radiation for diagnostic imaging
 3. Takes into account all human organs that may be vulnerable to radiation damage
 4. Occupational exposure—annual effective dose limit is 50 mSv (5 rem)
 5. Occupational exposure—annual equivalent dose limits for deterministic effects
   a. Lens of the eye—150 mSv (15 rem)
   b. Localized areas of skin, hands, feet—500 mSv (50 rem)

 6. Cumulative effective dose (CEfD) limit = Age (in years) × 10 mSv (1 rem)
 7. Students (older than age 18)—annual effective dose limit same as occupational exposure limit
 8. General public—annual effective dose limit for frequent exposure is 1 mSv (0.1 rem)
 9. General public—annual effective dose limit for infrequent exposure is 5 mSv (0.5 rem)
 10. Embryo-fetus—total equivalent dose for gestation is 5 mSv (0.5 rem)
 11. Embryo-fetus—equivalent dose limit per month is 0.5 mSv (0.05 rem)
 12. Level of negligible risk is 0.01 mSv (1 mrem per year)

KEY REVIEW POINTS
Annual Dose Limits

- Annual dose limits are published by the NCRP
- Effective dose limit is the upper boundary dose that can be absorbed, either in a single exposure or annually, with a negligible risk of somatic or genetic damage to the individual
- The ALARA (*as low as reasonably achievable*) principle means that radiographers do what is possible to keep doses to patients and themselves at minimal levels
- Linear-nonthreshold relationship states that no level of radiation can be considered completely safe, and the degree of response is directly proportional to the amount of radiation received
- Probabilistic effects are randomly occurring effects of radiation; the probability of such effects is proportional to the dose (not related to the severity of effects)
- Deterministic effects become more severe at high levels of radiation exposure but do not occur below a certain threshold dose
- NCRP Report #116 contains recommendations for annual dose limits
- Annual effective dose limit for occupational exposure is 50 mSv (5 rem or 5000 mrem)
- CEfD limit = age (in years) × 10 mSv (1 rem)
- Annual effective dose limit for the general public is 1 mSv (0.1 rem or 100 mrem) for frequent exposure and 5 mSv (0.5 rem or 500 mrem) for infrequent exposure
- Equivalent dose limit for the embryo or fetus for all of gestation is 5.0 mSv (0.5 rem or 500 mrem)

REVIEW OF THE CELL

CELL

A. Contains three main parts
 1. Cell membrane
 2. Cytoplasm
 3. Nucleus
B. Cell membrane
 1. Protects cell
 2. Holds in water and nucleus
 3. Allows water, nutrients, and waste products to pass into and out of the cell (it is semipermeable)

C. Cytoplasm
   1. Composed primarily of water
   2. Conducts all cellular metabolism
   3. Contains organelles
      a. *Centrosomes:* Participate in cell division
      b. *Ribosomes:* Synthesize protein
      c. *Lysosomes:* Contain enzymes for intracellular digestive processes
      d. *Mitochondria:* Produce energy
      e. *Golgi apparatus:* Combines proteins with carbohydrates
      f. *Endoplasmic reticulum:* Acts as a transportation system to move food and molecules within the cell
D. Nucleus
   1. Contains deoxyribonucleic acid (DNA—the master molecule) and the nucleolus (with ribonucleic acid [RNA])
   2. DNA controls cell division
   3. DNA controls all cellular functions
E. Other cell components
   1. Proteins—15% of cell
   2. Carbohydrates—1% of cell
   3. Lipids—2% of cell
   4. Nucleic acids—1% of cell
   5. Water—80% of cell
   6. Acids, bases, salts (electrolytes)—1% of cell

CELL DIVISION

A. *Mitosis:* Somatic cells
   1. Interphase
      a. Cell growth before mitosis
      b. Consists of three phases: G_1, S, G_2
      c. G_1—pre-DNA synthesis
      d. S—DNA synthesis
      e. G_2—post-DNA synthesis, preparation for mitosis
   2. Four subphases
      a. Prophase—nucleus enlarges
      b. Metaphase—nucleus elongates
      c. Anaphase—two complete sets of chromosomes
      d. Telophase—separates the two sets of genetic material; division complete; 46 chromosomes in each new somatic cell
B. *Meiosis:* Cell division of sperm or ovum (germ cells) that halves the number of chromosomes in each cell
   1. Replication division
      a. G_1
      b. S
      c. G_2
      d. M
   2. Reduction division
      a. G_1
      b. No S phase
      c. G_2
      d. M

   3. *Note:* Sperm and ovum unite to return the number of chromosomes in each cell of the new individual to 46

BIOLOGICAL EFFECTS OF IONIZING RADIATION

A. As LET of radiation increases, so does biological damage
B. *Relative biologic effectiveness (RBE):* Ability to produce biological damage; varies with LET
C. The W_R used to calculate rem is a measure of the RBE of the radiation being used
D. Ionizing radiation may change the molecular structure of a cell, affecting its ability to function properly
E. Somatic cell exposure may result in a disruption in the ability of the organism to function
F. Reproductive (germ) cell exposure may result in changes, called *mutations,* being passed on to the next generation
G. Basically, radiation striking a cell deposits energy in either the DNA (a direct effect) or water in the cytoplasm (an indirect effect) if an interaction occurs
H. Most radiation passes through the body without interacting because atoms are composed mainly of empty space

DIRECT EFFECT

A. Occurs when radiation transfers its energy directly to the DNA (the master molecule) or RNA
B. As these macromolecules are ionized, cell processes may be disrupted
C. Some of this damage may be repaired
D. If the DNA structure incurs sufficient damage, particularly to its nitrogenous bases, a mutation may result
E. *Mutation:* Erroneous information passed to subsequent generations via cell division
F. Results of the direct effect
   1. No effect—most common result
   2. Disruption of chemical bonds, causing alteration of cell structure and function
   3. Cell death
   4. Cell line death: Death of the tissues or organs that would have been produced from continued cell division had a cell survived; particularly significant if it results in the failure of a major organ or system to develop
   5. Faulty information passed on in the next cell division; possible results include mutations, cancer, and abnormal formations

INDIRECT EFFECT

A. Because water is the largest constituent of the cell, the probability that it will be struck by radiation is greater

B. *Radiolysis of water:* Occurs as radiation energy is deposited in the water of the cell
C. The result of radiolysis is an ion pair in the cell: a positively charged water molecule (HOH^+) and a free electron
D. Several possibilities exist for chemical reactions at this point; most reactions create further instability in the cell
E. If the two ions recombine, no damage occurs
F. Positive and negative water molecules may be formed and then break into smaller molecules such as free radicals
G. *Free radicals:* Highly reactive ions that have an unpaired electron in the outer shell
H. Free radicals may cause biological damage by transferring their excess energy to surrounding molecules or disrupting chemical reactions
I. Some free radicals may chemically combine to form hydrogen peroxide (H_2O_2)
J. Hydrogen peroxide is a poison that causes further damage to the cell
K. The DNA in the cell may be affected by the free radicals or H_2O_2
L. Such action is called indirect because the DNA itself is not struck by the radiation
M. Indirect effect results from ionization or excitation of water molecules
N. Results of indirect effect
   1. No effect—most common response
   2. Formation of free radicals
   3. Formation of H_2O_2
O. Most damage to the body occurs as a result of the indirect effect because most of the body is water, and free radicals are readily mobile in water

TARGET THEORY

A. Each cell has a master molecule (DNA) that directs cell activities
B. If the DNA is the target of radiation damage and is inactivated, the cell dies
C. DNA may be inactivated by either direct or indirect effects
D. All photon-cell interactions occur by chance
E. Whether a given cell death was the result of direct or indirect effects cannot be determined

RADIOSENSITIVITY OF CELLS

A. *Law of Bergonié and Tribondeau:* Cells are most sensitive to radiation when they are immature, undifferentiated, and rapidly dividing
B. If cells are more oxygenated, they are more susceptible to radiation damage (known as the *oxygen enhancement ratio [OER]*)
C. As cells mature and become specialized, they are less sensitive to radiation

D. *Blood cells:* Whole-body dose of 25 rads depresses blood count
   1. Caused by irradiation of bone marrow
   2. Lymphocytes are the most radiosensitive blood cells in the body
   3. Stem cells in bone marrow are especially radiosensitive
E. *Epithelial tissue:* Highly radiosensitive, divides rapidly, lines body tissue
F. *Muscle:* Relatively insensitive because of high specialization and lack of cell division
G. *Adult nerve tissue:* Requires very high doses (beyond medical levels) to cause damage, is very specialized, has no cell division, is relatively insensitive to radiation
H. Reproductive cells
   1. *Immature sperm cells:* Very radiosensitive, divide rapidly, unspecialized, require 10 rads or more (which is beyond most commonly used diagnostic levels) to increase chances of mutation
   2. Ova in female fetus and child are very radiosensitive
   3. Ovarian radiosensitivity decreases until near middle age, then increases again

SOMATIC EFFECTS OF RADIATION

A. Somatic effects are evident in the organism being exposed
B. Doses causing these effects are much higher than the levels of radiation used in diagnostic radiography
C. Caused when a large dose of radiation is received by a large area of the body (can also be caused by local areas of the body receiving high doses of radiation during radiation therapy)
D. Examples of early somatic effects of radiation (acute radiation syndrome)
   1. *Hematopoietic syndrome:* Decreases total number of all blood cells; can result in death
   2. *GI syndrome:* Causes total disruption of GI tract structure and function and can result in death
   3. *Central nervous system syndrome:* Causes complete failure of nervous system and results in death
E. Examples of late somatic effects
   1. *Carcinogenesis:* Causes cancer
   2. *Cataractogenesis:* Causes cataracts to form; follows a nonlinear-threshold dose-response curve
   3. *Embryologic effects:* Most sensitive during the first trimester of gestation
   4. *Thyroid:* Very radiosensitive organ; late somatic effect may be cancer or cessation of function
   5. *Shortening of life span:* Does not occur in modern radiation workers

GENETIC EFFECTS OF RADIATION

A. Caused by damage to DNA molecule, which is passed to the next generation

B. Follows a linear-nonthreshold dose-response curve; no such thing as a safe gonadal dose; any exposure can represent a genetic threat

C. Usually causes recessive mutations, so generally not manifested in the population

D. *Doubling dose:* Amount of radiation that causes the number of mutations in a population to double (is approximately 50 to 250 rads for humans)

E. Genetic mutations do not cause defects that are not already present in humans from other causes; that is, no defects are unique to radiation exposure

---

KEY REVIEW POINTS
Cell

- Main parts of the cell are the cell membrane, cytoplasm, and nucleus
- Nucleus contains DNA
- Cytoplasm contains the organelles and water
- *Interphase:* Portion of the cellular life cycle that occurs before mitosis
- *Mitosis:* Somatic cell division; comprises four phases: prophase, metaphase, anaphase, and telophase
- When mitosis is complete, each new cell contains 46 chromosomes
- *Meiosis:* Germ (sperm or ovum) cell division; halves the number of chromosomes in each cell so that the union of two germ cells produces a new cell with 46 chromosomes
- *LET:* Amount of energy deposited per unit length of travel of radiation passing through matter
- An increase in LET results in an increase in the potential for biological damage
- *RBE:* Ability of radiation to produce biological damage; it varies with LET
- *Direct effect:* Occurs when radiation transfers its energy directly to the DNA (the master molecule) or RNA
- *Mutation:* Erroneous information passed to subsequent generations via cell division
- *Indirect effect:* Occurs when radiation transfers its energy to the water in the cytoplasm; may cause radiolysis and produce free radicals or H_2O_2
- *Law of Bergonié and Tribondeau:* Cells are most sensitive to radiation when they are immature, undifferentiated, and rapidly dividing
- *OER:* If cells are more oxygenated, they are more susceptible to radiation damage
- As cells mature and become specialized, they are less sensitive to radiation
- Lymphocytes are the most radiosensitive blood cells in the body
- Stem cells in bone marrow are especially radiosensitive
- *Epithelial tissue:* Highly radiosensitive
- *Muscle:* Relatively insensitive to radiation
- *Adult nerve tissue:* Requires very high doses of radiation (beyond medical levels) to cause damage; is relatively insensitive to radiation
- *Immature sperm cells:* Very radiosensitive
- *Ova in female fetus and child:* Very radiosensitive
- Ova radiosensitivity decreases until near middle age, then increases again
- Somatic effects manifest in the individual being exposed

- *Early somatic effects:* Hematopoietic syndrome, GI syndrome, central nervous system syndrome
- *Late somatic effects:* Carcinogenesis, cataractogenesis, embryologic effects, life span shortening
- *Genetic effects:* Manifest in the next generation because of damage to the DNA; follow a linear-nonthreshold curve
- *Doubling dose:* Amount of radiation that causes the number of mutations in a population to double; 50 to 250 rads for humans

---

PATIENT EXPOSURE AND PROTECTION

The heart of radiation protection for the patient lies in the concept of ALARA. It is primarily the radiographer's responsibility to see that ALARA is in practice so that patients are properly protected. Taking adequate histories, communicating clearly, using proper immobilization, and conducting radiographic and fluoroscopic examinations calmly and professionally add to the level of safety your patients will encounter while under your care. This section reviews the many technical aspects of the radiographer's practice that contribute to ALARA for the patient.

BEAM LIMITATION

Beam limitation protects the patient by limiting the area of the body and the volume of tissue being irradiated.

A. Collimator
  1. Variable aperture device
  2. Contains two sets of lead shutters placed at right angles to each other
  3. Higher set of lead shutters is placed near the x-ray tube window to absorb off-stem (off-focus) radiation
  4. Lower set of lead shutters is placed near the bottom of the collimator box to restrict the beam further as it exits
  5. Accuracy of the collimator is subject to strict quality control standards (see Chapter 3)
  6. Collimation should be no larger than the size of the image receptor being used
  7. Collimators that automatically restrict the beam to the size of the image receptor have a feature called *positive beam limitation* (PBL), also called *automatic collimation*
  8. PBL responds when an image receptor is placed in the tray containing sensors that measure its size

B. Cylinder cones
  1. Metal cylinders that attach to the bottom of the collimator
  2. Used to restrict the beam tightly to a small circle
  3. Diameter of the far end of the cone determines field size
  4. Cones may be extended an additional 10 to 12 inches by a telescoping action for even tighter restriction of the beam

5. Cones may be used for examination of the os calcis, various skull projections, and cone-down views of vertebral bodies
6. Use of cones results in a restriction of the x-ray beam by cutting out a major portion of the beam
7. When cones are used, mAs must always be increased to make up for the rays attenuated by the cone
8. Cylinder cones do not work by focusing the x-ray beam down the cone; x-rays cannot be focused

C. Aperture diaphragm
   1. Flat piece of lead with a circle or square opening in the middle
   2. Placed as close to the x-ray tube window as possible
   3. Has no moving parts

FILTRATION

A filter is placed in the x-ray beam to remove long-wavelength (low-energy) x-rays. Low-energy x-rays contribute nothing to the diagnostic image but increase patient dose through the photoelectric effect. As low-energy rays are removed, the beam becomes "harder" (predominantly short-wavelength, high-energy). This process of removing low-energy rays results in a lower patient dose.

A. Two types of filtration: inherent and added
B. Inherent filtration
   1. Glass envelope of the x-ray tube
   2. Insulating oil around the tube
C. Added filtration
   1. Aluminum sheets placed in the path of the beam near the x-ray tube window
   2. Mirror placed in the collimator head
D. Total filtration
   1. Equals inherent plus added filtration
   2. Must equal 2.5-mm aluminum equivalent for x-ray tubes operating at greater than 70 kVp
E. *Half-value layer*: Amount of filtration that reduces the intensity of the x-ray beam to half of its original value—measured at least annually by a qualified radiation physicist
F. The radiographer never adjusts added filtration; if it is suspected that the filtration has been altered, the x-ray tube must not be used until checked by a radiation physicist

GONADAL SHIELDS

Gonadal shields are used to protect gonads from unnecessary radiation exposure. They should be used whenever they do not obstruct the area of clinical interest.

A. Gonadal shielding may reduce female gonad dose by up to 50%
B. Gonadal shielding may reduce male gonad dose by up to 95%

C. Proper collimation may also greatly reduce gonadal dose and should be used in conjunction with gonadal shields
D. Most commonly used gonadal shields
   1. *Flat contact shield*: Flat piece of lead or a lead apron placed over the gonads
   2. *Shadow shield*: Suspended from the x-ray tube housing and placed in the x-ray beam light field; requires no contact with the patient; especially useful during procedures requiring sterile technique

EXPOSURE FACTORS

Exposure technique determines the quantity and quality of x-rays striking the patient.

A. Use optimal kVp for the part being radiographed
B. Use the lowest possible mAs to reduce the amount of radiation striking the patient
C. The part being radiographed should be measured with calipers
D. A reliable technique chart should be consulted to determine the proper exposure factors to use
E. Use of automatic exposure controls (AEC) reduces the number of repeat radiographs

FILM-SCREEN COMBINATIONS – IF USING

Faster film-screen combinations reduce patient dose by allowing the use of fewer x-ray photons (i.e., lower mAs) to produce a diagnostic image. The efficient conversion of x-ray energy to light energy through the intensifying screens provides the same information with far less radiation exposure to the patient.

A. Use fastest practical film-screen combination for imaging a particular body part
B. Take into account the region of the body being irradiated, age of the patient, and requirements for recorded detail

PROCESSING – IF USING

The automatic processor should be a constant in the production of a visible radiographic image. Elimination of repeat films because of optimal processor performance reduces the dose to the patient and the radiographer.

A. Subject to strict quality control standards to eliminate retakes caused by processor malfunction (see Chapter 4)
B. Exercise care in loading and unloading cassettes
C. Prevent unnecessary exposure of film to safelight

GRIDS

A. Result in an increase in patient dose because increased mAs are required

B. Use appropriate type and ratio of grid for part being radiographed and examination being performed

REPEAT EXPOSURES

A. Always result in an increase in radiation dose to the patient
B. Must be kept to a minimum
C. Should be tracked via a departmental repeat exposure analysis
D. Reasons for repeat exposures should be documented
E. In-service education for areas of frequent repeat exposures should be conducted by qualified radiographers or radiologists

TECHNICAL STANDARDS FOR PATIENT PROTECTION

A. Minimum source-to-skin distance for portable radiography: at least 12 inches
B. Fluoroscopy
  1. Use of intermittent fluoroscopy (as opposed to a constant beam-on condition)
  2. Tight collimation of the beam
  3. High kVp
  4. Source-to-tabletop distance for fixed fluoroscopes: not less than 15 inches
  5. Source-to-tabletop distance for portable fluoroscopes: not less than 12 inches
  6. Proper filtration of the beam
  7. Fluoroscopy timer that sounds alarm after 5 minutes (300 seconds) of beam-on time
  8. Fluoroscopy timer should not be reset before alarm goes off; fluoroscopist must be made aware of time that the patient and other persons in the room were exposed
  9. Exposure switch must be dead-man type
  10. Limit dose at the tabletop to no more than 10 R per minute
  11. Limit use of high-level-control fluoroscopy (HLCF) during interventional procedures to no more than 20 rads per minute
  12. Long exposure times (>30 minutes) can lead to skin effects; the patient should be informed of the possibility of skin injury (e.g., erythema, epilation)
  13. Fluoroscopy times should be recorded
  14. Image intensifier should be moved as close as possible to the patient during fluoroscopy to achieve ALARA patient skin doses
  15. Pulsed fluoroscopy or low-dose modes should be used when possible to achieve ALARA objectives
  16. Personnel during fluoroscopy should stand on the image intensifier side of the C-arm during lateral or oblique projections
  17. When possible, use the C-arm with the x-ray tube below the patient for anteroposterior and posteroanterior projections
  18. During fluoroscopy, the radiographer should always wear radiation dosimeter outside of the lead apron at the level of the collar
  19. Avoid use of electronic magnification modes on the image intensifier when possible because this increases the dose to the patient and other persons in the room

OTHER FACTORS RELATING TO PATIENT DOSE

A. Measuring patient dose
  1. Skin entrance dose
  2. *Mean marrow dose (MMD):* Average dose to active bone marrow
B. *Genetically significant dose (GSD):* Radiation dose that, if received by the entire population, would cause the same genetic injury as the total of doses received by the persons actually being exposed; the average gonadal dose to the childbearing-age population
C. *Pediatrics:* Children need to be carefully protected from unnecessary exposure; high-speed image receptors should be used along with adequate immobilization
D. Pregnant patients
  1. It is the responsibility of the referring physician to determine whether a diagnostic examination involving x-rays is necessary; the benefit should outweigh the risk; if the abdomen or pelvis is involved, the radiologist should communicate the risk of the examination to the referring physician and the patient
  2. Most diagnostic x-ray examinations have fetal doses of less than 5 rads
  3. Radiation doses of less than 10 rads to the embryo or fetus are considered low risk; the NCRP states that fetal doses greater than 15 rads carry increased risk

---

KEY REVIEW POINTS
Patient Exposure and Protection

- Always observe the ALARA principle
- *Beam limiters:* Collimator, cylinder cones, aperture diaphragms
- *PBL:* Positive beam limitation, or automatic collimation
- *Beam filtration:* Removes long-wavelength rays; total filtration must be at least 2.5-mm aluminum equivalent
- *Gonadal shielding:* May reduce female gonad dose by up to 50%; may reduce male gonad dose by up to 95%
- *Exposure factors:* Use optimum kVp for the part; use lowest practical mAs
- Use fastest practical film-screen system for lowest dose

- Grids remove scatter radiation from exit beam; increase total dose to the patient because of the increased mAs needed
- Maintain a minimum of 12 inches source-to-skin distance for portable radiography
- Use intermittent fluoroscopy
- Maintain a minimum of 15 inches source-to-tabletop distance for fixed fluoroscopes
- Maintain a minimum of 12 inches source-to-tabletop distance for portable fluoroscopes (15 inches preferred)
- Monitor fluoroscopy timer that must sound alarm after 5 minutes (300 seconds) of beam-on time
- Fluoroscopy foot switch must be dead-man type
- Fluoroscopy dose at the tabletop is limited to no more than 10 R per minute
- *MMD:* Average dose to active bone marrow
- *GSD:* Radiation dose that, if received by the entire population, would cause the same genetic injury as the total of doses received by the persons actually being exposed; the average gonadal dose to the childbearing-age population

RADIATION WORKER EXPOSURE AND PROTECTION

The ALARA concept applies to radiographers as well as to patients. Many of the steps taken to reduce the dose to the patient also reduce the dose to the radiographer. However, additional steps may be taken to protect the radiation worker further. Agency standards also apply to the equipment used by radiographers. This section reviews practices and standards used to protect occupationally exposed individuals. As you study the factors involved in protecting the radiation worker, reexamine the annual effective dose limits covered previously.

CARDINAL PRINCIPLES OF RADIATION PROTECTION

A. *Time:* Amount of exposure is directly proportional to duration of exposure
B. *Distance:* Most effective protection from ionizing radiation
   1. Dose is governed by the inverse square law
   2. The greater the distance from the radiation, the lower the dose
   3. Dose varies inversely according to the square of the distance; for example, if the dose of radiation is 5 R at a distance of 3 feet, stepping back to a distance of 6 feet causes the dose to decrease to 1.25 R
   4. The inverse square law should always be used during fluoroscopy in which close contact with the patient is not required and during mobile radiography and fluoroscopy
C. *Shielding:* Lead-equivalent shielding absorbs most of the energy of the scatter radiation
   1. A lead apron of at least 0.25-mm lead equivalent *must* be worn (0.5-mm lead equivalent *should* be

worn) during exposure to scatter radiation; a thyroid shield of at least 0.5-mm lead equivalent *should* be worn for fluoroscopy
2. The radiographer should never be exposed to the primary beam
3. If exposure of the radiographer to the primary beam is unavoidable, the examination should not be performed
4. Family members of the patient, nonradiology employees, or radiology personnel not routinely exposed should be the first choices to assist with immobilization of the patient for an examination when all other types of immobilization have proved inadequate
5. The radiographer should be the last person chosen to assist with immobilization during an exposure
6. Radiographers and student radiographers should not be viewed as quick and easy-to-use immobilization devices
7. Thickness recommendations for lead devices have been determined by NCRP Report #102

SOURCE OF RADIATION EXPOSURE TO RADIOGRAPHER

A. Source of radiation exposure to the radiographer is scatter radiation produced by Compton interactions in the patient
B. Greatest exposure to the radiographer occurs during fluoroscopy, portable radiography, and surgical radiography
C. Photons lose considerable energy after scattering
D. Scattered beam intensity is about $\frac{1}{1000}$th the intensity of the primary beam at a 90-degree angle at a distance of 1 m from the patient
E. Beam collimation helps reduce the incidence of Compton interactions, resulting in decreased scatter from the patient
F. The use of high-speed image receptors may reduce the amount of scatter produced further because of decreased quantity of radiation needed for exposure

STRUCTURAL PROTECTIVE BARRIERS

A. Primary protective barriers
   1. Consist of $\frac{1}{16}$-inch lead equivalent
   2. Located where primary beam may strike the wall or floor
   3. If in the wall, extend from the floor to a height of 7 feet
B. Secondary protective barriers
   1. Consist of $\frac{1}{32}$-inch lead equivalent
   2. Extend from where primary protective barrier ends to the ceiling, with $\frac{1}{2}$-inch overlap
   3. Located wherever leakage or scatter radiation may strike

4. X-ray control booth is also a secondary protective barrier
   a. Exposure switch must have cord short enough that the radiographer has to be behind the secondary protective barrier to operate the switch
   b. Lead window by control booth is usually 1.5-mm lead equivalent
C. Determinants of barrier thickness
   1. *Distance:* Between the source of radiation and the barrier
   2. *Occupancy:* Who occupies a given area
      a. *Uncontrolled area:* Areas where personnel are not provided radiation exposure monitors (dosimeters) or radiation safety training should be shielded to ensure an effective dose limit to the general public of 0.1 rem
      b. *Controlled area:* Occupied by persons trained in radiation safety and wearing personnel monitoring devices; shielded to keep exposure under the annual effective dose limit of 5 rem
   3. *Workload:* Measured in mA minutes per week (mA min/wk); takes into account the volume and types of examinations performed in the room
   4. *Use factor:* Amount of time the beam is on and directed at a particular barrier

X-RAY TUBE HOUSING

A. X-rays may leak through the housing during an exposure
B. Patient and all others present in the room must be protected from excess leakage radiation
C. Leakage radiation may not exceed 100 mR per hour at a distance of 1 m from the housing

FLUOROSCOPIC EQUIPMENT

A. *Exposure switch:* Must be dead-man type
B. *Protective curtain:* Minimum 0.25-mm lead equivalent
C. *Bucky slot shield:* Minimum 0.25-mm lead equivalent
D. 5-minute timer with audible alarm

PORTABLE RADIOGRAPHIC EQUIPMENT AND PROCEDURE

A. Exposure switch must be on a cord at least 6 feet long
B. Lead aprons must be worn if mobile barriers are unavailable
C. Least scatter is at a 90-degree angle from patient
D. Apply the inverse square law to reduce dose by using exposure cord at full length
E. Radiographer should never hold the image receptor in place for a portable examination because of possible exposure to the primary beam
F. Commercial image receptor holders, pillows, and sponges should be used to hold the image receptor in place

---

📱 KEY REVIEW POINTS
Radiation Worker Exposure and Protection

- *Cardinal principles of radiation protection:* Time, distance, shielding; distance is the best protection
- Dose is governed by the inverse square law
- *Lead apron:* Must be at least 0.25-mm lead equivalent; should be at least 0.5-mm lead equivalent
- The radiographer must never be exposed to the primary beam
- Source of radiation exposure to radiographer is scatter radiation produced by Compton interactions in the patient during fluoroscopy, portable radiography, and surgical radiography
- Scattered beam intensity is about $\frac{1}{1000}$th the intensity of the primary beam at a 90-degree angle at a distance of 1 m from the patient
- Beam collimation helps reduce the incidence of Compton interactions, resulting in decreased scatter from the patient
- *Primary protective barriers:* Must be at least $\frac{1}{16}$-inch lead equivalent and extend from the floor to a height of 7 feet
- *Secondary protective barriers:* Must be at least $\frac{1}{32}$-inch lead equivalent and extend from the primary protective barrier to the ceiling with a $\frac{1}{2}$-inch overlap
- *Determinants of barrier thickness:* Distance, occupancy, workload, use
- *Uncontrolled area:* General public areas such as waiting rooms and stairways
- *Controlled area:* Occupied by persons trained in radiation safety and wearing personnel monitoring devices
- *X-ray tube leakage:* May not exceed 100 mR per hour at a distance of 1 m from the housing
- *Fluoroscopic protective curtain:* Minimum 0.25-mm lead equivalent
- *Bucky slot shield:* Minimum 0.25-mm lead equivalent
- Portable x-ray machine exposure switch must be on a cord at least 6 feet long

---

MONITORING RADIATION EXPOSURE

MONITORING PERSONNEL EXPOSURE

A. Optically stimulated luminescence (OSL) dosimeters
   1. Use aluminum oxide to record dose
   2. Radiation absorbed causes electrons to be trapped
   3. Aluminum oxide layer is stimulated by a laser beam after wear period
   4. Electrons release energy as visible light
   5. Light is in direct proportion to the amount of radiation received
   6. Sensitive to exposures of 1 mrem
   7. Relatively unaffected by temperature and humidity
   8. Can be worn 3 months at a time
   9. Can be reanalyzed multiple times, if necessary
B. Thermoluminescent dosimeters (TLDs)
   1. Use lithium fluoride crystals instead of film to record dose
   2. Electrons of crystals are excited by radiation exposure and release this energy on heating

3. Energy released is visible light, which is measured by a photomultiplier tube
4. Light is in direct proportion to the amount of radiation received
5. TLDs are used mainly in ring badges worn by nuclear medicine technologists
6. Sensitive to exposures of 5 mrem
7. Relatively unaffected by temperature and humidity
8. Can be worn for longer periods than film badges
9. TLDs and equipment used to read them are expensive

C. Film badges - not often used
1. Consist of plastic case, film, and filters
2. Plastic case holds film and filters and provides a clip for attaching to clothing
3. Film used is similar to dental x-ray film and measures doses of 10 mrem
4. Film is sensitive to extremes in temperature and humidity
5. Filters made of aluminum and copper measure intensity and type of radiation striking the film badge
6. Film badges are usually developed monthly, with readings returned to the institution via a film badge report
7. Film badge report indicates wearer's name, ID number, and radiation dose (expressed in millirem for deep and shallow doses)
8. Badge reading of *M* indicates exposure below sensitivity of film

MONITORING AREA EXPOSURE

A. Handheld ionization chamber
1. Used to measure radiation in an area (e.g., a fluoroscopic room), storage areas for radioisotopes, doses traveling through barriers, and patients who have radioactive sources within them
2. Not used to monitor short exposure times
3. Measures exposure rates of 1 mR per hour
4. Operates on a principle similar to the pocket ionization chamber, with internal gas being ionized when struck by radiation

B. Geiger-Mueller detector
1. Used to detect radioactive particles in nuclear medicine facilities
2. Sounds audible alarm when struck by radiation, with sound increasing as radiation becomes more intense
3. Meter reads in counts per minute

KEY REVIEW POINTS
Monitoring Radiation Exposure

- *OSL dosimeters:* Aluminum oxide layer stores energy that is released when exposed to a laser; correlate to dose; sensitive to exposures of 1 mrem; insensitive to environmental factors
- *TLDs:* Store energy in lithium fluoride crystals that is released when heated; correlate to dose; measure doses of 5 mrem; insensitive to environmental factors
- *Film badges:* Use small piece of x-ray film; measure doses of 10 mrem; sensitive to extremes in temperature and humidity
- *Handheld ionization chamber:* Used to measure radiation in an area; measures doses of 1 mR per hour
- *Geiger-Mueller detector:* Used to detect radioactive particles; meter reads in counts per minute

REVIEW QUESTIONS

1. According to NCRP Report #160, natural background radiation represents what percentage of humans' radiation exposure?
   a. 21%
   b. 50%
   c. 82%
   d. 5%
2. According to NCRP Report #160, the greatest source of natural background radiation exposure is:
   a. Cosmic rays
   b. Radioactive materials
   c. The body itself
   d. Radon gas
3. Cosmic radiation:
   a. Is present only in space
   b. Is a source of exposure only to persons who lie in the sun
   c. Is of concern only to space travelers
   d. Is greater at higher altitudes because of a thinner atmospheric shield
4. Radon gas:
   a. Presents a danger when undetected
   b. Is present in doses proportional to other sources
   c. Is entirely human-made
   d. Is the source of 100% of annual background dose
5. X-rays and gamma rays used in diagnostic imaging are:
   a. Not of concern because the beam is filtered
   b. Part of the natural background dose
   c. Part of an artificial background radiation dose
   d. An insignificant dose to the general population because they are used safely
6. A personnel monitoring device that is accurate to 1 mrem is the:
   a. Thermoluminescent dosimeter
   b. Film badge
   c. Optically stimulated luminescence dosimeter
   d. Pocket ionization chamber
7. The greatest source of human-produced radiation exposure is:
   a. Radon gas
   b. Medical x-ray and gamma ray imaging procedures

   c. MRI scans

   d. Sonograms

8. Which of the following is *not* part of background radiation?

   a. Dental x-rays

   b. Microwave ovens

   c. Radon gas

   d. Weapons testing

9. Which of the following occurs at greater than 1.02 million electron volts?

   a. Photoelectric interaction

   b. Compton interaction

   c. Classic scatter

   d. Pair production

10. Which of the following is also known as "coherent scattering"?

   a. Photoelectric interaction

   b. Compton interaction

   c. Classic scatter

   d. Pair production

11. Which of the following photon-tissue interactions does *not* occur in diagnostic radiography?

   a. Photoelectric interaction

   b. Compton interaction

   c. Coherent scatter

   d. Pair production

12. Which of the following is responsible for producing contrast on the radiograph?

   a. Photoelectric interaction

   b. Compton interaction

   c. Coherent scatter

   d. Pair production

13. Which of the following produces scatter radiation that exits the patient and may fog the radiograph?

   a. Photoelectric interaction

   b. Compton interaction

   c. Coherent scatter

   d. Pair production

14. Which of the following produces scatter as a result of vibration of orbital electrons?

   a. Photoelectric interaction

   b. Compton interaction

   c. Coherent scatter

   d. Pair production

15. Which of the following results in total absorption of an incident x-ray photon?

   a. Photoelectric interaction

   b. Compton interaction

   c. Classic scatter

   d. Pair production

16. Which of the following is the only photon-tissue interaction that does *not* result in ionization?

   a. Photoelectric interaction

   b. Compton interaction

   c. Coherent scatter

   d. Pair production

17. Which of the following involves interaction between an incident photon and an atomic nucleus?

   a. Photoelectric interaction

   b. Compton interaction

   c. Coherent scatter

   d. Pair production

18. Which of the following photon-tissue interactions primarily involves *K*-shell electrons?

   a. Photoelectric interaction

   b. Compton interaction

   c. Coherent scatter

   d. Pair production

19. Which of the following primarily involves loosely bound outer-shell electrons?

   a. Photoelectric interaction

   b. Compton interaction

   c. Coherent scatter

   d. Pair production

20. Which of the following results in the production of a photoelectron that is ejected from the atom?

   a. Photoelectric interaction

   b. Compton interaction

   c. Coherent scatter

   d. Pair production

21. Which of the following photon-tissue interactions necessitates the use of a grid?

   a. Photoelectric interaction

   b. Compton interaction

   c. Coherent scatter

   d. Pair production

22. Which of the following may result in occupational exposure for a radiographer?

   a. Photoelectric interaction

   b. Compton interaction

   c. Coherent scatter

   d. Pair production

23. What is the traditional unit of measurement that equals 100 ergs of energy deposited per gram of tissue?

   a. Roentgen

   b. Rad

   c. Rem

   d. Curie

24. What is the traditional unit of measurement that is derived from multiplying rad by a radiation weighting factor?

   a. Roentgen

   b. Gray

   c. Rem

   d. Curie

25. Which of the following units would be used to describe the radiation present in a fluoroscopic room?

   a. Roentgen

   b. Rad

   c. Rem

   d. Curie

26. The amount of energy deposited by radiation per unit length of tissue being traversed is:
    a. LET, which determines the use of a W_R when the equivalent dose is being calculated
    b. Linear energy transfer
    c. Higher for wave radiations than for particulate radiations
    d. LET, which is expressed as a W_R when absorbed dose is being calculated

27. What agency publishes radiation protection standards based on scientific research?
    a. Nuclear Regulatory Commission (NRC)
    b. American Society of Radiologic Technologists (ASRT)
    c. National Council on Radiation Protection and Measurements (NCRP)
    d. Bureau of Radiological Health (BRH)

28. The agency that enforces radiation protection standards relating to radioactive material at the federal level is the:
    a. Nuclear Regulatory Commission (NRC)
    b. International Commission on Radiation Protection (ICRP)
    c. National Council on Radiation Protection and Measurements (NCRP)
    d. Bureau of Radiological Health (BRH)

29. Effective dose limit is defined as the upper boundary dose that:
    a. Can be absorbed annually with a negligible risk of somatic or genetic damage to the individual
    b. Can be absorbed, either in a single exposure or annually, with no risk of damage to the individual
    c. Can be absorbed, either in a single exposure or annually, with no risk of somatic or genetic damage to the individual
    d. Can be absorbed, either in a single exposure or annually, with a negligible risk of somatic or genetic damage to the individual

30. *ALARA* is an acronym for:
    a. *As long as reasonably achievable*
    b. *As little as reasonably achievable*
    c. *As long as radiologist allows*
    d. A radiation protection concept that encourages radiation users to keep the dose to the patient *as low as reasonably achievable*

31. What are graphs called that show the relationship between dose of radiation received and incidence of effects?
    a. Nonlinear-nonthreshold effect
    b. Linear-nonthreshold effect
    c. H & D curves
    d. Dose-response curves

32. Which of the following is the basis for all radiation protection standards?
    a. Nonlinear-nonthreshold effect
    b. Linear-nonthreshold effect

    c. Linear-threshold effect
    d. Nonlinear-threshold effect

33. Which of the following means there is no safe level of radiation, and the response to the radiation is not directly proportional to the dose received?
    a. Nonlinear-nonthreshold effect
    b. Linear-nonthreshold effect
    c. Linear-threshold effect
    d. Nonlinear-threshold effect

34. Which of the following means there is no safe level of radiation, and the response to the radiation is directly proportional to the dose received?
    a. Nonlinear-nonthreshold effect
    b. Linear-nonthreshold effect
    c. Linear-threshold effect
    d. Nonlinear-threshold effect

35. Which of the following means there is a safe level of radiation for certain effects, and those effects are directly proportional to the dose received when the safe level is exceeded?
    a. Nonlinear-nonthreshold effect
    b. Linear-nonthreshold effect
    c. Linear-threshold effect
    d. Nonlinear-threshold effect

36. Which of the following means there is a safe level of radiation for certain effects, and those effects are not directly proportional to the dose received when the safe level is exceeded?
    a. Nonlinear-nonthreshold effect
    b. Linear-nonthreshold effect
    c. Linear-threshold effect
    d. Nonlinear-threshold effect

37. Effects of radiation that occur randomly, with the probability of such effects being proportional to the dose received, are called:
    a. Dose-response curves
    b. Probabilistic effects
    c. Genetic effects
    d. Somatic effects

38. Effects of radiation that become more severe at higher levels of exposure once the threshold dose is exceeded are called:
    a. Dose-response curves
    b. Deterministic effects
    c. Genetic effects
    d. Somatic effects

39. What is the embryo or fetus equivalent dose limit per month?
    a. 5 rem
    b. 0.1 rem
    c. 0.5 rem
    d. 0.05 rem

40. Occupational cumulative exposure = age in years × what dose?
    a. 5 rem
    b. 0.1 rem

c. 0.5 rem
d. 1 rem

41. The annual occupational effective dose limit for stochastic effects is:
    a. 5 rem
    b. 0.1 rem
    c. 0.5 rem
    d. 0.05 rem

42. What is the annual effective dose limit for radiography students younger than age 18?
    a. 5 rem
    b. 0.1 rem
    c. 0.5 rem
    d. 0.05 rem

43. What is the annual effective dose limit for the general public, assuming infrequent exposure?
    a. 5 rem
    b. 0.1 rem
    c. 0.5 rem
    d. 0.05 rem

44. What is the embryo or fetus equivalent dose limit for gestation?
    a. 5 rem
    b. 0.1 rem
    c. 0.5 rem
    d. 0.05 rem

45. What is the annual effective dose limit for the general public, assuming frequent exposure?
    a. 5 rem
    b. 0.1 rem
    c. 0.5 rem
    d. 0.05 rem

46. What is the annual effective dose limit for the general public for the lens of the eye?
    a. 1.5 rem
    b. 0.1 rem
    c. 0.5 rem
    d. 0.05 rem

47. The W_R used in calculating rem takes into account which of the following?
    a. Meiosis
    b. Age
    c. LET
    d. Pregnancy

48. LET and biological damage are:
    a. Directly proportional
    b. Indirectly proportional
    c. Inversely proportional
    d. Unrelated

49. The ability of different types of radiation to produce the same biologic response in an organism is called:
    a. LET
    b. W_R
    c. RBE
    d. Doubling dose

50. The phases of the cellular life cycle, in order, are:

a. Prophase, metaphase, anaphase, telophase
b. Interphase, prophase, metaphase, anaphase, telophase
c. G_1, S, G_2, telophase
d. Interphase (G_1, S, G_2), prophase, metaphase, anaphase, telophase

51. The process of cell division for germ cells is called:
    a. Mitosis
    b. Spermatogenesis
    c. Organogenesis
    d. Meiosis

52. Which of the following occurs when radiation transfers its energy to DNA?
    a. Indirect effect
    b. Target theory
    c. Direct effect
    d. Mutations

53. Which of the following states that each cell has a master molecule that directs all cellular activities and that, if inactivated, results in cellular death?
    a. Indirect effect
    b. Target theory
    c. Direct effect
    d. Mutations

54. Which of the following describes the amount of radiation required to increase the number of mutations in a population by a factor of 2?
    a. Indirect effect
    b. Target theory
    c. Doubling dose
    d. Mutations

55. What occurs when radiation transfers its energy to the cellular cytoplasm?
    a. Indirect effect
    b. Target theory
    c. Direct effect
    d. Doubling dose

56. Which of the following induces radiolysis?
    a. Indirect effect
    b. Target theory
    c. Direct effect
    d. Doubling dose

57. What is the name for changes in genetic code passed on to the next generation?
    a. Indirect effect
    b. Target theory
    c. Direct effect
    d. Mutations

58. Which of the following is responsible for producing free radicals?
    a. Indirect effect
    b. Target theory
    c. Direct effect
    d. Doubling dose

59. What occurs when the master molecule is struck by radiation?
    a. Indirect effect

b. Target theory
c. Direct effect
d. Doubling dose

60. Which of the following poisons the cell with H_2O_2?
    a. Indirect effect
    b. Target theory
    c. Direct effect
    d. Doubling dose

61. Most of the damage to a cell occurs as a result of:
    a. Direct effect
    b. Mutations
    c. Law of Bergonié and Tribondeau
    d. Indirect effect

62. Cell radiosensitivity is described by the:
    a. Inverse square law
    b. Law of Bergonié and Tribondeau
    c. Reciprocity law
    d. Ohm's law

63. The law that states that cells are most sensitive to radiation when they are nonspecialized and rapidly dividing is the:
    a. Inverse square law
    b. Law of Bergonié and Tribondeau
    c. Reciprocity law
    d. Ohm's law

64. Cells are more radiosensitive when:
    a. Fully oxygenated
    b. Deoxygenated
    c. Slowly dividing
    d. Near the skin

65. Blood count can be depressed with a whole-body dose of:
    a. 25 rem
    b. 25 mrem
    c. 1 rem
    d. 10 rem

66. The most radiosensitive cells in the body are:
    a. Lymphocytes
    b. Epithelial cells
    c. Nerve cells
    d. Muscle cells

67. Cells that are least sensitive to radiation exposure include:
    a. Ova and sperm
    b. Epithelial cells
    c. Nerve and muscle cells
    d. Blood cells

68. Compared with younger and older women, ova in women of reproductive age are:
    a. More radiosensitive
    b. Less radiosensitive
    c. About the same

69. Most somatic effects occur:
    a. At doses delivered during diagnostic radiography
    b. At doses beyond doses used during diagnostic radiography

c. In middle age
d. In old age because of an increase in medical care

70. Somatic effects manifest in:
    a. The person who has been irradiated
    b. The next generation
    c. Newborns
    d. Imaging technologists

71. Which of the following is considered a late somatic effect?
    a. Carcinogenesis
    b. Genetic effect
    c. Alzheimer's disease
    d. Parkinson's disease

72. Which of the following is used to limit the area of the patient being irradiated?
    a. Grid
    b. Lead mask
    c. Collimator
    d. Compensating filter

73. Gonadal shields may reduce exposure to female gonads by up to:
    a. 50%
    b. 95%
    c. 10%
    d. 75%

74. Which of the following sets of exposure factors would result in the lowest dose to the patient?
    a. High mAs, low kVp, 400-speed system
    b. Low mAs, high kVp, 400-speed system
    c. Low mAs, high kVp, small focal spot, 100-speed system
    d. Low mAs, high kVp, large focal spot, 100-speed system

75. Which of the following is used as part of an effort to observe the ALARA concept?
    a. Grids
    b. Slow-speed system
    c. Collimation
    d. Thinner filtration

76. The cardinal rules of radiation protection include:
    a. Collimation, gonadal shielding, no repeats
    b. Collimation, short exposure time, no repeats
    c. Shielding, distance, time
    d. Time, distance, collimation

77. Which of the following is used to survey an area for radiation detection and measurement?
    a. TLD
    b. Film badge
    c. Handheld ionization chamber
    d. Geiger-Mueller detector

78. Which of the following is accurate as low as 10 mrem?
    a. TLD
    b. Film badge
    c. Pocket ionization chamber
    d. Handheld ionization chamber

79. Which of the following includes filters for measurement of radiation energy?
    a. TLD
    b. Film badge
    c. Pocket ionization chamber
    d. Handheld ionization chamber
80. Which of the following may be used to measure in-air exposures in a fluoroscopic room?
    a. TLD
    b. Film badge
    c. Handheld ionization chamber
    d. Geiger-Mueller detector
81. What detection device sounds an alarm to indicate the presence of radioactivity?
    a. TLD
    b. Film badge
    c. Pocket ionization chamber
    d. Geiger-Mueller detector
82. Which of the following is accurate as low as 5 mrem?
    a. TLD
    b. Film badge
    c. Pocket ionization chamber
    d. Handheld ionization chamber
83. Which of the following is a digital monitor that may be used to measure dose in an area?
    a. TLD
    b. Film badge
    c. Pocket ionization chamber
    d. Handheld ionization chamber
84. Which of the following may be used for 3 months at a time?
    a. TLD
    b. Film badge
    c. Pocket ionization chamber
    d. Geiger-Mueller detector
85. Which of the following is sensitive to extremes in environment?
    a. TLD
    b. Film badge
    c. Pocket ionization chamber
    d. Handheld ionization chamber
86. For any given examination, the mean marrow dose can be calculated. Which of the following is used to represent the mean marrow dose?
    a. GSD
    b. ALARA
    c. MMD
    d. MPD
87. The radiation dose that would cause the same genetic injury to the population as the sum of doses received by individuals actually being exposed is called:
    a. GSD
    b. ALARA
    c. MMD
    d. MPD

88. The timer used in fluoroscopy:
    a. Must be 3 minutes
    b. Should always be reset before the alarm sounds so that it does not annoy the radiologist
    c. Sounds an alarm after 3 minutes
    d. Is used to alert the fluoroscopist after 5 minutes of fluoroscopy scanning have elapsed
89. The most effective protection against radiation exposure for the radiographer is:
    a. Lead apron
    b. Lead gloves
    c. Lead glasses
    d. Distance
90. If the dose of scatter radiation in fluoroscopy to the radiographer is 10 mR at a distance of 2 feet from the table, where should the radiographer stand to reduce the dose to 2.5 mR?
    a. 8 feet from the table
    b. 4 feet from the table
    c. At the foot of the table
    d. Directly behind the fluoroscopist
91. Lead aprons used in fluoroscopy must be at least:
    a. 0.5-mm lead
    b. 0.25-mm lead
    c. 0.1-mm lead
    d. 0.25-mm lead equivalent
92. Which of the following is true concerning holding of patients for radiographic examinations?
    a. May be performed routinely to obtain a diagnostic examination
    b. Should be done only when absolutely necessary, and then the holding should be done by a competent radiographer so that a repeat will not be needed
    c. Should be done only when absolutely necessary, and then the holding should be done by a nonpregnant member of the patient's family
    d. May be performed using a student radiographer to hold because students are not exposed as often as staff radiographers
93. The factors that must be considered in the design of structural shielding for a radiology room or department include:
    a. Use, occupancy, workload
    b. Time, distance, shielding
    c. Occupational and nonoccupational exposure
    d. Number of employees and number of students
94. The lowest intensity of scatter radiation from the patient is located:
    a. At the head of the table
    b. At a 90-degree angle from the patient
    c. At a 180-degree angle from the patient
    d. At the foot of the table
95. A film badge reading of *M* means:
    a. A dose less than 10 mrem has been received
    b. A maximum dose has been received
    c. A mean (average) dose has been received
    d. Much radiation has been received

96. A reading of 200 mR with a handheld ionization chamber means:
a. 200 milliroentgens has been detected
b. At least 200 milliroentgens has been received
c. 200 millirads has been received
d. Roentgens have been received

97. Which of the following is the most accurate personnel monitoring device?
a. TLD
b. Film badge
c. OSL dosimeter
d. Geiger-Mueller detector

98. Minimum source-to-skin distance for mobile radiography must be:
a. 15 inches
b. 12 inches
c. 36 inches
d. 55 inches

99. Positive beam limitation is also known as:
a. Use of collimators
b. Beam limitation used for all examinations
c. Use of beam restrictors
d. Automatic collimation

100. Added filtration should be adjusted by the radiographer:
a. To "harden" the x-ray beam
b. To remove the soft rays from the x-ray beam
c. To exercise radiation protection
d. Never

3

Review of Equipment Operation and Quality Control

Persistence prevails when all else fails.

BASIC PHYSICS TERMINOLOGY

Matter has form or shape and occupies space

Mass amount of matter in an object; generally considered the same as weight

Energy ability to do work

Potential energy energy of position

Kinetic energy energy of motion

Chemical energy energy resulting from a chemical reaction

Electrical energy energy resulting from movement of electrons

Thermal energy heat energy resulting from movement of atoms or molecules

Nuclear energy energy resulting from the nucleus of an atom

Electromagnetic energy energy that is emitted and transferred through matter

Ionizing radiation electromagnetic radiation that is able to remove an electron from an atom

Ionization removal of an electron from an atom

Measurement Standards

Length meter

Mass kilogram

Time second

SI system meter, kilogram, second

MKS system meter, kilogram, second

CGS system centimeter, gram, second

British system foot, pound, second

Velocity (speed) how fast an object is moving

Acceleration rate of change of speed per unit of time

Work force applied on an object over a distance

Power rate of doing work (measured in watts)

Atomic Structure

Atomic nucleus contains protons (positive charges) and neutrons (no charge); contains most of the mass of an atom

Atomic mass number of protons plus number of neutrons; represented by the letter A

Electron shells contain orbital electrons (negative charges); represented by the letters $K, L, M, N, O, P,$ and Q; in a stable atom, the number of electrons and protons is equal

Atomic number of an atom equals the number of protons in the nucleus; represented by the letter Z; the atomic number determines the chemical element; all chemical elements are represented in the periodic table of elements

Isotopes atoms with the same number of protons but with a different number of neutrons

Electron-binding energy force that holds electrons in orbit around the nucleus

Octet rule outer shell of an atom may not contain more than eight electrons

Particulate radiation alpha particles (helium nucleus—two protons and two neutrons); beta particles (electronlike particles emitted from the nucleus of a radioactive atom)

Characteristics of Electromagnetic Radiation

Photon smallest amount of any type of electromagnetic radiation; also considered a bundle of energy called a *quantum*; travels at the speed of light; travels in waves in a straight path

Sine waves waves of electromagnetic radiation; wave height is called *amplitude*; distance between the peaks of waves is called *wavelength*; as photon wavelength decreases, photon energy increases

Frequency number of wavelengths passing a given point per unit time; measured in hertz (Hz)

Speed of travel electromagnetic radiation travels at the speed of light (186,000 miles per second); travel at the speed of light is constant regardless of wavelength or frequency; wavelength and frequency of electromagnetic radiation are inversely proportional

Gamma rays electromagnetic rays produced in the nucleus of radioactive atoms; x-rays and gamma rays differ only in their origin

Wave-particle duality concept that although x-ray photons exist as waves, they exhibit properties of particles

Attenuation partial absorption of the energy of an x-ray beam as it traverses an object

Inverse square law law that governs the intensity of x-radiation; states that the intensity of the x-ray beam is inversely proportional to the square of the distance between the source of the x-rays and the object

Law of conservation of matter matter cannot be created or destroyed; only changed in form

Law of conservation of energy energy cannot be created or destroyed; only changed in form

Principles of Electricity and Magnetism

Electrostatics stationary electrical charges (static electricity)

Electrification movement of electrons between objects

Laws of electrostatics unlike charges attract, and like charges repel; electrostatic charges reside on the outer surface of a conductor and are concentrated at the area of greatest curvature; only negative charges move

Methods of electrification friction, contact, and induction

Conductor material that allows the free flow of electrons

Insulator object that prohibits the flow of electrons

Electrical current movement of electrons along a conductor or pathway (electrical circuit); measured in amperes

Electromotive force (EMF) measured in volts; the force with which electrons move in an electrical circuit

Electrodynamics electrical charges in motion

Semiconductor material that may act as an insulator or conductor under different conditions

Electrical resistance measured in ohms

Ohm's law voltage in the circuit is equal to the current × resistance

Electrical circuits path along which electrons flow; may be wired as series circuits or parallel circuits

Alternating current (AC) electrical circuit in which the current of electrons oscillates back and forth

Direct current (DC) unidirectional flow of electrons in an electrical conductor

Sine wave representation of electron flow as alternating current

Magnetic field energy field surrounding an electrical charge in motion; can magnetize a ferromagnetic material, such as iron, if the material is placed in the magnetic field

Magnetic poles every magnet has a north pole and a south pole

Laws of magnetics like poles repel, and unlike poles attract; the force of attraction between poles is governed by the inverse square law

Electromagnetism movement of electrons in a conductor produces a magnetic field around the conductor; a coiled conductor (i.e., a wire), through which an electrical current is flowing, has overlapping magnetic fields

Solenoid stacks of wire coil through which electrical current flows, creating overlapping force field lines; a magnetic field is concentrated through the center of the coil

Electromagnet solenoid with an iron core that concentrates the magnetic field

Electromagnetic induction process of causing an electrical current to flow in a conductor when it is placed within the magnetic field of another conductor; two types of electromagnetic induction are self-induction and mutual induction

Self-induction opposing voltage created in a conductor by passing alternating current through it

Mutual induction inducing current flow in a secondary coil by varying the current flow through a primary coil

Electrical generator device that converts mechanical energy to electrical energy; usual output of an electrical generator is alternating current

Single-phase, two-pulse alternating current simplest type of current; voltage (and accompanying current) flows as a sine wave; voltage begins at zero, peaks at full value at the crest of the wave, returns to zero, reverses, and again peaks on the inverse portion of the cycle at the trough

Three-phase alternating current special wiring patterns ("wye," "star," "delta") used to create voltage waveforms that are placed 120 degrees out of phase with one another; these voltage waveforms are called *three-phase*; three-phase waveforms may have 6 pulses per cycle or 12 pulses per cycle; three-phase, 6-pulse waveforms contain 360 pulses per second; three-phase, 12-pulse waveforms contain 720 pulses per second; high-frequency generators produce high-frequency electricity (thousands of hertz)

Electrical motor device that converts electrical energy to mechanical energy

Transformer changes electrical voltage and current into higher or lower values; the transformer operates on the principle of mutual induction, so it requires alternating current

Step-up transformer transformer that increases voltage from the primary to the secondary coil and decreases current in the same proportion; a step-up transformer has more turns in the secondary than in the primary coil; a step-up transformer is used in the x-ray circuit to increase voltage to the kilovoltage level for x-ray production

Step-down transformer transformer that decreases voltage from the primary to the secondary coil and increases current in the same proportion; a step-down transformer has more turns in the primary than in the secondary coil; a step-down transformer is used in the filament portion of the x-ray circuit to increase current flow to the cathode

Autotransformer transformer that contains an iron core and a single winding of wire; an autotransformer is used in the x-ray circuit to provide a small increase in voltage before the step-up transformer; the kVp settings are made at the autotransformer

Rectification process of changing alternating current to direct current

Line voltage compensation x-ray circuit depends on a constant source of power; power coming into the radiology department may vary; line voltage compensator keeps incoming voltage adjusted to proper value; usually operates automatically but may be manually adjusted on older equipment

CONDITIONS NECESSARY FOR THE PRODUCTION OF X-RAYS

A. Source of electrons
B. Acceleration of electrons
C. Sudden stoppage of electrons against target material

EQUIPMENT USED IN THE PRODUCTION OF X-RAYS

A. Autotransformer (Figure 3-1)
   1. Also known as a *variable transformer*
   2. Provides for the variation of voltage flowing in the x-ray circuit and applied to the x-ray tube
   3. Single coil of wire with an iron core
   4. Source for selecting kVp
   5. Operates on the principle of self-induction
      a. Single winding of wire incorporates both the primary and the secondary coils of the transformer
   6. Primary turns are fed 220 V from the radiology department's incoming line
   7. Secondary turns (secondary taps) are selected by the radiographer using the kVp select control
   8. Voltage is stepped up or stepped down by only a small amount and sent to the primary side of the high-voltage step-up transformer
   9. The high-voltage step-up transformer boosts the voltage to the kVp that was selected
B. Prereading voltmeter
   1. The voltmeter in the x-ray circuit indicates the voltage that is selected
   2. Called *prereading* because it indicates the kilovoltage that will be flowing through the tube once the exposure is made

3. Placed in the circuit between the autotransformer and the high-voltage transformer
C. Timer
   1. Used to regulate the duration of x-ray exposure
   2. Wired in the circuit between the autotransformer and the high-voltage transformer
   3. mAs timer
      a. Provides the safest tube current in the shortest time possible
      b. Measures total tube current
      c. Located after the secondary coil of the high-voltage transformer
      d. Used with falling load generators
   4. Electronic timer
      a. Microprocessor controlled
      b. Contained in most radiographic equipment
      c. Allows exposure times of 1 ms (0.001 second)
   5. Automatic exposure control (AEC)
      a. Used to provide consistency of radiographic quality
      b. Relies on excellent positioning skills and extensive knowledge of surface and internal anatomy because the part being radiographed must be accurately positioned over ionization sensors
      c. Consists of a flat ionization chamber that is located between the patient and the image receptor
      d. As radiation passes through the ionization chamber, it ionizes the gas contained inside
      e. Level of ionization is directly proportional to the density that will appear on the image
      f. When a predetermined level of ionization is reached (allowing time for a sufficient amount of radiation to pass through to strike the image receptor), an electronic switch terminates the exposure

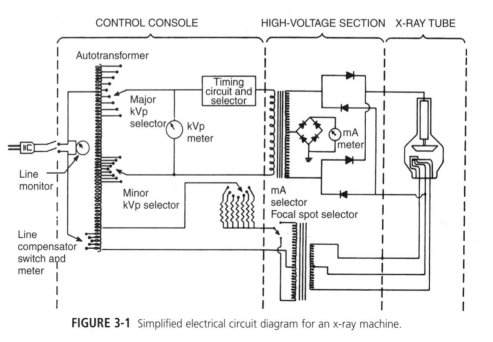

FIGURE 3-1 Simplified electrical circuit diagram for an x-ray machine.

g. Backup timer must be set to terminate the exposure in the event of a malfunction

h. Backup timer protects the patient from overexposure and the x-ray tube from overheating

i. *Minimum response time:* Shortest time possible with an AEC because of the time it takes to operate

j. Shortest time with an AEC is 1 ms (0.001 second)

6. Falling load generator

a. Modern generator that takes advantage of extremely short time capabilities and tube heat-loading potential

b. Radiographer sets mAs and kVp

c. Falling load generator calculates the most efficient method of obtaining the required mAs

d. X-ray tube current starts at highest level possible for first portion of the exposure

e. When the maximum heat load of the tube has been reached for that mA, the generator decreases the mA to the next lower level that the tube can handle

f. The exposure continues at progressively lower levels of mA for the shortest times possible until the desired mAs is reached

g. Falling load generator always uses the shortest times possible to obtain a given mAs

h. *Disadvantages:* Examinations in which long exposure times are used (e.g., breathing techniques for lateral thoracic spine); rapid-sequence exposures in which heat buildup in the tube may cause exposure times to increase

D. Step-up transformer (high-voltage transformer)

1. Consists of primary coils and secondary coils

2. Requires alternating current to operate

3. Primary coil receives voltage from the autotransformer

4. Operates on principle of mutual induction

a. Magnetic field surrounding a wire with electricity flowing through it induces (causes) electricity to flow in a second wire placed within the force field

5. Voltage in the primary coil is boosted to the kilovoltage level (thousands of volts) in the secondary coil

a. Number of turns of the wire in the primary coil compared with the number of turns of the wire in the secondary coil is called the *turns ratio*

b. Turns ratio determines how much the voltage is stepped up

c. The greater the turns ratio, the higher the resulting kilovoltage

d. Voltage is being induced in the secondary coil, which has many more wire turns than the primary coil

6. The turns ratio may be 500 to 1000, depending on the machine

7. Voltage is varied at the autotransformer and sent to the high-voltage transformer

8. Turns ratio in the step-up transformer is not varied

E. Rectifier

1. X-ray tube requires direct current to operate properly

2. Rectifier changes alternating current coming from the step-up transformer to direct current

3. Rectifiers are solid-state semiconductor diodes

a. Consist of silicon-based n-type and p-type semiconductors

4. Located between the step-up transformer and the x-ray tube

5. Unit with four diodes provides full-wave rectification for single-phase generator

a. Full-wave rectification produces pulsating direct current

b. Resultant waveform contains two pulses per cycle (120 pulses per second)

c. Uses both portions of rectified alternating current

d. Results in 100% ripple, with voltage dropping to zero 120 times per second

e. X-ray production ceases 120 times per second

6. Unit with 6 or 12 diodes provides full-wave rectification for three-phase equipment

a. Because three-phase current is used, voltage never drops to zero during the exposure

b. Voltage ripple for three-phase, 6-pulse is approximately 13%; the voltage actually used is about 87% of the kVp set

c. Voltage ripple for three-phase, 12-pulse is approximately 4%; the voltage actually used is about 96% of the kVp set

d. Voltage ripple for high-frequency generators is approximately 1%; the voltage actually used is about 99% of the kVp set

e. High-frequency units result in lower patient dose

f. Three-phase, full-wave rectified waveforms produce higher average photon energy (35% higher for three-phase, 6-pulse; 41% higher for three-phase, 12-pulse)

g. Three-phase and high-frequency units produce 12% to 16% more x-rays than single-phase units

h. kVp values used with single-phase equipment may be decreased 12% to 16% when the same examination is performed on three-phase or high-frequency equipment

F. Milliammeter (mA meter)

1. Measures tube current in milliamperes

2. Wired between the rectifier and x-ray tube

G. mA control (filament circuit)

1. Regulates the number of electrons available at the filament to produce x-rays

2. Voltage is provided by tapping windings of the autotransformer and varying the voltage being sent to the step-down transformer
   a. Step-down transformer reduces voltage and increases current in response to the use of variable resistors (rheostats) manipulated by the radiographer via the mA stations on the control panel
   b. Resultant high current is sent on to heat the filament
   c. A filament ammeter may also be connected
H. X-ray tube (Figure 3-2)
   1. *Cathode assembly:* Negative electrode in the x-ray tube
      a. Contains two filaments—small and large
      b. Filaments are made of tungsten (because of its high melting point); a small amount of thorium is added to reduce vaporization and prolong tube life
      c. Filaments are heated slightly when the x-ray machine is turned on; no electrons are ejected at this low level of heating
      d. During x-ray exposure, one filament is heated to a level that causes electrons to be "boiled off" in preparation for x-ray production (which is known as *thermionic emission*)
      e. Over time, filaments vaporize and coat the inner surface of the x-ray tube with tungsten, leading to tube failure
      f. Cathode assembly also includes the focusing cup
      g. The focusing cup surrounds the filaments on three sides
      h. The focusing cup has a negative charge applied, which tends to concentrate electrons boiling off the filaments into a narrower stream and repels them toward the anode
      i. Electron concentration keeps the electrons aimed at a smaller area of the anode
      j. Some x-ray tubes use the focusing cup as an electronic grid that can turn the tube current

on and off rapidly, allowing very short and precise exposure times, such as times needed for rapid serial exposures (referred to as a *grid-controlled tube*)
   2. *Anode:* Positive electrode in the x-ray tube
      a. Consists of a metal target made of a tungsten-rhenium alloy (because of its high melting point and high atomic number) embedded in a disk (or base) of molybdenum with a motor to rotate the target
      b. Must be able to tolerate extremely high levels of heat produced during x-ray production
      c. Anode rotates from 3300 to 10,000 rpm, depending on tube design
      d. Rotation is achieved by the use of an induction motor located outside the x-ray tube, which turns a rotor located inside the x-ray tube; the target is attached at the end of the rotor
      e. Rotation of the target allows greater heat dissipation
      f. Rotation of the target is stopped by a braking action provided by the induction motor
      g. X-ray machine should never be shut off immediately after an exposure; machine should not be shut off until the target has stopped rotating
      h. Without the braking action, the target may spin for 30 minutes, causing great strain on the bearings
      i. Electrons strike the target on the focal track (sometimes called the *focal spot*)
      j. Focal track is beveled, producing the target angle
      k. Target angle allows for a larger actual focal spot (area bombarded by electrons), while producing a smaller effective focal spot (the area seen by the image receptor)
      l. The larger the actual focal spot, the greater the heat capacity; the smaller the effective focal spot, the greater the radiographic image sharpness
      m. This effect is called the *line-focus principle*
      n. Target angle may be 7 to 20 degrees, depending on tube design
      o. Exposure switch should be activated in one continuous motion, activating the rotor and then the exposure button
      p. The equipment allows the rotor to come up to speed before making the exposure
      q. Radiographer does not control this by activating the rotor and waiting to press the exposure button
      r. Activating the rotor and allowing it to operate by itself results only in unnecessary heating of the filament and wear on the induction motor, shortening tube life

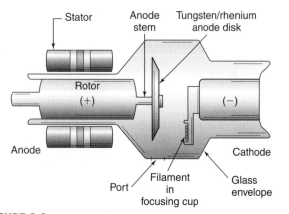

FIGURE 3-2 Structure of a typical x-ray tube, including the major operational parts.

3. Glass envelope with window
   a. Cathode and target are inside the glass envelope; some models use a partial metal envelope
   b. Glass envelope also contains a vacuum so that electrons from the filament do not collide with atoms of gas
   c. *Tube window:* Thinner section of glass envelope that allows x-rays to escape
4. *Tube housing:* Encases the x-ray tube
   a. Made of aluminum with lead lining
   b. Supports and protects the tube, restricts leakage radiation during exposure, and provides electrical insulation
   c. Also contains oil in which the x-ray tube is immersed to assist with cooling and additional electrical insulation

X-RAY PRODUCTION

A. Overview of the x-ray circuit
   1. The x-ray machine is turned on, and a small amount of current is sent to the filament to warm it and ready it for much higher current
   2. Radiographer takes equipment through warm-up exposures to warm the filament further and warm the anode
   3. Radiographer chooses exposure factors on control console for the examination to be performed
   4. Electricity coming into the radiology department is adjusted by the line voltage compensator in the x-ray equipment to maintain it at a constant level
   5. When making the exposure, the radiographer presses the rotor switch and exposure switch in one continuous motion
   6. The induction motor begins spinning the anode; the filament gets hotter
   7. When the exposure switch is closed, the voltage selected by the mA control flows from the autotransformer, through the variable resistors, and into the step-down transformer in the filament circuit
   8. The filament heats considerably, boils off electrons (thermionic emission), and creates a space charge or electron cloud around the filament
   9. At the same time, the alternating current and voltage the radiographer selects by choosing taps off the autotransformer are sent to the primary coils of the high-voltage step-up transformer, where they are boosted to kilovoltage levels
   10. After leaving the secondary coils of the step-up transformer, the voltage and alternating current are sent through the rectifier, which changes the alternating current to pulsating direct current
   11. The kilovoltage creates a high potential difference in the x-ray circuit, making the anode less negative (relatively positive) and the cathode highly negative

12. This high potential difference causes the electrons to move at very high speed (approximately half the speed of light) from the cathode to the anode
13. The collision of these projectile electrons with the atoms of the target material causes a conversion of the kinetic energy of the electrons (100%) to heat (99.8%) and x-rays (0.2%)
14. Heat is produced when the projectile electrons strike the outer shell electrons of the target material and place them in an excited state, which causes them to emit infrared radiation
15. The production of x-rays comes from two interactions with the anode

B. Bremsstrahlung (brems) radiation (Figure 3-3)
   1. A projectile electron misses outer shell electrons in the target and moves in close to the nucleus
   2. Because the nucleus is positive and the electron is negative, it is slowed or braked
   3. The reduction in kinetic energy causes the electron to slow and release energy as an x-ray photon
   4. The resultant x-rays are called *bremsstrahlung* (braking) x-rays because they are produced by the slowing (braking) of projectile electrons
   5. At diagnostic levels, most x-rays produced are from brems interaction

C. Characteristic radiation (Figure 3-4)
   1. A projectile electron collides with an inner shell electron of a target atom
   2. It removes the inner shell electron from orbit and ionizes the atom
   3. A hole exists in the inner shell from the vacated electron
   4. An electron from an outer shell falls in to fill the hole

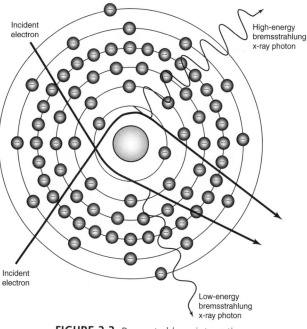

Incident electron

High-energy bremsstrahlung x-ray photon

Incident electron

Low-energy bremsstrahlung x-ray photon

FIGURE 3-3 Bremsstrahlung interaction.

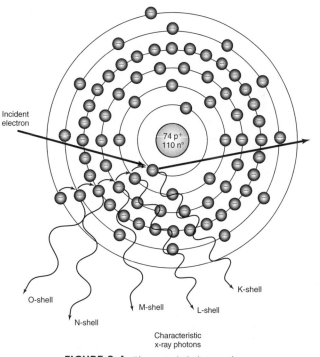

Incident electron

74 p$^+$
110 n°

O-shell

N-shell

M-shell

L-shell

K-shell

Characteristic
x-ray photons

FIGURE 3-4 Characteristic interaction.

5. As the electron falls in, energy is given off in the form of an x-ray photon
6. This creates a hole in its shell of origin, and an electron from the next outer shell falls in to fill this vacancy; this continues until the atom is stable again
7. Each time an electron falls in to fill a hole, an x-ray photon is given off
8. Each x-ray photon has a specific energy, equal to the difference in the binding energies of the two shells involved
9. Only x-rays produced at the *K*-shell are of sufficient energy to be used in diagnostic radiography
10. Because the x-rays possess energy characteristic of the specific binding energies of the atom involved, they are called *characteristic x-rays*
11. Characteristic x-rays are produced at kVp levels greater than 70 but only in small numbers

D. X-ray properties
1. Part of the electromagnetic radiation spectrum
2. Highly penetrating
3. Invisible
4. Travel at the speed of light (186,000 miles per second)
5. Travel in straight lines as waves
    a. *Wavelength of diagnostic x-rays:* 0.1 to 0.5 angstroms (Å) (1 Å × 10^{-10} m, which is one 10-billionth of a meter)
    b. Wavelength is the distance from crest to crest or trough to trough, or the distance covered by one complete sine wave

c. *Frequency:* The number of waves passing a given point per unit time
d. Wavelength and frequency are inversely proportional to one another; as wavelength increases, frequency decreases, and as wavelength decreases, frequency increases
e. Short-wavelength rays are more penetrating; long-wavelength rays are less penetrating

6. Invisible to the human eye
7. Have characteristics of waves and particles; travel in bundles or packets of energy called *photons*
8. Exist in a wide range of wavelengths and energies
9. Can ionize matter and gases
10. Cause fluorescence of phosphors
11. Unable to be focused by a lens
12. Liberate a small amount of heat when passing through matter
13. Electrically neutral
14. Affect photographic film
15. Cause biological and chemical changes through excitation and ionization
16. Scatter and produce secondary radiation

E. X-ray beam characteristics
1. Because x-rays are produced by brems and characteristic interactions at the anode, the resultant x-ray beam contains many different energies
2. An x-ray beam containing many different energies is called *heterogeneous*
3. The collection of all different energies (wavelengths) of x-rays is called the *x-ray emission spectrum*
4. *Discrete x-ray spectrum:* Produced by characteristic x-rays because energies involved are specific to the target atom and are predictable
5. *Continuous x-ray spectrum:* Produced by brems radiation because these energies all are different (from the peak electron energy down to zero energy)
6. The maximum energy an x-ray photon can have corresponds to the kVp that was used
7. Beam characteristics may be altered by using filtration
    a. A filter is usually a sheet of aluminum placed in the primary beam just as it exits the x-ray tube and before it reaches the collimator
    b. The oil and glass envelope of the x-ray tube offer inherent filtration
    c. Total beam filtration equals inherent filtration plus added filtration
    d. Total filtration must be at least 2.5-mm aluminum equivalent
    e. Filtration removes the low-energy (long-wavelength, "soft") rays from the beam
    f. The result of removing soft rays from the beam is a lower patient skin dose

g. Other types of filters that directly affect the radiographic image may be used, known as *compensating filters* (e.g., wedge, boomerang)

h. *Half-value layer:* Amount of filtration that reduces the beam intensity by half

F. Heat units and their management

1. Heat units are a calculation of the total heat produced during an x-ray exposure

2. Heat units are calculated using the following equations:

a. *Single-phase, full-wave rectified equipment:* kVp × mAs

b. *Three-phase, 6-pulse, full-wave rectified equipment:* kVp × mAs × 1.35 (*Remember:* This equipment produces x-ray photons with 35% higher average photon energy)

c. *Three-phase, 12-pulse, full-wave rectified equipment:* kVp × mAs × 1.41 (*Remember:* This equipment produces x-ray photons with 41% higher average photon energy)

3. X-ray tubes and tube housing are constructed to absorb certain levels of heat units

4. Most modern x-ray equipment automatically prevents the user from making an exposure capable of producing too much heat in the tube; this is indicated on some control panels by the warning "technique overload," a red light, or a failure to get a green light indicating that the anode is ready

5. Most modern x-ray equipment prevents overloading of the tube during a series of exposures and does not allow additional exposures until the tube has cooled sufficiently

---

KEY REVIEW POINTS
Conditions Necessary for the Production of X-rays

- *Needed for x-ray production:* Source of electrons, acceleration of electrons, sudden stoppage of electrons
- *Autotransformer:* A variable transformer; operates on the principle of self-induction; allows the manipulation of kVp and mA
- *Prereading voltmeter:* Indicates the kVp that will flow through the x-ray tube during exposure
- *Timer:* Regulates duration of x-ray exposure; electronic timer accurate at 1/1000 second
- *AEC:* Ionization chamber that provides consistency of radiographic quality; placed between the patient and the image receptor
- *Falling load generator:* Provides extremely short exposure times by taking advantage of tube heat-loading potential
- *Step-up transformer (high-voltage transformer):* Operates on principle of mutual induction; steps up voltage, steps down current
- *Rectifier:* Changes AC to DC
- *Milliammeter (mA meter):* Measures tube current

- *Step-down transformer:* Operates on principle of mutual induction; steps down voltage, steps up current
- *X-ray tube:* Consists of two electrodes—cathode (negative) and anode (positive)
- *Cathode:* Contains filaments, the source of electrons for exposure
- *Focusing cup:* Attempts to narrow the stream of electrons as it leaves the cathode filament
- *Anode:* Metal target where electron energy is converted to x-ray energy and heat energy
- *Focal spot (focal track):* Area on anode where electrons strike, from where x-rays emanate
- *Exposure switch:* Consists of rotor (begins rotation of the anode and boiling electrons off of filament) and exposure button (closes circuit allowing flow of electrons through the x-ray tube)
- *Leaded glass envelope:* Encircles the anode and cathode and provides a vacuum inside the x-ray tube
- *Tube housing:* Encases the x-ray tube; aluminum lined with lead
- *X-ray production:* Occurs when current inside the x-ray tube flows from the cathode and is suddenly stopped at the anode
- More than 99% of electrons' energy is converted to heat; less than 1% is converted to x-rays
- *Brems:* X-rays produced by slowing of incoming electrons by the target atoms; slowing releases energy in the form of x-rays
- *Characteristic:* X-rays produced when incoming electrons at the anode dislodge orbital electrons from the target material, and outer shell electrons fall in to fill the hole created; this movement releases energy in the form of x-rays
- *X-ray properties:* Highly penetrating; invisible; travel at the speed of light (186,000 miles per second); travel in straight lines as waves; have diagnostic wavelengths of 0.1 to 0.5 Å; travel as bundles of energy called *photons*; can ionize matter; can cause fluorescence; electrically neutral
- *Wavelength:* Distance from crest to crest or trough to trough of a sine wave
- *Frequency:* Number of waves passing a given point per unit time
- Wavelength and frequency are inversely proportional to each other
- Short-wavelength rays are more penetrating; long-wavelength rays are less penetrating
- *X-ray emission spectrum:* Collection of all different energies (wavelengths) of x-rays in a typical x-ray beam
- *Beam filtration:* Removes long-wavelength rays; total filtration must be at least 2.5-mm aluminum equivalent
- *Heat units:* Calculation of the total heat produced during an x-ray exposure

---

DEDICATED IMAGING EQUIPMENT

A. Fluoroscopy (conventional, nondigital)

1. Provides dynamic visualization of internal structures

2. Consists of an x-ray table to hold the patient, with x-ray tube inside the table, the spot film device and image intensifier (image receptors) over the table, and a television monitor nearby

3. Spot film device allows the fluoroscopist to take radiographs of an area of interest as it is seen "live" on the television monitor

4. X-ray tube and image receptors are connected with a C-arm to keep them the appropriate distance apart, regardless of the movement of the equipment
5. X-ray tube for fluoroscopy is operated at 3 to 5 mA
6. Regulation of kVp and mA for fluoroscopy depends on the part being examined
7. kVp and mA determine the brightness level of the fluoroscopic image
   a. kVp and mA are automatically adjusted during fluoroscopy by a process known as *automatic brightness control* (ABC)
   b. Also called *automatic brightness stabilization*
   c. Also called *automatic gain control*
8. Visible image on the television monitor is a result of image intensification
9. Image-intensifier tube converts x-ray energy into visible light and then into an electronic signal that is displayed as an image on the monitor
10. Image-intensifier tube consists of the following parts (Figure 3-5)
    a. *Input phosphor:* Made of cesium iodide; receives exit rays from the patient and converts them into visible light
    b. Visible light from input phosphor strikes the photocathode, a thin layer next to the input phosphor; it releases electrons in amounts directly proportional to the visible light striking it
    c. The electrons are concentrated and directed toward the other end of the image-intensifier tube (anode) by a series of electrostatic lenses and by 25 kVp applied through the tube
    d. The electrons strike the output phosphor, which is made of zinc cadmium sulfide
    e. The energy of the electrons is converted by the phosphors to visible light in amounts 50 to 75 times greater than at the photocathode
    f. This increase in brightness caused by acceleration of the electrons is called *flux gain*

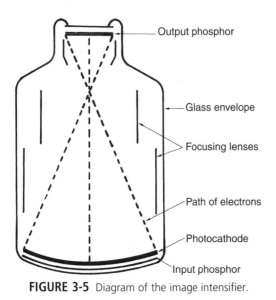

FIGURE 3-5 Diagram of the image intensifier.

(labels on figure: Output phosphor; Glass envelope; Focusing lenses; Path of electrons; Photocathode; Input phosphor)

g. The output phosphor is smaller than the input phosphor, resulting in an increase in brightness called *minification gain*
h. Total brightness gain is a product of minification gain and flux gain
i. Total brightness gain ranges from 5000 to 20,000 and decreases as the tube ages
j. Magnification is possible only with dual-focus or trifocus tubes, which result in increased patient dose
k. Varying the voltage flowing through the image-intensifier tube changes the size of the area on the input phosphor or photocathode being used; this results in the ability to perform magnification during fluoroscopy
11. Viewing and recording of fluoroscopic image
    a. Image may be sent to various viewing and recording devices using an image distributor located near the output phosphor
    b. The signal may be sent to a television monitor for viewing by using Vidicon or Plumbicon video tubes or a charge-coupled device (CCD)
    c. The fluoroscopic image may be recorded on videotape or magnetic disk
    d. Digital fluoroscopy provides computerized images from the output phosphor
B. Digital fluoroscopy (Figure 3-6)
   1. X-ray equipment is similar to conventional fluoroscopy
   2. An operating console and computer workstation are added
   3. The x-ray beam is pulsed to keep patient dose and heat units at a minimum
   4. Initial image is obtained in a manner similar to the technique of conventional fluoroscopy and sent to the monitor
   5. The analog signal is sent through an analog-to-digital converter to convert information into numerical data
   6. Viewing should take place on a high-resolution monitor to take advantage of the digital capabilities
   7. Postprocessing manipulation of the image is possible because the image is in digital format (subtraction is an especially useful postprocessing technique, whereby bone and soft tissue are removed from the image)
   8. "Overhead" postfluoroscopy images are usually eliminated with digital fluoroscopy
C. Mobile radiographic and fluoroscopic units
   1. Mobile fluoroscopic units are usually called *C-arms*
      a. X-ray tube and image intensifier are located on opposite cusps of the "C" just as in stationary fluoroscopy
      b. Mobile units are capable of providing stationary images (using a last-image-hold feature) and dynamic images
      c. Mobile units are used primarily in surgery

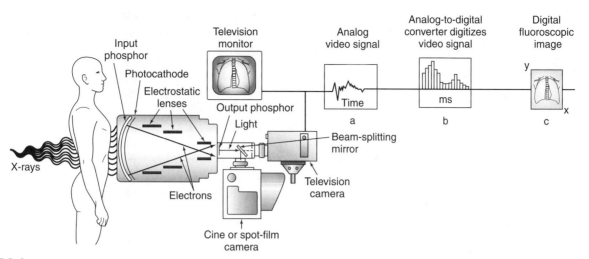

FIGURE 3-6 Analog and digital signals in fluoroscopy. The video signal from the television camera is analog, wherein the voltage signal varies continuously. This analog signal is sampled *(a)*, producing a stepped representation of the analog video signal *(b)*. The numerical values of each step are stored *(c)*, producing a matrix of digital image data. *(Courtesy Eastman Kodak Company.)*

2. Mobile radiographic units allow radiography to be performed under almost any conditions
   a. Most common mobile radiographic units operate on nickel-cadmium batteries
   b. These batteries are recharged by plugging the machine into an outlet
   c. The batteries provide power to propel the unit and operate the x-ray tube
   d. Capacitor-discharge mobile radiographic units must be plugged into a wall outlet for power, and the capacitor must be charged before each exposure
   e. High-frequency mobile radiographic units are smaller and provide ripple-free output
D. *Mammographic equipment:* Used exclusively for performing mammograms
E. *Panoramic tomography equipment:* Used to obtain dental survey and complete images of the mandible, from one temporomandibular joint (TMJ) to the other
F. Tomographic equipment
   1. Uses motion of x-ray tube and image receptor to blur unwanted structures from the image
   2. X-ray tube and image receptor are connected by a rigid rod that pivots around a fulcrum
   3. Position of fulcrum corresponds to level in the body that will appear in focus on the radiograph (called the *objective plane*)
   4. Structures above and below the objective plane are blurred beyond recognition
   5. Angle of arc through which the x-ray tube travels is called the *exposure angle*
      a. Exposure angle determines thickness of tomographic cut
      b. Wider angles provide thin cuts
      c. Narrower angles provide thick cuts
   6. Primary use of tomography is nephrotomography
   7. Tomography has largely been displaced by CT

KEY REVIEW POINTS
Dedicated Imaging Equipment

- *Fluoroscopy:* Provides dynamic visualization of internal structures
- X-ray tube for fluoroscopy is operated at 3 to 5 mA
- *ABC:* In fluoroscopy, adjustment of mA and kVp to provide optimal image
- *Image-intensifier tube:* Consists of input phosphor, photocathode, electrostatic lenses, output phosphor
- *Input phosphor:* Converts x-ray energy to light energy
- *Photocathode:* Converts light energy to electron energy
- *Electrostatic lenses:* Keep electron beam narrowed as it travels toward output phosphor
- *Output phosphor:* Converts electron energy to light energy for viewing
- *Total brightness gain:* Product of flux gain and minification gain
- *Flux gain:* Gain in brightness caused by acceleration of electronic beam inside image-intensifier tube
- *Minification gain:* Gain in brightness caused by minification of the image at the output phosphor compared with the input phosphor
- *Mammographic equipment:* Used exclusively for performing mammography
- *Panoramic tomography equipment:* Used to obtain dental survey and complete images of the mandible, from TMJ to TMJ
- *Tomographic equipment:* Uses motion of x-ray tube and film to blur unwanted structures from the image; provides images of "slabs" of tissue; largely replaced by CT
- *Digital fluoroscopy:* Uses conventional fluoroscope with an added operating console and computer workstation

QUALITY CONTROL OF X-RAY–PRODUCING EQUIPMENT

A. Quality control and assurance
   1. *Quality assurance:* Complete program in a radiology department that addresses all aspects of quality, including customer service, image interpretation,

accuracy of diagnosis, and distribution of radiologists' reports

2. *Quality control:* Program that specifically addresses the safe and reliable operation of equipment

3. A quality control program is required by The Joint Commission

4. A quality control program is the responsibility of radiologists, radiology managers, radiation physicists, quality control technologists (sometimes a separate position and sometimes a staff radiographer's duties; this depends on the size of the radiology department)

5. Many different tests may be performed as part of a quality control program

6. *Filtration-beam quality:* Tested using a digital dosimeter; half-value layer measurement is required

7. *Collimator:* Must be accurate to within 2% of the source-to-image receptor distance (SID)

8. *Effective focal-spot size:* Measured using the slit camera, pinhole camera, or star test pattern; should be within 50% of size stated in equipment specifications

9. *KVp:* Tested using the Wisconsin kVp test cassette or similar devices or using a digital kVp meter; kVp must be accurate to within 4 kVp of that chosen

10. Timer
    a. Timer on single-phase equipment may be tested with a spinning top test; one dot appears on radiograph for each $\frac{1}{120}$-second exposure (assuming full-wave rectification)
    b. Timer on three-phase equipment may be tested with a motorized spinning top, which indicates an arc on the finished radiograph; amount of arc in degrees (fractions of 360 degrees) indicates exposure time
    c. Timer on three-phase equipment may also be tested with a digital testing device

11. *Exposure linearity:* Tested with a digital dosimeter; various mA-time combinations for a given mAs are checked; adjacent mA stations should be within 10% of one another

12. *Exposure reproducibility:* Tested with a digital dosimeter; tests kVp, mA, and time in successive exposures; variation in measured radiation intensity should not be more than 5%

13. *AEC:* Tested to verify reproducibility of exposure using phantoms to simulate variations in patient thickness

14. *Fluoroscopy exposure rate:* Tested with a digital dosimeter; entrance skin dose should not be more than 10 rads per minute

15. *ABC on image intensifier:* Checked to ensure that radiation dose hitting the input phosphor is constant

16. *Resolution of television system:* Tested by use of resolution test patterns

---

📱 KEY REVIEW POINTS
Quality Control of X-Ray-Producing Equipment

- *Quality assurance:* Complete program in a radiology department that addresses all aspects of quality, including customer service, image interpretation, accuracy of diagnosis, and distribution of radiologists' reports
- *Quality control:* Program that specifically addresses the safe and reliable operation of equipment
- *Filtration-beam quality:* Tested using a digital dosimeter; half-value layer measurement is required
- *Collimator:* Must be accurate to within 2% of SID
- *Effective focal-spot size:* Should be within 50% of size stated in equipment specifications
- *kVp:* Must be accurate to within 4 kVp of that chosen
- *Timer:* May be tested by use of a spinning top test (single-phase) or digital devices
- *Exposure linearity:* Various mA-time combinations for a given mAs are checked; adjacent mA stations should be within 10% of one another
- *Exposure reproducibility:* Tests kVp, mA, and time in successive exposures; variation in measured radiation intensity should not be more than 5%
- *AECs:* Tested to verify reproducibility of exposure, with phantoms used to simulate variations in patient thickness
- *Fluoroscopy exposure rate:* Entrance skin dose should not be more than 5 rads per minute
- *ABC on image intensifier:* Checked to ensure that radiation dose hitting the input phosphor is constant

---

REVIEW QUESTIONS

1. In many cases, digital fluoroscopy eliminates which of the following?
   a. The need for a radiographer
   b. Postprocedure "overhead" images
   c. Image acquisition
   d. Accurate positioning

2. What is the smallest particle of an element that retains the characteristics of the element?
   a. Mole
   b. Atom
   c. Molecule
   d. Quark

3. In digital fluoroscopy, the image must be turned into digital form by what device?
   a. Digital-to-analog converter
   b. Flux capacitor
   c. Analog-to-digital converter
   d. DVD-ROM

4. X-rays travel as bundles of energy called:
   a. Energy waves
   b. Phasers
   c. Electromagnetic bursts
   d. Photons

5. What is atomic mass?
   a. The number of protons plus the number of neutrons
   b. The number of photons
   c. The number of electrons
   d. The number of protons plus the number of electrons

6. What device may be used to ensure consistency of radiographic quality from one exposure to the next?
   a. Electronic timer
   b. Step-up transformer
   c. Automatic exposure control
   d. High frequency generator

7. When a predetermined level of ionization is reached in the ionization chamber, what does the machine do?
   a. The unit shuts off as a result of a malfunction
   b. The maximum allowable time has been reached
   c. The highest allowable dose to the patient has been reached
   d. The exposure is terminated

8. What type of x-ray machine uses a continually decreasing mA for the shortest times possible?
   a. Ionization chamber
   b. Portable
   c. C-arm
   d. Falling load generator

9. What type of current is required for proper operation of the x-ray tube?
   a. Direct
   b. Falling load
   c. Alternating
   d. Fluctuating

10. The law stating that the outer shell of an atom can contain no more than eight electrons is called:
    a. Ohm's law
    b. Octet rule
    c. Octagon rule
    d. Electron binding energy

11. Examples of particulate radiation are:
    a. X-rays, gamma rays, and cosmic rays
    b. Helium nuclei and beta particles
    c. Electrons, protons, and meteorites
    d. X-rays and quarks

12. Electromagnetic radiation travels:
    a. In waves along a straight path
    b. In circles
    c. Back and forth
    d. As electrons in waves along a straight path

13. Electromagnetic radiation travels in bundles of energy called:
    a. Protons
    b. Phasers
    c. Electrons
    d. Photons

14. At what speed do x-rays travel?
    a. The speed of light—186,000 miles per hour

    b. The speed of the incident electrons—93,000 miles per second
    c. The speed of light—186,000 miles per second
    d. Infinite speed

15. Waves of radiation are called:
    a. Sine waves
    b. Strong waves
    c. Signal waves
    d. Current waves

16. Wavelength is defined as the distance from:
    a. The x-ray tube to the patient
    b. The cathode to the anode
    c. The bottom of a wave to the top
    d. Peak to peak of the wave

17. Frequency is defined as:
    a. Synonymous with wavelength
    b. The number of waves passing a point per unit time
    c. The number of waves striking the patient
    d. The number of exposures needed during an examination

18. The speed of x-rays is based on:
    a. mAs
    b. kVp
    c. Size of the patient
    d. The fact that they are a form of electromagnetic radiation

19. Wavelength and frequency are:
    a. Directly proportional to each other
    b. Inversely proportional to each other
    c. Inversely proportional to the square of their distance
    d. Unrelated to each other

20. The x-ray beam changes as it travels through the patient by a process called:
    a. Filtration
    b. Attenuation
    c. Electrification
    d. Annihilation

21. The intensity of radiation is inversely proportional to the square of the distance between the source of radiation and the person receiving it. This describes the:
    a. Square law
    b. Reciprocity law
    c. Inverse square law
    d. Octet law

22. As radiation strikes matter:
    a. The energy of the rays is destroyed
    b. The energy of the rays is increased as they acquire the energy of the atoms
    c. The energy is transferred to the atoms according to the law of conservation of energy
    d. The energy is converted to matter according to Einstein's theory

23. Which of the following statements are true regarding electrostatic charges?
    1. Electrostatics is the study of electric charges at rest

2. The movement of electrons from one object to another is called *ionization*
3. Like charges attract, and unlike charges repel
4. Electrostatic charges concentrate on a conductor in the area of greatest curvature
5. Friction, contact, and induction are methods of ionization
   a. 2, 3, 5
   b. 1, 4
   c. 1, 2, 3
   d. 2, 4, 5

24. Which of the following statements are false?
    1. A magnetic field always surrounds an electrical charge in motion
    2. Current flows back and forth in AC
    3. Current flows in one direction in DC
    4. The volt is the unit of electrical current
    5. A conductor allows the free flow of electrons
    6. The ampere is the unit of electromotive force
    7. The volt is the unit of potential difference
    8. The path of electrical current is called the *circuit*
    9. Ohm's law is calculated using the equation $VI = R$
    10. A semiconductor is a material that may act as a conductor under some conditions and as an insulator under other conditions
        a. 4, 6, 9
        b. 1, 2, 3, 5, 7, 8, 10
        c. 1, 7, 10
        d. 4, 6, 9, 10

25. Electromagnetic induction is the process of causing an electrical current to flow in a conductor:
    a. When it is placed in contact with another conductor
    b. When it is placed in contact with an insulator
    c. When it is placed in contact with a superconductor
    d. When it is placed in the magnetic field of another conductor

26. The two types of electromagnetic induction are:
    a. Autoinduction and mutual induction
    b. Self-induction and mutual induction
    c. Generated induction and self-induction
    d. Current induction and voltage induction

27. Self-induction is used in the operation of what device?
    a. Step-up transformer
    b. Autotransformer
    c. Step-down transformer
    d. Electronic timer

28. The strength of the magnetic fields in a transformer is increased by:
    a. Coiling the wires and placing them in adjoining machines
    b. Coiling the wires and letting their magnetic fields overlap
    c. Keeping the wires very straight, increasing their effectiveness
    d. Replacing the wires with diodes

29. Electricity is supplied to the imaging department by a:
    a. Motor
    b. Rectifier
    c. Generator
    d. Voltmeter

30. The electricity provided to the radiology department is:
    a. 110 Hz or 220 Hz DC
    b. 110 Hz or 220 Hz DC
    c. 60 Hz AC
    d. 60 Hz DC

31. The electricity provided to the radiology department operates at:
    a. 120 pulses per second
    b. 60 pulses per second
    c. 110 pulses per second
    d. 220 pulses per second

32. High-frequency power:
    a. Is less effective than single-phase power
    b. Has almost no ripple
    c. Has more ripple than three-phase power
    d. Is yet unproved

33. The primary advantage of three-phase power is that:
    a. Voltage drops to zero only 6 times per second
    b. Voltage drops to zero only 12 times per second
    c. Voltage never drops to zero
    d. Voltage is always at peak value

34. A variable transformer that is used to select kVp for the x-ray circuit is the:
    a. Step-up transformer
    b. Autotransformer
    c. Step-down transformer
    d. Rectifier

35. A transformer that has more turns in the secondary coil than in the primary coil is called a:
    a. Step-up transformer
    b. Solenoid
    c. Step-down transformer
    d. Filament transformer

36. What is the transformer used to boost voltage to kilovoltage levels called?
    a. Autotransformer
    b. Step-down transformer
    c. Step-up transformer
    d. Low-voltage transformer

37. Voltage coming to the x-ray machine is kept constant through the use of a(n):
    a. Autotransformer
    b. Step-down transformer
    c. Rectifier
    d. Line voltage compensator

38. A step-down transformer:
    a. Steps down voltage
    b. Steps down current
    c. Steps up voltage
    d. Steps up resistance

39. Where does thermionic emission occur?
   a. Step-down transformer
   b. Rectifier
   c. Cathode
   d. Timer

40. Which of the following devices is prereading?
   a. Step-down transformer
   b. Rectifier
   c. Timer
   d. kVp meter

41. Which device reduces voltage and provides current to produce an electron cloud or space charge at the filament?
   a. Step-down transformer
   b. Rectifier
   c. Cathode
   d. Timer

42. Which device is electronic, with increments of 0.001 second?
   a. Step-down transformer
   b. Rectifier
   c. Cathode
   d. Timer

43. What changes AC to DC?
   a. Step-down transformer
   b. Rectifier
   c. Cathode
   d. Timer

44. Which of the following is surrounded by a negatively charged focusing cup?
   a. Step-down transformer
   b. Rectifier
   c. Filament
   d. Timer

45. Which of the following is composed of solid-state, silicon-based diodes?
   a. Step-down transformer
   b. Rectifier
   c. Cathode
   d. Timer

46. What regulates the duration of x-ray production?
   a. Step-down transformer
   b. Rectifier
   c. Cathode
   d. Timer

47. What is located in the x-ray circuit between the high-voltage transformer and the x-ray tube?
   a. Step-down transformer
   b. Rectifier
   c. Cathode
   d. Timer

48. Which of the following measures tube current?
   a. Anode
   b. mA meter
   c. Ionization chamber
   d. Falling load generator

49. What device spins at 3300 to 10,000 rpm?
   a. Anode
   b. mA meter
   c. Ionization chamber
   d. Step-up transformer

50. What device uses maximum heat storage ability of the tube to deliver mAs?
   a. Anode
   b. mA meter
   c. Ionization chamber
   d. Falling load generator

51. What is the source of bremsstrahlung and characteristic rays?
   a. Anode
   b. mA meter
   c. Falling load generator
   d. Step-up transformer

52. What device increases voltage approximately 500 times?
   a. Anode
   b. mA meter
   c. Ionization chamber
   d. Step-up transformer

53. What is the most commonly used AEC?
   a. Anode
   b. mA meter
   c. Ionization chamber
   d. Falling load generator

54. What device always delivers the shortest exposure time possible?
   a. Anode
   b. mA meter
   c. Ionization chamber
   d. Falling load generator

55. What device is turned by a rotor?
   a. Anode
   b. mA meter
   c. Ionization chamber
   d. Step-up transformer

56. Which of the following is located between the patient and the image receptor?
   a. Anode
   b. mA meter
   c. Ionization chamber
   d. Falling load generator

57. The filament is kept warm by:
   a. A standby current from the time the x-ray machine is turned on
   b. Insulating oil
   c. Lead housing
   d. Current produced only during exposures

58. Activating the rotor:
   a. Accelerates a procedure
   b. Reduces tube life
   c. Keeps it oiled
   d. Keeps the cooling fan activated

59. When making an exposure, the radiographer should:
    a. Hold the rotor for several seconds before pressing "expose"
    b. Activate the rotor and exposure switch in one continuous motion
    c. Begin the rotor while a student is still positioning the patient
    d. Activate the rotor while estimating how fast the anode is spinning

60. The process of thermionic emission causes:
    a. Electrons to boil off the anode
    b. The anode to spin
    c. The cathode to cool quickly
    d. Electrons to boil off the filament

61. The electron stream passes from cathode to anode because of _____ passing through the x-ray tube.
    a. Current
    b. Kilovoltage
    c. Tungsten
    d. Heat

62. Heat is produced in the x-ray tube as:
    a. Electrons break apart while striking the anode
    b. Electrons interact with the target material
    c. The anode stops spinning
    d. The rectifier operates

63. Most of the energy conversion in the x-ray tube produces:
    a. X-rays
    b. Light
    c. Heat
    d. Current

64. X-rays are produced as incident electrons interact with target atoms by a process called:
    a. Classical
    b. Photoelectric
    c. Bremsstrahlung
    d. Compton

65. X-rays are produced as incident electrons interact with inner shell electrons in target atoms by a process called:
    a. Characteristic
    b. Photoelectric
    c. Bremsstrahlung
    d. Compton

66. What percentage of energy in the x-ray tube is converted to x-rays?
    a. 99%
    b. 75%
    c. 1%
    d. 100%

67. Which of the following are properties of x-rays?
    1. Electrically negative
    2. Affect film emulsion
    3. Scatter and produce secondary radiation
    4. Invisible to the human eye
    5. Travel at the speed of light (186,000 miles per hour)
    6. Possess wavelengths between 1 Å and 5 Å
    7. Travel in bundles of energy called *photons*
    8. Can ionize matter and gases
    9. Can be focused by collimators
    10. Cause phosphors to fluoresce
        a. 2, 3, 7, 8
        b. 2, 3, 4, 7, 8, 10
        c. 1, 5, 6, 9
        d. 2, 3, 4, 6, 8, 9, 10

68. The x-ray beam is:
    a. Heterogeneous—all rays possess the same energy
    b. Homogeneous—all rays possess the same energy
    c. Monoenergetic—all energies correspond to the kVp
    d. Heterogeneous or polyenergetic—consisting of many different energies (wavelengths)

69. The x-ray emission spectrum consists of:
    a. Brems and characteristic rays
    b. Discrete spectrum (produced by brems rays) and continuous spectrum (produced by characteristic rays)
    c. Discrete spectrum (produced by characteristic rays) and continuous spectrum (produced by brems rays)
    d. X-rays and electrons, both part of the electromagnetic spectrum

70. The *primary* purpose of filtration is:
    a. Radiation protection
    b. Removal of short-wavelength (soft) rays
    c. Hardening the beam for imaging
    d. Removal of long-wavelength (hard) rays

71. The amount of material needed to reduce the intensity of the beam by $\frac{1}{10}$ is called:
    a. Half-value layer
    b. Tenth-value layer
    c. Total filtration
    d. Inherent filtration

72. Which of the following statements regarding filtration is true?
    a. Total filtration must not be less than 2-mm aluminum equivalent
    b. Total filtration must remove all soft rays from the beam
    c. Total filtration (added+compensating) must not be less than 2.5-mm aluminum equivalent
    d. Total filtration (not less than 2.5-mm aluminum equivalent)=inherent filtration (glass envelope, tube housing, oil)+added filtration (aluminum)

73. Calculating heat units for three-phase, 12-pulse equipment requires the use of _____ as a constant; calculating heat units for single-phase equipment requires the use of _____ as a constant; calculating heat units for three-phase, 6-pulse equipment requires the use of _____ as a constant.
    a. 1, 1.35, 1.41
    b. 1.35, 1, 1.41

c. Calculating heat units does not require the use of a constant because all x-rays possess the same ionizing potential

d. 1.41, 1, 1.35 because average photon energy is different with each type of equipment

74. When a quality control test is performed to ensure that the penetrating ability of the x-ray beam is accurate, the result must be within what amount of the control panel setting?
a. 2% of SID
b. 4%
c. 10%
d. 4

75. The primary type of grid used in diagnostic imaging is:
a. Crosshatch
b. Parallel
c. Rhombic
d. Focused

76. The portion of the image-intensifier tube that converts electron energy to visible light is the:
a. Output phosphor
b. Photocathode
c. Input phosphor
d. Brightness gain

77. The portion of the image-intensifier tube that converts visible light to an electronic image is the:
a. Output phosphor
b. Photocathode
c. Input phosphor
d. Brightness gain

78. The input phosphor of the image-intensifier tube converts:
a. Electron energy to x-ray energy
b. X-rays and heat to visible light
c. X-ray energy to visible light
d. X-ray energy to an electronic image

79. Total brightness gain achieved using an image intensifier equals:
a. Flux gain times minification gain
b. Diameter of input phosphor times diameter of output phosphor
c. Intensification factor—brightness without an image intensifier divided by brightness with an image intensifier
d. Total light emitted at the photocathode

80. Single-phase, full-wave rectification produces:
a. Direct current
b. Pulsating direct current
c. Pulsating direct current with 120 pulses per second
d. Pulsating direct current with 120 pulses per second and 100% ripple

81. Three-phase, 6-pulse full-wave rectification produces:
a. Direct current with 13% ripple
b. Direct current with 4% ripple
c. Direct current with 100% ripple
d. Alternating current with 13% ripple

82. Three-phase, 12-pulse full-wave rectification produces:
a. Direct current with 13% ripple
b. Direct current with 4% ripple
c. Direct current with 100% ripple
d. Alternating current with 13% ripple

83. The increase in average photon energy when using three-phase, 6-pulse equipment compared with single-phase equipment is:
a. 1.35%
b. 41%
c. 1.41%
d. 35%

84. The increase in average photon energy when using three-phase, 12-pulse equipment compared with single-phase equipment is:
a. 1.35%
b. 41%
c. 1.41%
d. 35%

85. Programs that deal with the safe and reliable operation of equipment and programs that address all aspects of the delivery of radiology services are called:
a. Quality assurance and quality control
b. Total quality improvement
c. Quality control and quality assurance
d. Total quality management

86. Examples of dedicated x-ray equipment include:
a. Mammography units
b. Tomography units
c. Mobile x-ray machines
d. All of the above

87. The collimator must be accurate to a level of:
a. 4
b. 5%
c. 2% of SID
d. 10%

88. kVp must be accurate to within:
a. 4
b. 5%
c. 2% of SID
d. 10%

89. Exposure linearity must be accurate to within:
a. 4
b. 5%
c. 2% of SID
d. 10%

90. Exposure reproducibility must be accurate to within:
   a. 4
   b. 5%
   c. 2% of SID
   d. 10%

91. When a spinning top test is performed on single-phase equipment, a radiograph exhibiting four dots would indicate:
   a. An accurate timer, if set on 1/20 second
   b. A malfunctioning timer, if set on 1/3 second
   c. An accurate timer, if set on 1/30 second
   d. b and c

92. When a spinning top test is performed on three-phase equipment, a timer setting of 1/60 second should indicate the following on the resultant radiograph:
   a. 2 dots
   b. 60 dots
   c. 6-degree arc
   d. 90-degree arc

93. The test that measures the accuracy of adjacent mA stations is:
   a. Exposure reproducibility
   b. Spinning top test
   c. Pinhole camera
   d. Exposure linearity

94. The test that measures the accuracy of successive exposures is:
   a. Exposure reproducibility
   b. Spinning top test
   c. Pinhole camera
   d. Exposure linearity

95. Effective focal-spot size may be measured using the following tool(s):
   a. Slit camera
   b. Star test pattern
   c. Pinhole camera
   d. All of the above

96. Resolution of the television system may be measured using the following tool(s):
   a. Wire mesh test
   b. Line pairs-per-millimeter resolution tool
   c. Resolution test pattern
   d. All of the above

97. AECs may be tested using:
   a. Phantoms
   b. Images of real patients
   c. Analog meters
   d. Fluoroscopic screens

98. The amount of mA used for fluoroscopy is:
   a. 300 to 500
   b. 3 to 5
   c. 10 to 12
   d. 100 to 300

99. Marks on the focal track of the anode resulting from bombardment of electrons are called:
   a. Melts
   b. Bullet marks
   c. Pitting
   d. Cracks

100. Effective quality control and quality assurance programs are required for accreditation by:
   a. The Joint Commission
   b. Joint Review Committee on Education in Radiologic Technology
   c. American Healthcare Radiology Administrators
   d. Starfleet Academy

Image Acquisition and Evaluation

Accept the challenges so that you may feel the exhilaration of victory.

PHOTOGRAPHIC PROPERTIES OF THE RADIOGRAPHIC IMAGE

DENSITY (BRIGHTNESS)

A. Amount of blackness on a given area of a radiograph
B. Controlled by the number of exit (remnant) rays striking the image receptor and window level

Factors Controlling and Influencing Density (Brightness)

A. mAs
  1. Controls the number of electrons passing from cathode to anode in the x-ray tube
  2. Controls the quantity of x-rays produced at the anode
  3. Controls the amount of radiation exiting the x-ray tube
     a. This is a directly proportional relationship
     b. As mAs is increased, density increases in the same amount
     c. As mAs is decreased, density decreases in the same amount
  4. Directly controls the number of x-ray photons that emerge from the patient as exit rays
  5. Directly controls the number of x-rays that eventually strike the image receptor as exit rays
  6. Governed by the reciprocity law
     a. Any combinations of mA and time that produce the same mAs value result in the same density on the radiograph
     b. Sometimes expressed by the equation: mAs = mAs
B. kVp
  1. Directly controls the energy or quality of the x-rays produced
     a. As the kVp increases, a greater potential difference exists between the cathode and the anode
     b. As the potential difference increases, the electrons from the cathode strike the anode in greater numbers and with greater energy

c. This results in an increased level of production of short-wavelength, high-energy radiation
  2. Directly affects density, although not in a directly proportional relationship
     a. As kVp increases, density increases
     b. As kVp decreases, density decreases
     c. Governed by the 15% rule (an increase in kVp of 15% doubles density; a decrease in kVp of 15% halves density)
  3. Determines the penetrating ability of the x-ray beam
     a. As kVp is increased, wavelength decreases, and x-rays become more penetrating
     b. As kVp is decreased, wavelength increases, and x-rays become less penetrating
  4. Penetrating ability of the x-rays also determines the number of x-rays exiting the patient to strike the image receptor
C. Distance
  1. Inverse square law
     a. Beam intensity (and ultimately radiographic density, which is a function of beam intensity) are governed by the inverse square law
     b. *Inverse square law:* Intensity of the x-ray beam is inversely proportional to the square of the distance between the source of x-rays and the image receptor
     c. Intensity is measured in roentgens (traditional) or coulombs/kilogram (SI)
     d. Expressed as: $I_{old}/I_{new} = D_{new}^2/D_{old}^2$ (old intensity over new intensity equals new SID squared over old SID squared)
     e. This equation describes changes in beam intensity (and radiographic density, which is a function of beam intensity) when SID is changed and no changes are made in exposure technique
     f. If SID is doubled, intensity (density) decreases four times; if distance is halved, intensity (density) increases four times
     g. Variation in intensity is the result of the divergence of the x-ray beam as it travels through space

2. Density maintenance formula
   a. Expressed as: $mAs_{old}/mAs_{new} = D_{old}^2/D_{new}^2$ (old mAs over new mAs = old SID squared over new SID squared)
   b. Used to calculate changes in mAs needed to maintain density when dealing with a change in SID
   c. If SID is doubled, mAs must be increased four times to maintain the same density as a radiograph taken at the old distance; if distance is halved, mAs must be decreased four times to maintain the same density as a radiograph taken at the old distance
D. Grids
   1. Decrease amount of scatter radiation striking the image receptor
   2. Density decreases when grids are used, unless mAs is increased to compensate for the loss of scatter fog
E. Beam restriction
   1. Decreases density by limiting the size of the x-ray beam, unless mAs is increased to compensate
   2. Decreases density by limiting the area of the patient being struck by x-rays
   3. Reduces the amount of scatter radiation being produced, reducing density on the image caused by fog; necessary for proper image processing with digital imaging
F. Anatomy and pathology
   1. Anatomy affects density through its variation of atomic number, tissue thickness, and tissue density
   2. Pathologic changes affect density by altering tissue integrity, atomic number, tissue density, and tissue thickness (see Chapter 5 for specific pathological conditions and their effects on radiographic technique)
G. Anode heel effect
   1. X-ray intensity varies along the longitudinal axis of the x-ray beam
      a. Density is greater near the cathode end of the x-ray beam
      b. Density is less near the anode end of the x-ray beam because of absorption of x-rays by the "heel" of the anode
   2. Thicker anatomy should be placed under the cathode side of the x-ray tube to take advantage of the anode heel effect
H. Filtration
   1. Negligible effect on density; its purpose is primarily for radiation protection
   2. Radiation protection is due to the reduction in the number of soft, long-wavelength rays being absorbed in the patient
   3. Has an impact on contrast because the average wavelength of the filtered beam is shorter than the nonfiltered beam
   4. Compensating filters even out density of irregular anatomy

---

KEY REVIEW POINTS
Density (Brightness)

- *Density:* The amount of blackness on a given area of a radiographic image (brightness)
- Density is directly controlled by mAs—mAs controls the current through the x-ray tube and, consequently, the number of x-rays produced at the anode; also controlled by window level
- *kVp:* Controls the energy of x-rays produced; also has a direct impact on density, although not proportional; governed by the 15% rule
- *SID:* Affects density through the inverse square law
- *Grids:* Absorb scatter radiation; this has an impact on the density of the image
- *Beam restriction:* Limits the size of the x-ray beam; affects density by reducing the amount of scatter produced
- *Anatomy and pathology:* Affect density through variations of atomic number, tissue thickness, and tissue density
- *Anode heel effect:* Has some effect on density when a large field is being exposed

---

CONTRAST

A. Differences in adjacent densities on the radiograph
B. Primary function is to make the detail visible
C. *High contrast:* Few gray tones, mainly black and white image; may also be referred to as *short-scale contrast*
D. *Low contrast:* Many gray tones on image; may also be referred to as *long-scale contrast*

Factors Controlling and Influencing Contrast

A. kVp
   1. Directly controls contrast by controlling the differential absorption of the x-ray beam in the body; ultimately, image contrast is controlled by window width and bit depth
   2. Controls differential absorption of the x-ray beam by the body because of its control of x-ray beam energy (Figure 4-1)
      a. As kVp is increased, contrast decreases (becomes lower or longer scale) because the shorter wavelength rays more uniformly penetrate anatomical parts
      b. As kVp is decreased, contrast increases (becomes higher or shorter scale) as a result of greater absorption of lower energy rays by the anatomical parts (increased photoelectric interaction)
   3. High kVp = low contrast = long-scale contrast = many gray tones
   4. Low kVp = high contrast = short-scale contrast = few gray tones (mainly black and white tones)

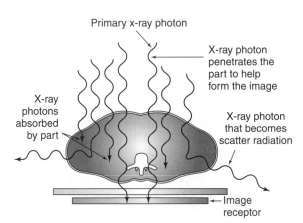

FIGURE 4-1 As the primary x-ray beam interacts with the anatomical part, photons are absorbed, scattered, and transmitted. The differences in the absorption characteristics of the anatomical part create an image that structurally represents the anatomical part.

B. Grids
   1. Reduce the amount of scatter reaching the image receptor
   2. Less scatter fog results in fewer gray tones, which increases contrast
C. Beam restriction
   1. Limits area being irradiated
   2. Produces less scatter by reducing number of Compton's interactions taking place
   3. Less scatter fog reduces the number of gray tones on the radiograph, increasing contrast
D. Filtration (Figure 4-2)
   1. As filtration is increased, beam becomes harder (average photon striking the patient has shorter wavelength)
   2. Contrast decreases as filtration increases
E. Anatomy and pathology
   1. Also known as subject contrast
   2. Control contrast with variations in the following
      a. *Atomic number:* Higher atomic number— increase in contrast owing to photoelectric effect
      b. *Tissue density:* As tissue density increases, contrast decreases owing to Compton interaction
      c. *Tissue thickness:* As tissue thickness increases, contrast decreases owing to Compton interaction
      d. Use of a contrast agent increases contrast owing to photoelectric effect
F. Cause differential absorption of x-ray photons, which results in contrast

---

📱 **KEY REVIEW POINTS**
Contrast

- *Contrast:* Differences in adjacent densities on the radiographic image
- Primary function is to make detail visible
- Produced by photoelectric effect

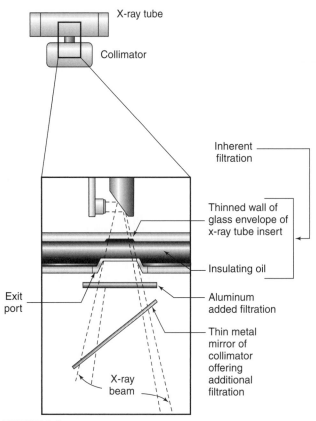

FIGURE 4-2 Aluminum added filtration is shown at the port of the x-ray tube. The inherent filtration of the glass envelope and the oil and the collimator mirror are shown.

- *High contrast:* Few gray tones, mainly black and white image; may also be referred to as *short-scale contrast*; produced at lower kVp
- *Low contrast:* Many gray tones on image; may also be referred to as *long-scale contrast*; produced at higher kVp
- Contrast is controlled by kVp—kVp controls differential absorption of the x-ray beam by the body because of its control of x-ray beam energy
- Ultimately controlled by window width and bit depth
- *Grids:* Reduce the amount of scatter reaching the film, so contrast is increased
- *Beam restriction:* Limits area being irradiated, so less scatter is produced, and contrast is increased
- *Subject contrast:* Controlled by anatomy and pathology; affects contrast through variations of atomic number, tissue thickness, and tissue density

---

GEOMETRIC PROPERTIES OF THE RADIOGRAPHIC IMAGE

RECORDED DETAIL - SPATIAL RESOLUTION

A. Sharpness with which anatomical structures are displayed on an image receptor
B. May be described as the geometric representation of the part being radiographed
C. May also be referred to as *detail sharpness, definition, image resolution,* or *spatial resolution*

Factors Controlling and Influencing Recorded Detail

A. Object-to-image receptor distance (OID)
   1. Distance from the anatomical part being imaged to the image receptor
   2. Shortest possible OID should be used
   3. Increased OID causes magnification of the image, resulting in loss of recorded detail
B. Source-to-image receptor distance (SID)
   1. Distance from the source of radiation (usually anode in the x-ray tube) to the image receptor
   2. Longest practical SID should be used
   3. Shorter SID causes magnification of the image, resulting in loss of recorded detail
C. Focal-spot size (Figure 4-3)
   1. Use small focal spot when possible
   2. Use of large focal spot decreases sharpness of recorded detail
   3. Decreased sharpness is caused by x-rays emanating from a larger area of the anode; adds to image blur
D. Motion
   1. Any motion results in image blur and subsequent loss of recorded detail
   2. Motion may be caused by the following
      a. Patient motion (voluntary and involuntary)
      b. X-ray tube motion
      c. Excessive motion from reciprocating grid
E. Pixel pitch

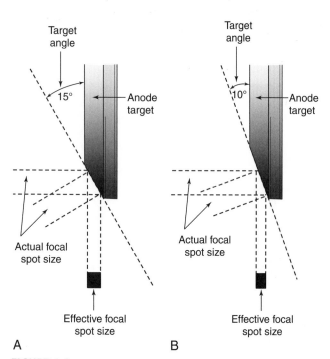

FIGURE 4-3 The line focus principle states that a large target angle produces a large effective focal-spot size (**A**) and that a small target angle produces a small effective spot size (**B**). Both actual focal-spot sizes are the same, meaning that they can withstand the same heat loading from the same exposure factors.

DISTORTION

A. Any geometric misrepresentation of an anatomical structure on an image receptor
B. Two types of distortion—size and shape

Factors Controlling Distortion

A. Size
   1. Magnification
   2. Caused by excessive OID
   3. Caused by insufficient SID
   4. Causes anatomical structure to appear larger on the image than in reality
B. Shape (Figure 4-4)
   1. Elongation
      a. Causes anatomical structure to appear longer than in reality

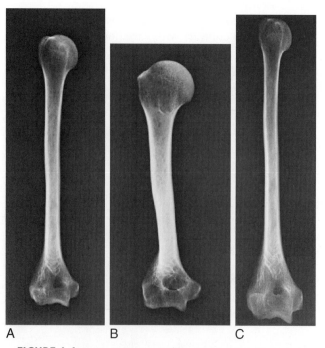

FIGURE 4-4 **A,** No distortion. **B,** Foreshortened. **C,** Elongated.

b. Caused by improper tube, part, or image receptor angulation or alignment

c. Caused by angulation along the long axis of the part

2. Foreshortening

a. Causes anatomical structure to appear shorter than in reality

b. Caused by improper tube, part, or image receptor angulation

c. Caused by angulation against the main axis of the part

KEY REVIEW POINTS
Distortion

- Distortion — any misrepresentation of an anatomic structure on an image receptor that alters its size and/or shape
- Size distortion — magnification; caused by excessive object-to-image distance (OID) or insufficient source-to-image distance (SID)
- Shape distortion — elongation or foreshortening
- Elongation — causes anatomic structure to appear longer than in reality; caused by improper tube, part, or film angulation or alignment, with angulation along the long axis of the part
- Foreshortening — causes anatomic structure to appear shorter than in reality; caused by improper tube, part, or film angulation or alignment, with angulation against the main axis of the part

---

AUTOMATIC EXPOSURE CONTROLS

A. Use fixed kVp while machine controls mAs

B. Require proper ionization chambers to be selected for part being radiographed

C. Part being radiographed must be placed exactly over ionization chamber

D. Varying kVp when using automatic exposure control (AEC) does not alter density, although contrast changes

E. Varying kVp serves to alter penetrating ability of the beam, resulting in faster or shorter exposure time

F. Changing density controls on AEC allows density to be increased or decreased; each step represents a change of 25% in density

---

KEY REVIEW POINTS
Automatic Exposure Controls

- *Ionization chamber:* Placed between the patient and the image receptor
- *Image quality:* Consistent from examination to examination
- Radiographer sets optimal kVp; machine controls mAs
- *Requirements:* Proper chambers selected; exact positioning
- Varying kVp serves to alter penetrating ability of the beam, resulting in faster or shorter exposure time; does not change density
- Changing density controls on AEC allows density to be increased or decreased; each step represents a change of 25% in density

---

GRIDS

A. Use

1. Reduce the amount of scatter radiation reaching the image receptor

a. Scatter travels in divergent paths compared with image-producing rays (Figure 4-5)

b. More likely to be absorbed in the grid

2. Generally used when part thickness is 10 cm or greater or using greater than 60 kVp

B. Construction

1. Lead strips separated by aluminum interspacers

2. Grid ratio

a. Grid ratio is the height of the lead strips divided by the distance between the lead strips: grid ratio = H/D

b. Ratios range from 4:1 to 16:1

3. Grid frequency

a. Number of lead strips per inch (or centimeter)

b. As grid frequency increases, lead strip thickness decreases and becomes less visible

c. Ranges from 60 to 150 lines per inch

C. Grid types

1. Linear

a. Lead strips are parallel to one another

b. X-ray tube may be angled along the length of the grid without cutoff

c. *Grid cutoff:* Decreased density along the periphery of the image caused by absorption of image-forming rays

d. Used primarily with large SID or small field

2. Focused grids (Figures 4-6 and 4-7)

a. Lead strips are angled to coincide with divergence of x-ray beam

b. Used within specific ranges of SID

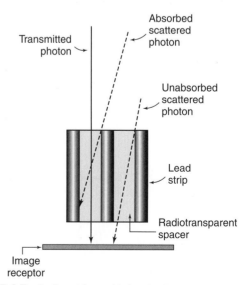

FIGURE 4-5 Ideally, grids would absorb all scattered radiation and allow all transmitted photons to reach the film. In reality, however, some scattered photons are allowed to pass through to the film, and some transmitted photons are absorbed.

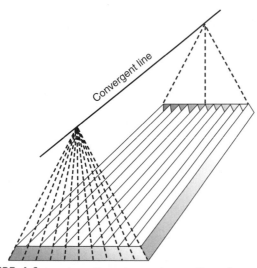

FIGURE 4-6 Imaginary lines drawn above a linear focused grid from each lead line meet to form a convergent line.

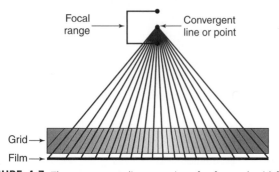

FIGURE 4-7 The convergent line or point of a focused grid falls within a focal range.

    c. *Grid radius:* Distance at which focused grid may be used (also called *focal distance* or *focal range*)
    d. Focal range is wide for low-ratio grids
    e. Focal range is narrow for high-ratio grids
    f. Focal range is stated on the front of the grid
  3. Crossed grids (Figure 4-8)
    a. Also called *crosshatch grids*
    b. Consist of two linear grids placed perpendicular to each other
    c. Superior scatter cleanup
    d. Allow no angulation of x-ray beam
    e. Require perfect positioning and centering

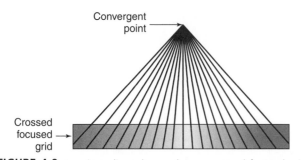

FIGURE 4-8 Imaginary lines drawn above a crossed focused grid from each lead line meet to form a convergent point.

D. Grid characteristics
  1. Contrast improvement factor
    a. Measure of ability of a grid to increase contrast
    b. Expressed as the ratio of the contrast with a grid to the contrast without a grid
  2. Grid selectivity
    a. Expressed as the ratio of primary radiation transmitted through the grid to secondary radiation transmitted through the grid
    b. The higher the grid frequency and grid ratio, the more selective the grid
    c. High selectivity indicates high efficiency of scatter cleanup
  3. Grid conversion factor (GCF)
    a. Also called *Bucky factor*
    b. Amount of exposure increase necessary to compensate for the absorption of image-forming rays and scatter in the cleanup process
    c. Used to indicate the increase in mAs needed when converting from nongrid to grid status (multiply mAs by GCF)
    d. Used to indicate the decrease in mAs when converting from grid to nongrid status (divide mAs by GCF)
    e. Factors used at 120 kVp—5:1 grid, 2; 6:1 grid, 3; 8:1 grid, 4; 12:1 grid, 5; 16:1 grid, 6
E. Grid motion
  1. Stationary grids
    a. Do not move during the exposure
    b. Grid lines may be seen
  2. Moving grids
    a. Reciprocate (move back and forth) during exposure
    b. Eliminate the visibility of grid lines
    c. Grid must begin moving just before the exposure and continue until just after the exposure to blur grid lines.
F. *Grid errors: Focused grids*
  1. Upside down
    a. Result is normal density in the middle of the radiograph with decreased density on the sides
    b. Focused grid must be placed with labeled tube side facing x-ray tube
  2. Off-level
    a. Result is image-forming rays absorbed all across the radiographic field, with cutoff (decreased density) visible over the entire radiograph
    b. Grid must be perpendicular to the central ray
  3. Lateral decentering
    a. Central ray does not strike the grid in the center
    b. Cutoff visible, more to one side of the radiograph
  4. Grid-focus decentering
    a. Violation of the grid radius when a focused grid is used
    b. Normal density in the middle of the radiograph with cutoff visible on the sides

G. Air gap technique
   1. Uses increased OID
   2. Increased OID allows scatter (which travels in widely divergent paths) to exit the patient and miss the image receptor
   3. *Example:* Lateral cervical spine
      a. Distance from spine to shoulder causes gap
      b. Eliminates need for grid (gap is similar to using a 10:1 grid)
      c. Use of grid with air gap increases patient dose and is unnecessary
H. Radiographic quality and grids
   1. Produce higher contrast by absorbing Compton scatter rays, which produce fog if they strike the image receptor

---

KEY REVIEW POINTS
Grids

- Use of grids reduces the amount of scatter radiation reaching the film
- *Construction:* Lead strips separated by aluminum interspacers
- *Grid ratio:* The height of the lead strips divided by the distance between the lead strips: grid ratio = H/D
- *Grid frequency:* Number of lead strips per inch (or centimeter)
- *Linear grids:* Lead strips are parallel to one another
- *Focused grids:* Lead strips are angled to coincide with divergence of the x-ray beam
- *Grid cutoff:* Decreased density along the periphery of the film caused by absorption of image-forming rays
- *Grid radius:* Distance at which focused grid may be used (also called *focal distance* or *focal range*)
- *Contrast improvement factor:* Measure of grid's ability to enhance contrast
- *Grid selectivity:* Expressed as the ratio of primary radiation transmitted through the grid to secondary radiation transmitted through the grid
- *GCF:* Amount of mAs exposure increase necessary to compensate for the absorption of image-forming rays and scatter in the cleanup process (also called *Bucky factor*)
- *GCFs:* At 120 kVp—5:1 grid, 2; 6:1 grid, 3; 8:1 grid, 4; 12:1 grid, 5; 16:1 grid, 6
- *Stationary grids:* Do not move during the exposure
- *Moving grids:* Reciprocate (move back and forth) during exposure; eliminate the visibility of grid lines
- *Upside-down grid:* Result is normal density in the middle of the radiograph with decreased density on the sides
- *Off-level grid:* Result is image-forming rays absorbed all across the radiographic field, with cutoff (decreased density) visible over the entire radiograph
- *Lateral decentering:* Cutoff visible, more to one side of the radiograph
- *Grid-focus decentering:* Normal density in the middle of the radiograph with cutoff visible on the sides

Table 4-1 summarizes variables and how they affect the radiographic image.

TABLE 4-1 Variables and Their Effect on Photographic and Geometric Properties of the Radiographic Image

| Radiographic Variables | Photographic Properties | | Geometric Properties | |
	Density	Contrast	Recorded Detail	Distortion
↑ mAs*	↑	0	0	0
↓ mAs	↓	0	0	0
↑ kVp	↑	↓	0	0
↓ kVp	↓	↑	0	0
↑ SID	↓	0	↑	↓
↓ SID	↑	0	↓	↓
↑ OID†	↓	↑	↓	↓
↓ OID	↑	↓	↑	↓
↑ Grid ratio	↓	↑	0	0
↓ Grid ratio	↑	↓	0	0
↑ Film-screen speed	↑	0	↓	0
↓ Film-screen speed	↓	0	↑	0
↑ Collimation	↓	↑	0	0
↓ Collimation	↑	↓	0	0
↑ Focal-spot size	0	0	↓	0
↓ Focal-spot size	0	0	↑	0
↑ Central ray angle	↓	0	↓	↑

↑, Increased effect; ↓, decreased effect; *0*, no effect; *OID*, object-to-image receptor distance; *SID*, source-to-image receptor distance.
*The mAs has no significant effect on contrast as long as densities remain within diagnostic range.
†The amount of OID needed to affect contrast depends on the type of anatomical part being imaged.
From Fauber TL: *Radiographic imaging and exposure,* ed 4, St Louis, 2012, Mosby.

TECHNIQUE CHARTS

A. Measurement
   1. Part thickness should always be measured using calipers
   2. Caliper measurement is used to consult the technique chart
B. Types of technique charts
   1. Fixed kVp–variable mAs
      a. Assumes optimal kVp for the part being radiographed
      b. Except for exceptionally large patients, kVp never changes for a given projection
      c. mAs is varied according to the part thickness as measured with the calipers
      d. Based on the assumption that thicker parts absorb more rays and more rays must be placed in the primary beam

2. Variable kVp–fixed mAs
   a. kVp is varied according to part thickness as measured with the calipers
   b. Based on the assumption that thicker parts require a beam with shorter wavelength rays that are more penetrating
3. Variable technique (vary both mAs and kVp)
   a. Provides for alteration of routine techniques because of pathological conditions, patient age, ability to cooperate, casts, or contrast media

KEY REVIEW POINTS
Technique Charts

- *Primary purpose:* Radiation protection through decreased repeat exposures; more consistent image quality
- Part thickness should always be measured using calipers
- *Types of technique charts:* (1) fixed kVp–variable mAs, (2) variable kVp–fixed mAs, (3) variable kVp–variable mAs

DIGITAL IMAGING*

B. Computed radiography (CR) (Figure 4-9)
   1. Radiographer selects exposure factors, as in conventional radiography
   2. Accurate positioning remains critical
   3. Image receptor is an imaging plate (IP)
      a. Made of a photostimulable phosphor (PSP) that is applied to a semirigid support layer
      b. PSP are struck by the remnant rays exiting the patient
      c. Remnant rays transfer their energy to electrons in the phosphors, placing the electrons in a higher level conductive layer where they are trapped until placed in the reader
      d. IP can store the image for several hours; after that, the energy slowly dissipates, and the latent image fades; plates should be processed within 8 hours
      e. The x-ray exposure must fall within a range that allows the appropriate number of x-ray photons to strike the CR plate
   4. Reader unit accepts the cassette and removes the IP so that it may be scanned with a laser
      a. Laser beam scans PSPs
      b. Laser scanning allows the electrons to relax into lower energy levels in the phosphors
      c. As the electrons relax into lower energy levels, a visible blue light is emitted

---

*Note: The American Registry of Radiologic Technologists (ARRT) addresses digital imaging equipment and digital image characteristics as topics in separate sections of the content specifications (see Chapter 1). Given the newness and complexity of digital imaging, the topic is presented in its entirety here to make your review more logical and thorough and the subject easier to understand.

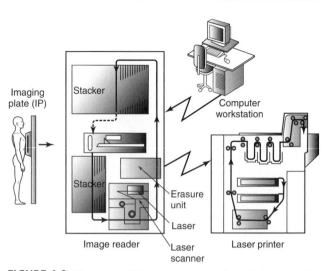

FIGURE 4-9 The exposed IP is placed in a reader unit to release the stored image, convert the analog image to a digital image, and send the data to a computer monitor or a laser printer. The reader unit also erases the exposed IP in preparation for the next exposure. *(Courtesy Fuji Medical Systems.)*

   d. Blue light energy is amplified by a photomultiplier and then converted from analog to digital form and sent to the computer for processing
   5. The radiographer must be very familiar with the equipment being used, the manufacturer's terminology for exposure indication (e.g., s-number, exposure index), and whether the exposure indication is directly or indirectly proportional to the number of photons striking the CR plate
   6. Viewing of the digital image takes place on a computer monitor, normally a flat panel liquid crystal display (LCD) screen
C. Direct digital radiography (DR) (Figure 4-10)
   1. Differs from CR by using flat panel detectors that communicate directly with a computer workstation; detectors may be wired or wireless
   2. The flat panel DR systems produce an image more quickly than CR
   3. Patient throughput generally is higher than with CR
   4. Flat panel DR system may use either direct or indirect detectors
      a. Direct detectors convert exit radiation directly into electrical charges, speeding image construction
      b. Indirect detectors convert exit radiation first to visible light and then to electrical charges
   5. Electrical signals from either direct or indirect detectors are converted from analog to digital
   6. Viewing of the digital image takes place on a computer monitor, normally a flat panel LCD screen
D. CR and DR image characteristics
   1. Wider exposure latitude than with film radiography
   2. Exhibits better visualization of soft tissue and bone
   3. Digital image is composed of numerical values indicating the variety of tissue thicknesses, densities,

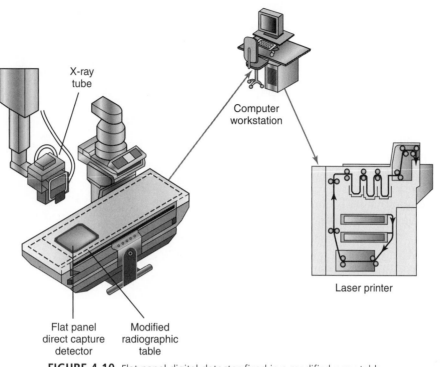

X-ray
tube

Computer
workstation

Flat panel
direct capture
detector

Modified
radiographic
table

Laser printer

FIGURE 4-10 Flat panel digital detector fixed in a modified x-ray table.

and atomic numbers through which the x-ray photons were attenuated

4. Digital image is composed of rows and columns called a *matrix*
   a. Smallest component of the matrix is the *pixel* (picture element)
   b. Each pixel corresponds to a shade of gray representing an area in the patient called a *voxel* (volume element)
5. A *histogram* (graphic display) is constructed to show the radiographer the distribution of pixel values (indicating low, proper, or high exposure)
6. The correct processing algorithm (mathematical formula) must be chosen so that the computer can reconstruct the image specific to the examination that was performed
7. As a digital image, the information can be manipulated through various postprocessing steps (subtraction, edge enhancement, contrast enhancement, and black/white reversal)
   a. *Subtraction:* Removal of superimposed or unwanted structures from the image
   b. *Contrast enhancement:* Altering of image to display varying brightnesses
   c. *Edge enhancement:* Improves visibility of small high-contrast areas
   d. *Black/white reversal:* Reversal of the gray scale in the image
8. Postprocessing can compensate for overexposures or underexposures of considerable degree (−100% to +500%)
   a. Because radiographers comply with the *as* *low* *as* *reasonably* *achievable* (ALARA) concept, patients should never be overexposed with the intention of correcting the resultant images in the postprocessing mode (dose creep)
9. Image may be printed onto film with a laser camera
10. Resolution is finer with DR than with CR because DR involves less conversion of the information
11. In both CR and DR, visibility of the resolution depends on the monitor being used to display the image
12. Changing the window level (midpoint of densities) adjusts the image brightness throughout the range of densities; this is a direct relationship
    a. As window level increases, image brightness increases
    b. As window level decreases, image brightness decreases
13. Changing the window width adjusts the radiographic contrast in postprocessing mode; this is an inverse relationship
    a. As window width decreases, contrast increases (shows fewer gray tones)
    b. As window width increases, contrast decreases (shows more gray tones)
14. *Spatial frequency resolution:* Level of detail or sharpness on the CR image
15. *Look-up table (LUT):* Histogram of brightness level values from image acquisition that can be used to correct, or enhance, luminance values

16. Quantum mottle ("grainy" or "noisy" image)
    a. Is a source of noise in the image, as in conventional radiography
    b. Caused by too few x-ray photons hitting the image receptor
17. Artifacts may be present in digital radiography
    a. May be caused by a dirty or damaged plate (Figures 4-11 through 4-13)
    b. May be caused by dirty light guide in the plate reader (Figures 4-14 through 4-17)
    c. Improper use of grids may cause a Moiré pattern (Figure 4-18)
    d. Scatter radiation is easily imaged in digital imaging; control of scatter is critical
    e. Equipment malfunction (Figures 4-19 through 4-21)
18. DR may be part of an integrated system of images and written data
    a. *Picture archiving and communications system (PACS)*
    b. *Digital imaging and communications in medicine (DICOM):* A standard protocol used for blending PACS and various imaging modalities

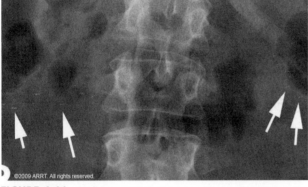

FIGURE 4-11 Appearance of dust *(arrows)* inside the CR cassette on the PSP plate. *(From Online Digital Imaging Academy (ODIA), © 2009 ARRT.)*

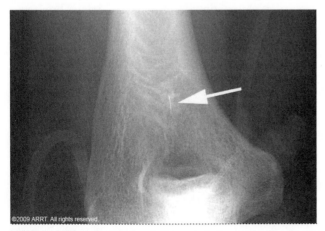

FIGURE 4-12 Appearance of dirt or hair *(arrow)* inside the CR cassette on the PSP plate. *(From Online Digital Imaging Academy (ODIA), © 2009 ARRT.)*

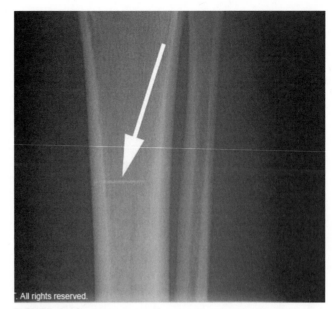

FIGURE 4-13 Appearance of a scratch *(arrow)* on the PSP plate. *(From Online Digital Imaging Academy (ODIA), © 2009 ARRT.)*

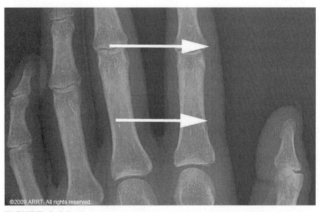

FIGURE 4-14 Line *(arrows)* caused by a dirty light guide in the plate reader. *(From Online Digital Imaging Academy (ODIA), © 2009 ARRT.)*

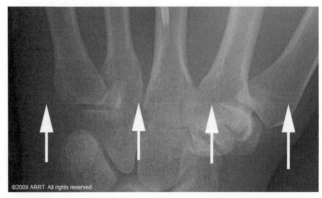

FIGURE 4-15 Very faint line *(arrows)* caused by dirty light guide in the plate reader. *(From Online Digital Imaging Academy (ODIA), © 2009 ARRT.)*

The American Society of Radiologic Technologists (ASRT) developed "Appendix for Digital Image Acquisition and Display" as a study guide for students and practitioners. The appendix is provided here in its original

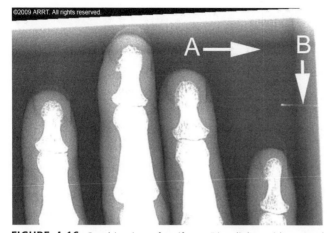

FIGURE 4-16 Combination of artifacts. Dirty light guide caused line *A*; scratch on the PSP plate caused line *B*. *(From Online Digital Imaging Academy (ODIA), © 2009 ARRT.)*

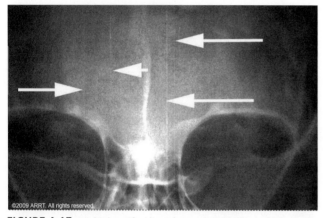

FIGURE 4-17 Multiple artifact lines *(arrows)* caused by multiple specks of dirt. *(From Online Digital Imaging Academy (ODIA), © 2009 ARRT.)*

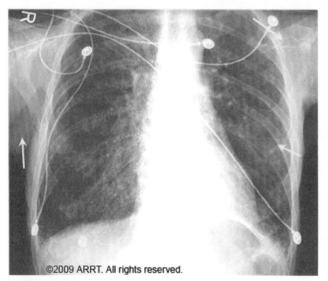

FIGURE 4-18 Moiré pattern *(arrow)* caused by improper use of a grid. *(From Online Digital Imaging Academy (ODIA), © 2009 ARRT.)*

format with minor editing; the format differs from the format used elsewhere in this text. The information contained in the appendix is the most current available on this topic as of publication.

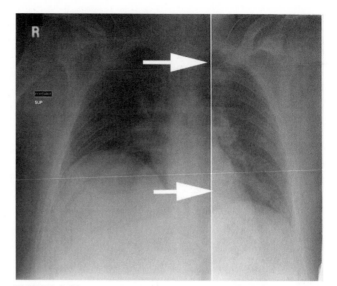

FIGURE 4-19 Reader malfunctioning when the plate was stopped and then restarted as it was read. The bright line artifact *(arrow)* is the area on the plate where it was paused. *(From Online Digital Imaging Academy (ODIA), © 2009 ARRT.)*

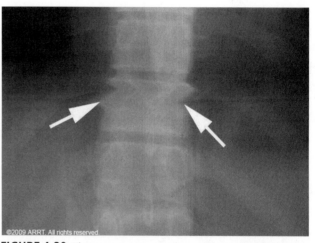

FIGURE 4-20 The wavy appearance *(arrow)* shows that the laser or the plate was disturbed when the plate was being read. Data samples from that region of the plate mixed across the entire plate. *(From Online Digital Imaging Academy (ODIA), © 2009 ARRT.)*

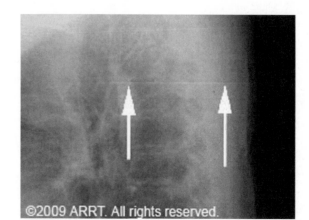

FIGURE 4-21 Illustration of the effect of the loss of a row of DELs *(arrow)* on flat panel detector. *(From Online Digital Imaging Academy (ODIA), © 2009 ARRT.)*

TABLE 4-2   American Registry of Radiologic Technologists (ARRT) Standard Definitions

Term	Film-Screen Radiography	Term	Digital Radiography
Recorded detail	Sharpness of the structural lines as recorded in the radiographic image	Recorded detail	Sharpness of the structural edges recorded in the image
Density	Degree of blackening or opacity of an area in a radiograph caused by accumulation of black metallic silver after exposure and processing of a film $\text{Density} = \text{Log} \dfrac{\text{Incident light intensity}}{\text{Transmitted light intensity}}$	Brightness	Measurement of the luminance of a monitor calibrated in units of candela (cd) per square meter on a monitor or soft copy Density on a hard copy is the same as film
Contrast	Visible differences between any two selected areas of density levels within the radiographic image Scale of contrast refers to the number of densities visible (or the number of shades of gray) *Long scale* is the term used when slight differences between densities are present (low contrast), but the total number of densities is increased *Short scale* is the term used when considerable or major differences between densities are present (high contrast), but the total number of densities is reduced	Contrast	Image contrast of display contrast is determined primarily by processing algorithm (mathematical codes used by the software to provide the desired image appearance); default algorithm determines the initial processing codes applied to the image data Scale of contrast is synonymous to gray scale and is linked to the bit depth of the system; *gray scale* is used instead of *scale of contrast* when referring to digital images
Film latitude	Inherent ability of the film to record a long range of density levels on the radiograph Film latitude and film contrast depend on the sensitometric properties of the film and the processing conditions and are determined directly from the characteristic H and D curve	Dynamic range	Range of exposures that may be captured by the detector; the dynamic range for digital imaging is much larger than film
Film contrast	Inherent ability of the film emulsion to react to radiation and record a range of densities	Receptor contrast	Fixed characteristic of the receptor; most digital receptors have an essentially linear response to exposure; this is impacted by *contrast* resolution (the smallest exposure changed or signal differences that can be detected); ultimately, contrast resolution is limited by the dynamic range and the *quantization* (number of bits per pixel) of the detector
Exposure latitude	Range of exposure factors that produce a diagnostic radiograph	Exposure latitude	Range of exposure that produces quality images at appropriate patient dose
Subject contrast	Difference in the quantity of radiation transmitted by a particular part as a result of the different absorption characteristics of the tissues and structures making up that part	Subject contrast	Magnitude of the signal differences in the remnant beam

KEY REVIEW POINTS
Dedicated Imaging Equipment

- DR is produced when the analog signal is sent through an analog-to-digital converter (ADC) to convert information into numerical data
- Postprocessing manipulation of the fluoroscopic image is possible because the image is in digital format
- *CR:* Uses an IP made of a PSP; absorbs energy exiting the patient; IP is scanned with a laser; energy released is converted from analog to digital for postprocessing
- With CR, x-ray exposure must fall within a range that allows the appropriate number of x-ray photons to strike the IP
- *Direct DR:* Uses wired or wireless flat panel detectors that communicate directly with a computer workstation
- DR flat panel systems produce an image more quickly than CR
- Flat panel DR systems may use either direct or indirect detectors
- *DR direct detectors:* Convert exit radiation directly into electrical charges, speeding image construction
- *DR indirect detectors:* Convert exit radiation first to visible light and then to electrical charges
- Electrical signals from either direct or indirect detectors are converted from analog to digital; viewed on a monitor
- *CR and DR image characteristics:* Wider exposure latitude than with film radiography; better visualization of soft tissue and bone
- *Digital image:* Composed of rows and columns called a *matrix*
- *Pixel:* Picture element; smaller part of a digital image; is a shade of gray representing a voxel
- *Voxel:* Volume element; an area of tissue in the patient
- *Histogram (graphic display):* Shows the radiographer the distribution of pixel values (indicating low, proper, or high exposure)
- *Processing algorithm (mathematical formula):* Used by the computer to reconstruct the image specific to the examination that was performed
- *Postprocessing:* Subtraction, edge enhancement, contrast enhancement, black/white reversal
- *Subtraction:* Removal of superimposed or unwanted structures from the image
- *Contrast enhancement:* Altering of image to display varying brightnesses
- *Edge enhancement:* Improves visibility of small high-contrast areas
- *Black/white reversal:* Reversal of the gray scale in the image
- *Window level (midpoint of densities):* Adjusts the image brightness throughout the range of densities; this is a direct relationship
- *Window width:* Adjusts the radiographic contrast in postprocessing mode; this is an inverse relationship
- *Spatial frequency resolution:* Level of detail or sharpness on the CR image
- *LUT:* Histogram of brightness level values from image acquisition that can be used to correct or enhance luminance values
- *Quantum mottle ("grainy" or "noisy" image):* Source of noise in the image; caused by too few x-ray photons hitting the image receptor
- *Digital image artifacts:* May be caused by dust on the IP; improper use of grids may cause a Moiré pattern; scatter radiation is easily imaged in digital imaging
- *PACS:* Integrated system of images and information
- *DICOM:* Standard protocol used for blending PACS and various imaging modalities

Appendix for Digital Image Acquisition and Display

Note: The following content represents the development of this appendix by the curriculum revision project group at the time of posting.

Glossary of Terms

Amorphous selenium (a-Se)—Amorphous selenium layers have the same structure as single crystals over short distances but are less ordered over larger distances. As a result, amorphous selenium layers provide uniform x-ray detection over the large areas needed by flat-panel x-ray detectors. Direct-conversion detectors use amorphous selenium. The a-Se can be deposited onto amorphous-silicon TFT arrays.

Amorphous silicon (a-Si)—Amorphous materials make flat-panel detectors possible. Early semiconductor technology required single-crystal silicon, which limited the size of electronic devices to the largest single crystal that could be grown. The development of amorphous silicon materials, which have the same structure as single crystals over short distances but are less ordered over larger distances, has enabled fabrication of flat-panel thin-film transistor (TFT) arrays large enough to be used as the basis for all flat-panel x-ray detectors.

Automatic rescaling (Auto Ranging, rescaling, scaling, normalization)—Software function maps the gray scale to the values of interest (VOI) in the histogram. This feature provides image brightness that is at a prescribed level over a large range of exposure. With some digital systems the image brightness will be consistent for a $50 \times$ to $100 \times$ change in exposure.

Bit depth—The available gray scale for image acquisition and display. Bit depth is equal to 2n, where *n* is the number of bits. Bit depth cannot be changed after equipment is purchased and is a vendor-specific system characteristic (i.e., 8 bits = 256 shades of gray, 10 bits = 1024 shades of gray, 12 bits = 4096 shades of gray).

Complementary metal-oxide semiconductor (CMOS)—A photographic detector. None are in use except for intraoral dental imaging.

Contrast resolution—The smallest exposure change (signal difference) that can be captured by a detector. Ultimately, contrast resolution is limited by the dynamic range and the quantization (number of bits per pixel) of the detector. Increased contrast resolution is considered one of the major advantages of digital receptors and tends to counteract the lower spatial resolution of many digital systems.

Detective quantum efficiency (DQE)—An indicator of the potential "speed class" or dose level required to acquire an optimal image. The DQE performance is obtained by comparing the image noise of a detector with that expected for an "ideal" detector having the

KEY REVIEW POINTS
Film-Screen Imaging and Processing

Note to student and educator: A limited number of questions related to film-screen imaging and processing remain on the certification examination (see ARRT Content Specifications in Chapter 1). This Key Review Points box presents the main concepts that are listed there that *could* be included on the examination. Be certain to check www.arrt.org for any updates that may occur that affect the inclusion of film-screen topics on the examination.

A. Film
1. Made of polyester base and emulsion composed of silver halide crystals suspended in gelatin
2. Speed and contrast of film are based on the size of the silver halide crystals and thickness of the emulsion
3. Film should be stored at temperatures no greater than 68° F to 70° F with humidity 40% to 60%
4. Stored film should be protected from radiation, fumes, outdating, and light and placed on end
5. Care must be taken when handling film to prevent pressure marks and static

B. Intensifying Screens
1. Made of polyester base with an active layer containing phosphors that produce visible light when struck by x-rays
2. Normally mounted inside the cassette in pairs for use with double-emulsion film
3. Contact between the screens and the film must be perfect; poor contact results in localized loss of recorded detail and localized blurring on the image
4. Poor film-screen contact may be verified by radiographing a wire-mesh screen

C. Automatic Processing and Quality Assurance
1. Developer solution in developer tank converts exposed silver bromide crystals (latent image) to black metallic silver (visible image)
2. Fixer solution in fixer tank clears and removes unexposed silver bromide crystals, stops development, and hardens the emulsion
3. Water in the wash tank removes chemicals remaining on film; film is dried in dryer system
4. Processing systems
   a. *Transport system:* Moves film through the processor and agitates the chemistry
   b. *Replenishment system:* Adds fresh developer and fixer solution for each film as it is fed into the processor
   c. *Recirculation system:* Agitates and filters developer solution; stabilizes solution temperature; prevents stratification of chemicals in the tank
   d. *Dryer system:* Dries film at approximately 120° F after it leaves wash tank

5. Start-up procedure
   a. Close wash tank valve
   b. Turn on water source
   c. Turn on processor
   d. Wash crossover racks
   e. Put lid in place
   f. Run several 14- to 17-inch films through processor
   g. Check replenishment rates (also check several times throughout the day)
   h. Check developer temperature after warm-up
6. Shutdown procedure
   a. Turn off water source
   b. Turn off processor
   c. Open wash tank valve and drain tank
   d. Wash crossover racks
   e. Leave lid ajar several inches to prevent contamination of solutions resulting from condensation or algae formation
7. Cleaning and maintenance (recommended)
   a. *Daily:* Wash crossover racks twice daily (startup and shutdown or morning and evening); drain wash tank
   b. *Weekly:* Clean deep racks
   c. *Monthly:* Drain and clean by hand all tanks and dryer; put in fresh developer and fixer; change developer filter; change water filters
8. Processor and Handling Malfunctions and Artifacts
   a. *Artifacts:* Unwanted, irregular mark or density on the radiograph; may be caused by improper handling, pressure, or static discharge
   b. *Temperature fluctuations:* High developer temperature causes chemical fog and increased density
   c. *Contamination:* Fixer solution splashing into developer tank (1 mL) causes contamination with odor of ammonia; causes increased density on films known as *chemical fog*
   d. *Jamming:* Films caught during transport owing to rollers out of alignment or inadequate replenishment rate, depriving the film of hardener, which allows the emulsion to swell to the point at which it cannot pass between the rollers
9. *Photographic anomalies:* Causes and corrections
   a. *Dark films and fogged films:* May be caused by developer temperature too high, developer overreplenishment, fixer contamination of developer; white light leak; crack in safelight filter; outdated film
   b. *Light films:* May be caused by developer temperature too low; developer underreplenishment
   c. *Films appear milky:* May be caused by poor fixer replenishment
   d. *Films appear greasy:* May be caused by inadequate washing
   e. *Dark flakes:* May be caused by algae in wash water

same signal-response characteristics. The only source of noise in an ideal detector results from the incident x-ray quantum statistics.

Detector size or field of view (FOV)—The detector size and FOV describe the useful image acquisition area of an imaging device. Cassette-less digital systems have a fixed OV, which makes some projections difficult, while cassette-based CR systems have flexible FOVs like screen/film.

Detector element (DEL)—The detector element is the smallest resolvable area in a TFT- or CCD-based digital imaging device.

Dynamic range—The range of exposures over which a detector can acquire image data. Digital image acquisition systems are capable of capturing an image across a much larger range of exposures than film-screen. The increased dynamic range allows more anatomical structures to be captured during an exposure. Typical digital systems will respond to exposures as low as 100 μR and as high as 100mR. In order to visualize all of the anatomy, the image has to be displayed on a system that allows the viewer to manipulate the window and level. Dynamic range should not be confused with exposure latitude.

Exposure latitude—The range of receptor exposures that provides a quality, low-noise image at an appropriate patient exposure consistent with ALARA. Exposure latitude is not the exposure range, which will be rescaled to consistent image brightness.

Histogram—A data set, in a graphical form, of the pixel digital values versus the prevalence number of those values in the image. The horizontal axis represents pixel exposure; the vertical axis represents incidence of those values. The software has histogram models for all menu choices. The histogram models include values of interest (VOI) that determine what part of the data set should be incorporated into the displayed image.

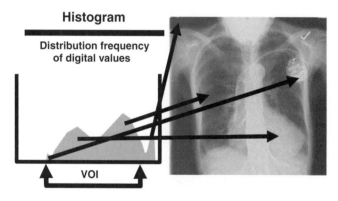

Image noise—All images have unwanted fluctuations in brightness that are unrelated to the object being imaged. These are collectively described as image noise. In addition to the x-ray quantum noise, which cannot be avoided, imaging systems contribute additional noise to an image. Underexposed digital images exhibit objectionable quantum noise. The electronic components of all digital detectors and displays also add noise. Indirect-conversion detectors may contribute additional noise via the improved conversion of photons to data.

Look-up table (LUT)—The default gradient curve applied to the data set of an image determining the initial display contrast. The LUT can be adjusted after the initial image processing has been applied.

Matrix size—The matrix size is the number of pixels that make up the image; this is normally expressed in terms of the number of pixels in two orthogonal directions (length and width of the image). The matrix size is dependent on VOV and pixel size. Matrix size also may be used to describe the number of detector elements that comprise the active FOV of a detector.

Modulation transfer function (MTF)—A measure of the ability of the imaging system to preserve signal contrast as a function of the spatial resolution. Every image can be described in terms of the amount of energy for each of its spatial frequency components. MTF describes the fraction of each component that will be preserved in the captured image. MTF often is regarded as the ideal expression of the image quality provided by a detector.

Nyquist frequency—The highest spatial frequency that can be recorded by a digital detector. The Nyquist frequency is determined by the pixel pitch. The pixel pitch is determined by sampling frequency for cassette-based PSP systems and by DEL spacing for TFT flat panel. The Nyquist frequency is half the number of pixels/mm. A digital system with a pixel density of 10 pixels/mm would have a Nyquist frequency of 5 line pair/mm.

Photodiode—An electronic element that converts light into charge. With indirect TFT detectors this is accomplished by a light-sensitive amorphous silicon photodiode on top of the TFT array.

Photoconductor—Amorphous selenium TFT detectors, the a-Se layer forms a continuous x-ray–sensitive photoconductor that converts x-ray energy directly to charge. This charge can be directly "read out" by the TFT array. A photodiode is not necessary with a-Se detectors.

Pixel—A "picture element," or pixel, the smallest area represented in a digital image. A digital radiography image consists of a matrix of pixels, which is typically several thousand pixels in each direction.

Pixel density—A term that describes the number of pixels/mm in an image. Pixel density is determined by the pixel pitch.

Pixel pitch—The space from the center of a pixel to the center of the adjacent pixel. It is measured in microns (μm). Pixel pitch is determined by the DEL size or the sampling frequency.

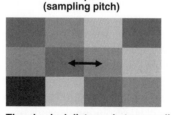

- **The physical distance between adjacent DEL's or between data samples**
- **Pixel pitch determines the maximum spatial resolution**
- **Nyquist's frequency**

Processing algorithm—The mathematical codes used by the software to generate the image appearance desired by the viewer. The processing algorithm includes gradient processing (brightness and contrast), frequency processing (edge enhancement and smoothing), and other more complex processing such as equalization. The processing algorithm also may be referred to as the default processing codes and is linked to the anatomical menu items (i.e., the body part and projection chosen on the user interface menu determines which processing algorithm will be applied to your image data). The software will try to match the histogram of your image data to the histogram model of the chosen examination and projection.

Quantization—All x-ray digital receptors respond smoothly and continuously to the incident exposure. Digital images require each pixel to be assigned a unique value (quantized), so that a unique gray shade is assigned to that pixel. The number of levels that can be represented digitally is determined by the system's bit depth. The bit depth for digital radiography systems ranges from 10 bits (1024 gray shades) to 14 bits (16,384 gray shades).

Sampling frequency—The frequency that a data sample is acquired from the exposed detector. Sampling frequency is expressed in pixel pitch and pixels per mm. Sampling frequency may be determined by receptor size, depending on the vendor. (As of 2006, Kodak, Konica, and Agfa have different sampling frequencies based on receptor size. As receptor size decreases, sampling frequency increases; therefore spatial resolution increases.)

Scintillator—A material that absorbs x-ray energy and re-emits part of that energy as visible light. Indirect TFT flat-panel detectors use a scintillator. Two modern high-efficiency x-ray scintillators are cesium iodide and gadolinium oxysulfide. Cesium iodide is hygroscopic and must be hermetically sealed to avoid water absorption or it will degrade rapidly. Gadolinium oxysulfide is commonly used in x-ray intensifying screens to expose film. It is a highly stable material, but has significantly more light spread than a layer of cesium iodide with equal x-ray absorption.

Signal-to-noise ratio (SNR)—Noise, especially quantum noise, ultimately limits our ability to see an object's edge (signal difference); SNR can be used to describe the edge conspicuity of a particular object under well-defined exposure conditions. DQE is a measure of the efficiency with which the SNR of the incident exposure is preserved in an image.

Spatial resolution—A characteristic of the imaging system. Maximum spatial resolution (Nyquist frequency—line pairs per millimeter or lp/mm) is equal to half the number of pixels/mm (i.e., if the sampling frequency is 5 pixels/mm, the maximum spatial resolution is 2.5 lp/mm). Spatial resolution depends on the sampling frequency for cassette-based systems and the detector element size for cassette-less systems. With TFT-based detectors, the actual spatial resolution is near the Nyquist frequency. With PSP-based CR systems, the spatial resolution is less than the Nyquist frequency to the light spread from the PSP plate during image extraction. Unlike screen film systems there is no correlation between exposure level and spatial resolution.

Structured (needle) phosphor—A phosphor layer with columnar phosphor crystals within the active layer. Resembles needles lined up on end and packed together.

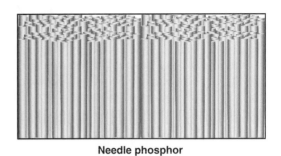

Needle phosphor

Thin-film transistor (TFT)—An electronic switch on flat-panel detectors commonly made of amorphous silicon. The TFT allows the charge collected at each pixel to be independently transferred to external electronics, where it is amplified and quantized.

Tiling—A process whereby several flat-panel detectors are joined to obtain one larger detector. Tiling results in segments that have unequal response requiring flat-field correction for flat-panel detectors.

Turbid phosphor—A phosphor layer with a random distribution of phosphor crystals within the active layer. This layer can be used in both cassette-based and cassette-less systems and is similar to a standard intensifying screen used with film (as of 2007 all cassette-based systems, except for the Agfa scan head, employ turbid structure).

Content (Numbering Matches ASRT Outline)

I. Basic Principles of Digital Radiography

A. Digital receptors—Cassette-based and cassette-less
1. TFT arrays
   a. Direct versus indirect—Direct uses amorphous selenium; x-rays are converted directly into electrons (only Hologic). Indirect uses a scintillator, which converts x-rays to light and then light is converted into electrons by a silicon layer just above the TFT (all other vendors).
   b. Turbid phosphor versus structured phosphor—Structured phosphor layer demonstrates less light spread than turbid.
2. CCD and CMOS systems—Both use a scintillator. These systems are cameralike, they both use lenses to focus the light onto a detector.

B. Comparison of detector properties and evaluatory criteria
1. DQE—Predicts how high or low the patient dose may be. Higher DQE means you may have lower patient doses. If DQE is too high, the image will be noisy as a result of low mAs. Factors that may influence the DQE are phosphor absorption efficiency and conversion efficiency.
2. System speed versus "speed class" operation—Because digital systems can be used at a wide range

of exposures, the term "speed" is an inappropriate descriptor (*Huda). Speed class refers to the operational exposure level at which a digital system is operated; you can have technique charts that will operate the system at a specific speed class. (You can operate at a 50 speed class or a 400 speed class with the exact same piece of equipment.) With screen/film, the relative speed determined the techniques used; with digital, the techniques used determine the speed class at which the equipment operates. As speed class increases, the likelihood of noise increases; as speed class decreases, the patient exposure increases.

C. Dynamic range versus latitude
  2. Latitude—Amount of error for optimal image acquisition. Automatic rescaling provides a false sense of very large latitude.
    a. Exposure latitude is the range of techniques that will produce an image that has an acceptable appearance and does not violate ALARA. It should be considered an ALARA violation if exposure is more than double the optimal.
    b. Beam-part-receptor alignment latitude— Collimation must be such that the software is able to detect collimated edges so that the histogram analysis is performed only on the data within the exposure field. If the exposure field is not recognized accurately, the histogram will contain data outside the exposure field, widening the histogram, resulting in a histogram analysis error followed by a rescaling error, resulting in a repeat being necessary. Newer software is more forgiving in this area.

II. Image Acquisition

A. and B. Image extraction
C. Histogram analysis—The software compares the histogram from your image data set to the histogram model you chose on the menu. If there is a significant difference between the image data set histogram and the model, a histogram analysis error may occur, resulting in a poor quality image displayed.
D. Exposure indicators
  1. Cassette-less
    a. DAP—Dose area product
      (1) Actual patient dose measured by a DAP meter embedded in the collimator. The DAP value is dependent on the exposure and field size and is expressed in cGy/m^2. DAP meters must be routinely calibrated to ensure accuracy.
  2. Cassette-based—represents exposure level to plate.
    a. Vendor-specific values
      (1) Sensitivity "S" (Fuji, Philips, Konica) inversely related to exposure—200 S# = 1 mR to the plate—optimal range 250 to 300 for trunk, 75 to 125 for extremities.

      (2) Exposure index (EI) (Kodak)—Directly related to exposure; has a logarithmic component (change of 300 in EI = factor of 2 [i.e., 1800 is exposed twice as much as 1500]); optimal range 1800 to 1900.
      (3) Log Mean (LgM) (Agfa)—Directly related to exposure; has a logarithmic component (change of 0.3 in LgM = factor of 2 [i.e., 2.3 is exposed twice as much as 2.0]); optimal range 1.9 to 2.1.
    b. Reader calibration—For exposure indicators to be meaningful readers must be recalibrated annually with a calibrated ion chamber by a medical physicist or qualified service engineer.
    c. Centering and beam collimation—Misalignment may cause a histogram analysis error; may lead to incorrect exposure indicators.

III. Image Acquisition Errors

A. Exposure field recognition—Inappropriate collimation margins or beam alignment may result in histogram analysis errors and rescaling errors.
B. Scatter control
  1. Grid use
    a. In order to limit patient dose, kVp should be used to compensate for grid use rather than mAs. Digital imaging changes in kVp will not greatly affect the radiographic contrast as kVp changes did with screen/film.

IV. Software (Default) Image Processing—Set by vendor. If images do not have desired appearance, default image processing codes need to be changed rather than routinely postprocessing to improve image appearance.

A. Frequency processing
  1. Smoothing—A software function to reduce the appearance of noise in your image. Applying smoothing software results in a loss of fine detail such as trabecular bone. This will not improve edge visibility (i.e., the image looks nicer but the information is not there).
  2. Edge enhancement—An artificial increase in display contrast at an edge.
B. Equalization—A software function designed to even the brightness displayed in the image. Light areas of the image (low exposures) are made darker, and dark areas of the image (high exposures) are made lighter.
C. Effects of excessive processing—Degrades visibility of specific anatomical structures and may create false information, resulting in missed diagnosis or misdiagnosis resulting from inappropriate default processing.

V. Fundamental Principles of Exposure

A. Exposure myths associated with digital systems
  1. mAs—*Myth:* Digital is mAs driven. *Truth:* Digital is exposure driven. The digital detector is unable

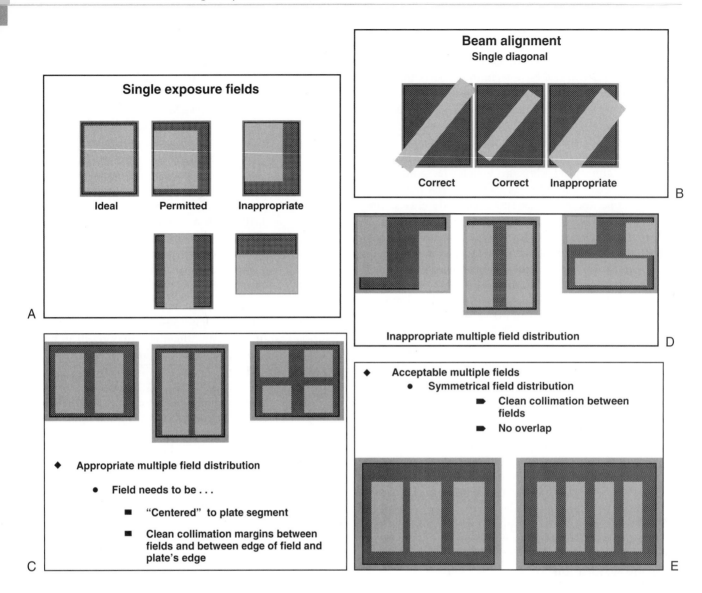

Single exposure fields

Ideal   Permitted   Inappropriate

A

Beam alignment
Single diagonal

Correct   Correct   Inappropriate

B

Inappropriate multiple field distribution

D

◆ Appropriate multiple field distribution

● Field needs to be . . .

■ "Centered" to plate segment

■ Clean collimation margins between fields and between edge of field and plate's edge

C

◆ Acceptable multiple fields

● Symmetrical field distribution

➡ Clean collimation between fields

➡ No overlap

E

to discriminate whether the exposure change was mAs or kVp. The only thing that matters is exposure to pixels.

2. kVp—*Myth:* Digital is kVp driven. *Truth:* See above.

3. Collimation—*Myth:* You cannot collimate. *Truth:* You can and should collimate. Inappropriate collimation will cause a histogram analysis error.

4. Grid—*Myth:* You cannot use grids and do not need them. *Truth:* Digital systems are sensitive to scatter just like film; in fact, they are more sensitive. Appropriate grid use is even more important. A grid should be used when the remnant beam is more than 50% scatter, chest larger than 24 cm, and anything else larger than 12 cm.

5. SID—*Myth:* Magnification does not occur with digital so SID is unimportant. *Truth:* Geometric rules of recorded detail and distortion are unchanged from film to digital.

6. Speed class—*Myth:* It is a 200 speed class; you need to double your mAs and increase your kVp by 10. *Truth:* This technique adjustment would be like changing to a 100 speed class from a 400 speed class. Also your digital system will operate at whatever speed class you choose.

7. Fog—*Myth:* Digital systems cannot be fogged by scatter or background radiation. *Truth:* Digital systems are more sensitive to both. *Myth:* Fluorescent lights fog PSP plates. *Truth:* That is not true.

B. Control patient exposure.

1. Higher kVp levels—May be 5 to 15 kVp higher than with screen/film. With corresponding mAs, adjustment is made to provide the same receptor exposure, and the image processing codes are changed to provide the appropriate contrast display.

2. Additional filtration—Use of 0.1 to 0.2 mm of copper is recommended to reduce patient dose.

C. Monitor patient exposure; see ASRT position statements from 2005.

VI. Image Evaluation
VII. Quality Assurance and Maintenance Issues
A. Initial acceptance testing—Just make the point that this needs to be done
B. Plate maintenance
   1. Cleaning and inspecting plates—Every 3 months is suggested or as needed due to conditions. Use only approved products.
   2. Erasing plates—Every 48 hours, if unused.
C. Uniformity of processing codes—All systems within a facility should use identical processing codes to ensure image appearance consistency.
VIII. Display
A. Monitor—It needs to be pointed out that in most facilities the technologists' workstations have significantly different monitors and viewing conditions than the radiologists. How it looks to you on the workstation in the brightly lit work area will be very different from how it looks on the radiologists' high-resolution monitors in the dark reading room.
B. Print to film
   1. Sacrifice dynamic range of digital image on monitor when printed to film.
   2. Thermal film degradation—Film is very sensitive to heat both before and after printing. If you leave a printed film in your hot car, the image will fog.
   3. Film storage—Heat and moisture are a larger issue than they were for an analog film.
C. PACS
   1. Terminology
   2. System components and functions
      a. Modalities—All modalities in a facility can be networked to the same PACS server.
      b. Short- and long-term archives—Make a note that this includes an off-site archive of images for disaster recovery that should be regularly updated.
      c. Display workstations.

Bibliography for this Section

Introduction to Digital Radiography: The Role of Digital Radiology in Medical Imaging. Rochester, NY: Eastman Kodak Company, Health Imaging Division; 2000. M1-412 ©Eastman Kodak Company, 2000. 11/00 CAT. NO 183 6998.

Samei E, Flynn MJ, eds. *2003 Syllabus, Advances in Digital Radiography: Categorical Course in Diagnostic Radiology Physics.* Oak Brook, IL: Radiological Society of North America; 2003. LC Control Number 2004275095.

Siebert JA, Filipow LJ, Andriole KP. *Practical Digital Imaging and PACS. AAPM Medical Physics Monograph No. 25.* Madison, WI: Medical Physics Publishing; 1999. ISBN 0944838200.

Burns CB, Barba J, Woodward A. Digital Radiography for Radiologic Science Educators [handout materials]. Chapel Hill, NC: University of North Carolina Division of Radiologic Science; 2005.

Personal contributions to this section by:

Anne Brittain, PhD, RT(R)(M)
Barry Burns, MS, RT(R), DABR
Darcy J. Nethery, PhD, RT(R)
Barbara Smith, BS, RT(R)(QM), FASRT

REVIEW QUESTIONS

1. Density may be defined as:
   a. Darkness on a radiographic image
   b. A combination of contrast and recorded detail
   c. The light areas of a radiographic image
   d. Differences in dark areas on a radiographic image
2. The radiographic image is formed by:
   a. Exit rays striking the image receptor
   b. Laser light
   c. Cosmic rays
   d. Electrons and heat
3. The primary controlling factors of density are:
   a. kVp and SID
   b. mAs and window level
   c. SID and OID
   d. OID and FSS
4. Which of the following describes the relationship between mAs and density?
   a. Density is directly proportional to mAs
   b. Density is inversely proportional to mAs
   c. Density is directly proportional to mAs^2
   d. mAs controls the number of electrons boiled off the anode and the number of x-rays produced
5. The number of electrons boiled off the cathode and consequently the number of x-rays produced are controlled by:
   a. kVp
   b. SID
   c. mAs
   d. OID
6. The law stating that any combinations of mA and time that produce the same mAs value will produce the same radiographic density is the:
   a. Inverse square law
   b. mAs-density law
   c. Reciprocity law
   d. 15% law
7. The active portion of a CR IP is(are):
   a. Calcium tungstate
   b. PSP

   c. Silver bromide crystals

   d. Rare earth phosphor

8. mAs directly controls:

   a. The energy of the x-ray emission spectrum

   b. The quality and quantity of x-rays produced at the cathode

   c. The quality and quantity of x-rays produced at the anode

   d. The quantity of x-rays produced

9. Differences in densities on a radiograph describe:

   a. Density

   b. Recorded detail

   c. Log relative exposure

   d. Contrast

10. The primary controlling factor(s) of contrast is(are):

   a. mAs, which controls the energy of the x-rays produced

   b. kVp, which primarily controls the quantity of x-rays produced at the target

   c. Focal-spot size, which controls the quantity and quality of x-rays produced

   d. kVp and window width

11. The relationship between kVp and density may be described as:

   a. Directly proportional

   b. Direct, although not proportional

   c. Governed by the 15-50 rule

   d. Controlled by x-ray tube current

12. The 15% rule states that:

   a. Density may be halved by decreasing kVp by 15%

   b. kVp should be 15% of the mAs selected

   c. Density may be halved by increasing kVp by 15%

   d. At least a 15% change in mAs is required to make a change visible

13. Which of the following statements are true concerning the role of kVp in radiograph production?

   1. As kVp is increased, penetrating ability of the x-rays increases

   2. As kVp is increased, more x-rays exit the patient to strike the IR

   3. As kVp is decreased, wavelength and density decrease

   4. As kVp increases, radiographic density increases

   5. As kVp decreases, radiographic density remains constant because mAs controls density

     a. 1, 2, 4

     b. 1, 2, 3

     c. 1, 3, 4

     d. 5

14. Given an original technique of 30 mAs and 80 kVp, which of the following would produce a radiograph with double the density?

   a. 60 mAs, 90 kVp

   b. 30 mAs, 92 kVp

   c. 15 mAs, 80 kVp

   d. 30 mAs, 70 kVp

15. Which of the following governs the relationship between SID and density?

   a. Reciprocity law

   b. 15% rule

   c. Inverse square law

   d. Ohm's law

16. If SID is doubled, what may be said about radiographic density?

   a. Density doubles

   b. Density is reduced by one-half

   c. Density is reduced by new mAs^2

   d. Density is reduced to one-fourth

17. If SID is reduced by one-half, what must be done to mAs to maintain a constant density?

   a. Reduce mAs to one-fourth its original value

   b. Reduce mAs to one-half its original value

   c. Increase mAs by four times its original value

   d. Increase mAs by two times its original value

18. Poorer recorded detail may be caused by which of the following factors?

   1. Long SID

   2. Long OID

   3. Large focal spot

   4. Small focal spot

   5. Patient motion

   6. Magnification

     a. 2, 3, 5, 6

     b. 2, 3

     c. 1, 4, 6

     d. 5, 6

19. In digital fluoroscopy, what equipment should be used to view the image?

   a. Conventional view box

   b. High-resolution monitor capable of displaying millions of pixels

   c. High-definition television

   d. Plasma television required

20. A primary advantage to digital fluoroscopy is:

   a. Postprocessing manipulation of the image

   b. Radiation dose to the patient is substantially lower

   c. No radiologist is needed

   d. Lower cost

21. Which of the following describes the relationship between radiographic density and the use of grids?

   a. Grids always reduce density

   b. Grids reduce density unless mAs is increased to compensate

   c. Grids reduce density by absorbing scatter radiation

   d. Density increases as grid ratio increases

22. The use of filtration:

   a. Greatly reduces radiographic density because of the absorption of short-wavelength x-rays

   b. Greatly reduces radiographic density because of the absorption of high-energy x-rays

c. Increases radiographic density by removing long-wavelength x-rays

d. Has little effect on density because x-rays removed from beam are not image-producing rays

23. As beam restriction increases (becomes tighter):
    a. Density increases
    b. Density increases as a result of focusing of x-rays
    c. Density decreases
    d. Density is not affected

24. Which of the following affects radiographic density?
    a. Atomic mass of the x-ray tube anode
    b. X-ray tube angle
    c. Atomic number of the cathode filament

25. The variation of x-ray intensity along the longitudinal axis of the x-ray beam describes:
    a. Beam collimation
    b. Positive beam limitation
    c. Anode heel effect
    d. X-ray emission spectrum

26. The thicker part of anatomy should be placed under which aspect of the x-ray tube?
    a. Central ray
    b. Cathode
    c. Anode
    d. Collimator

27. The function of contrast is to:
    a. Make the image appear sharper
    b. Compensate for uneven anatomical structures
    c. Brighten the image
    d. Make detail visible

28. A radiograph with few gray tones, primarily exhibiting black and white, would be described as having what type of contrast?
    1. Long scale
    2. Short scale
    3. Low
    4. High
        a. 2 and 4
        b. 1 and 3
        c. 1 and 4
        d. 2

29. Poorer recorded detail may be caused by which of the following factors?
    a. Short OID
    b. Long SID
    c. Small focal spot
    d. Pixel pitch wide

30. High kVp produces which of the following?
    1. High contrast
    2. Few gray tones
    3. Long-scale contrast
    4. Short-scale contrast
    5. Low contrast
    6. Many gray tones
        a. 1, 2, 4
        b. 3, 5, 6

c. 5
d. 1

31. Low kVp produces which of the following?
    1. High contrast
    2. Few gray tones
    3. Long-scale contrast
    4. Short-scale contrast
    5. Low contrast
    6. Many gray tones
        a. 1, 2, 4
        b. 3, 5, 6
        c. 5
        d. 1

32. More uniform penetration of anatomical structures occurs when what level of kVp is used?
    a. Low
    b. High
    c. kVp does not affect penetration
    d. Level at which photoelectric interaction predominates

33. Differential absorption of the x-ray beam is a function of:
    a. Compton interaction
    b. Atomic mass of anatomical structures
    c. mAs
    d. Photoelectric interaction

34. What effect does beam restriction have on contrast?
    a. Decreases contrast by focusing the x-ray beam
    b. Decreases contrast because of higher kVp level used
    c. Increases contrast by focusing the x-ray beam
    d. Increases contrast because of reduction in the number of Compton interactions that occur

35. The adjustment in technical factors required when using beam restriction is:
    a. Increase kVp
    b. Decrease kVp to reduce the number of Compton interactions taking place
    c. Decrease mAs to reduce the number of Compton interactions taking place
    d. Increase mAs to compensate for the number of rays removed from the primary beam

36. What effect does the use of radiographic grids have on contrast?
    a. Decreases contrast
    b. Increases contrast
    c. No effect on contrast
    d. Increases contrast by absorbing scatter radiation

37. As the amount of beam filtration is increased:
    a. Contrast increases
    b. There is no effect on contrast
    c. Contrast decreases
    d. Contrast increases because the beam is harder

38. The portion of contrast that is caused by variations in the anatomy or is secondary to pathological changes is called:
    a. Radiographic contrast

b. Anatomical contrast

c. Pathological contrast

d. Subject contrast

39. Recorded detail is:

a. Photographic representation of the part being radiographed

b. Controlled by kVp

c. Controlled by mAs

d. Geometric representation of the part being radiographed

40. Better recorded detail may be caused by which of the following factors?

1. Long SID

2. Long OID

3. Short SID

4. Short OID

5. Large focal spot

6. Small focal spot

   a. 2, 3, 5

   b. 1, 4, 6

   c. 1, 4, 6

   d. 2, 3, 6

41. Optimal recorded detail may be created using which of the following factors?

a. Large focal spot

b. Narrow pixel pitch

c. Long OID

d. Short SID

42. TFT is a:

a. Thin film transistor—a diode used in rectifiers

b. Thin film transistor—an electronic device used in CR cassettes

c. Thin film transistor—an electronic switch used on flat panel detectors

d. Thin film transistor—the electronics used with AECs

43. Distortion may be described as:

a. Misrepresentation of an anatomical structure on film

b. Foreshortening

c. Elongation

d. Magnification

44. Elongation and foreshortening are examples of:

a. Size distortion

b. Shape distortion

c. Motion

d. Distortion caused by short SID and long OID

45. Magnification is caused by:

1. Short SID

2. Long SID

3. Short OID

4. Long OID

   a. 2, 3

   b. 1, 4

   c. 1, 3

   d. 1 only

46. Distortion that occurs when the x-ray beam is angled against the long axis of a part is:

a. Elongation

b. Magnification

c. Minification

d. Foreshortening

47. Distortion that occurs when the x-ray beam is angled along the long axis of a part is:

a. Elongation

b. Magnification

c. Minification

d. Misrepresentation

48. The actual patient dose as measured by a meter embedded in the collimator is:

a. RAD—radiation absorbed dose

b. DAP—dose area product

c. REM—radiation equivalent man

d. Doubling dose

49. Quality assurance and maintenance of CR cassettes includes cleaning and inspecting the plates at least:

a. Daily

b. Every 48 hours

c. Every 3 months

d. Weekly

50. Quality assurance and maintenance of CR cassettes includes erasing plates at least:

a. Daily

b. Every 48 hours

c. Every 3 months

d. Weekly

51. Quality assurance of digital imaging requires the uniformity of processing codes to ensure:

a. Image appearance consistency

b. Faster throughput

c. Less heat loading on the anode

d. Smoother integration into PACS

52. A software function that evens the brightness displayed in the image is called:

a. Smoothing

b. Equalization

c. Postprocessing

d. Subtraction

53. Beam-part-receptor alignment latitude describes:

a. The latitude of collimation that still allows the software to detect collimated edges

b. The alignment that maintains ALARA requirements

c. Exposure latitude

d. Acceptable distortion of the image

54. Exposure technique in digital imaging may be adjusted by:

a. Lowering kVp

b. Increasing mAs

c. Shortening SID

d. Increasing kVp

55. Digital imaging is more sensitive to:
   a. Scatter and background radiation
   b. Fluorescent lights
   c. Free electrons
   d. Free radicals

56. Inappropriate collimation causes:
   a. A fogged image
   b. Pixel unresponsiveness
   c. DICOM incompatibility
   d. Histogram analysis error

57. The appearance of images on technologists' monitors is:
   a. The same as on radiologists' monitors
   b. Substantially better than on radiologists' monitors
   c. Not as good as on radiologists' monitors

58. Digital imaging is driven by:
   a. kVp
   b. mAs
   c. IR speed class
   d. Exposure

59. Digital systems operate at what speed class?
   a. 200
   b. 400
   c. 100
   d. The speed class chosen by the radiographer

60. An artificial increase in display contrast at an edge of the image is:
   a. Smoothing
   b. Edge enhancement
   c. Contrast resolution
   d. Spatial resolution

61. As speed class increases:
   a. The likelihood of noise increases
   b. The likelihood of noise decreases
   c. Patient exposure increases
   d. Sharpness increases

62. As speed class decreases:
   a. The likelihood of noise increases
   b. Noise is unaffected
   c. Patient exposure increases
   d. Sharpness decreases

63. Smoothing software may result in:
   a. Enhanced fine detail
   b. Less distortion
   c. Loss of fine detail
   d. Increased distortion

64. Excessive processing of the digital image may:
   a. Degrade visibility of anatomy
   b. Provide additional anatomical information
   c. Enhance visibility of desired anatomy
   d. Increase patient dose

65. A high SNR provides an image with:
   a. Poor spatial resolution
   b. Higher spatial resolution
   c. Poor contrast
   d. Higher distortion

66. Quantum noise limits ability to see:
   a. Detail
   b. Contrast
   c. Fatty tissue
   d. Additive pathologies

67. If the exposure field is not accurately recognized, the histogram will contain data:
   a. Outside the exposure field, narrowing the histogram
   b. Inside the exposure field, widening the histogram
   c. Outside the exposure field, widening the histogram
   d. Inside the exposure field, narrowing the histogram

68. Grid ratio is defined as:
   a. The ratio of the lead strips to the space between them
   b. The thickness of the lead strips divided by the thickness of the aluminum interspacers
   c. The ratio of the height of the lead strips over the distance between the lead strips
   d. The ratio of the distance between the lead strips over the height of the lead strips

69. Grid frequency is defined as:
   a. The same as grid ratio
   b. The amount of lead in the grid (expressed in terms of focusing distance)
   c. How often a grid is used
   d. The amount of lead in the grid (expressed as the number of lead strips per inch)

70. Which of the following statements concerning grids are true?
   1. Contrast improvement factor is the measure of the ability of a grid to enhance contrast
   2. Grid selectivity is the ratio of primary radiation transmitted through the grid to secondary radiation transmitted through the grid
   3. Grids are used when part thickness is less than 10 cm
   4. GCF is the amount of increase in kVp necessary when converting from nongrid to grid technique
   5. The primary purpose of grids is radiation protection
   6. The main function of grids is to prevent Compton scatter from reaching the film
   7. Grids prevent the production of scatter
   a. 1, 2, 6
   b. 1, 2, 4, 6
   c. 1, 2, 3, 5, 7
   d. 1, 2, 6, 7

71. A grid with lead strips and aluminum interspacers that are angled to coincide with the divergence of the x-ray beam is called a:
   a. Parallel grid
   b. Focused grid

c. Crosshatch grid
d. Rhombic grid

72. The range of SIDs that may be used with a focused grid is called:
    a. Grid ratio
    b. Objective plane
    c. Anticutoff distances
    d. Grid radius

73. The best scatter cleanup is achieved with the use of:
    a. Air gap technique
    b. Focused grids
    c. Crosshatch grids
    d. Parallel grids

74. Grid cutoff may be described as:
    a. Decreased density in the middle of the radiograph caused by the use of a parallel grid inserted upside down
    b. Decreased density on a radiograph as a result of absorption of image-forming rays
    c. Increased density in the center of a radiograph caused by the use of a focused grid inserted upside down
    d. Decreased density on the edges of a radiograph only

75. When a nongrid technique using 10 mAs and 75 kVp is changed to a 12:1 grid using 75 kVp, what new mAs must be used to maintain the same density as the original film?
    a. 50 mAs
    b. 2 mAs
    c. 40 mAs
    d. 120 mAs

76. Use of the air gap technique:
    a. Works because x-rays are absorbed in the air between the patient and the film
    b. Should occur when possible
    c. May cause some magnification because of decreased OID
    d. Works because scatter radiation travels in divergent paths and misses the IR as a result of increased OID

77. Use of technique charts:
    a. Is unnecessary for any examination because of AECs
    b. Does not require that the part thickness be measured with calipers
    c. Is usually based on fixed mAs and variable kVp
    d. Is helpful when manual techniques are used

78. When AEC is used, increasing the kVp:
    a. Increases density proportionately
    b. Increases radiographic contrast
    c. Increases exposure time
    d. Has no effect on density

79. Materials that make flat panel detectors possible are:
    a. Silicon dioxide
    b. Amorphous silicon
    c. Diodes
    d. Pixels

80. Which of the following maintains image brightness over a wide range of exposures?
    a. AEC
    b. Bit depth
    c. Automatic rescaling
    d. Detector size

81. The available gray scale of an imaging system is determined by:
    a. Pixel pitch
    b. Bit depth
    c. Exposure latitude
    d. Image latitude

82. The smallest exposure change able to be captured by a detector is called:
    a. Spatial resolution
    b. Exposure latitude
    c. Pixel
    d. Contrast resolution

83. An indicator of the dose level needed to acquire an optimal image is:
    a. Detective quantum efficiency
    b. Dose area product
    c. Field of view
    d. Dynamic range

84. The useful image acquisition area of an image receptor is:
    a. Detector element
    b. Detector size
    c. TFT size
    d. Dynamic range

85. The smallest resolvable area in a digital imaging device is:
    a. Detector size
    b. Detector element
    c. Matrix size
    d. Focal spot size

86. What allows more anatomical structures to be captured during an exposure?
    a. Contrast resolution
    b. Spatial resolution
    c. Dynamic range
    d. MTF

87. The range of receptor exposures that provides a quality image is called:
    a. Detector latitude
    b. Exposure latitude
    c. Histogram
    d. Dynamic range

88. Which of the following is a graphical representation of pixel values?
    a. Dynamic range
    b. Luminance
    c. Look-up table
    d. Histogram

89. Undesirable fluctuations in brightness are called:
   a. MTF
   b. Image noise
   c. Quantization
   d. Scintillation

90. The number of pixels making up the digital image is the:
   a. Pixel depth
   b. Matrix size
   c. Pixel pitch
   d. Field of view

91. The expression of image quality provided by a detector is called:
   a. MTF
   b. Matrix size
   c. SNR
   d. Nyquist frequency

92. Which of the following terms describes the highest spatial frequency that can be recorded by a digital detector?
   a. Spatial resolution
   b. Contrast resolution
   c. MTF
   d. Nyquist frequency

93. What converts light into a charge?
   a. Diode
   b. Cathode
   c. AC to DC converter
   d. Photodiode

94. The smallest area represented in a digital image is the:
   a. Image matrix
   b. Pixel
   c. Voxel
   d. Bit

95. The number of pixels/mm in an image is called:
   a. Pixel density
   b. Bit depth
   c. Pixel pitch
   d. Matrix depth

96. The space from the center of a pixel to the center of the adjacent pixel is called:
   a. Pixel density
   b. Bit depth
   c. Pixel pitch
   d. Matrix depth

97. Mathematical codes used to generate the digital image are called:
   a. Binary codes
   b. Algorithms
   c. Binary digits
   d. Bytes

98. The process of assigning a value to each pixel to represent a gray tone is called:
   a. Quantization
   b. Scintillating
   c. Nyquist frequency
   d. Sampling

99. A material that absorbs x-ray energy and emits part of that energy as visible light is called:
   a. Diode
   b. Scintillator
   c. TFT
   d. Cathode

100. Bit depth is equal to:
   a. 2n (*n* equals the number of bits)
   b. 4096 shades of gray
   c. Pixel pitch
   d. Bits times bytes

5

Review of Imaging Procedures: Anatomy, Positioning, Procedures, Pathology, Terminology

Some people dream of worthy accomplishments, while others stay awake and do them.

BASIC PROCEDURES AND POSITIONING TERMINOLOGY

Anterior or ventral forward or front

Caudal inferior, away from the head

Central midarea

Cranial cephalic, superior, toward the head

Distal farthest from the origin or point of reference

Lateral away from the median plane of the body or the middle of a part

Medial toward the median plane of the body or the middle of a part

Posterior dorsal; back of a part (not used to describe the foot)

Proximal nearer origin or point of reference

Dorsal recumbent supine, lying on back

Ventral recumbent prone, lying face down

Right lateral recumbent lying on right side

Left lateral recumbent lying on left side

Projection path of the central ray

Position placement of the body or part

View image as seen by the image receptor (opposite of projection)

Oblique body rotated from supine, prone, or lateral

Right anterior oblique (RAO) angle that places right anterior portion of the body closest to the image receptor

Left anterior oblique (LAO) angle that places left anterior portion of the body closest to the image receptor

Left posterior oblique (LPO) angle that places left posterior part of the body closest to the image receptor

Right posterior oblique (RPO) angle that places right posterior portion of the body closest to the image receptor

Decubitus position patient lying down; central ray parallel to the floor (horizontal)

Left or right lateral decubitus patient lying on left or right side; central ray parallel to the floor (horizontal); anteroposterior (AP) or posteroanterior (PA) projection

Dorsal decubitus patient lying on back; central ray parallel to the floor (horizontal), lateral projection

Ventral decubitus patient lying on abdomen; central ray parallel to the floor (horizontal), lateral projection

Tangential central ray skims between body parts or skims body surface; shows profile of body part, free of superimposition

Axial longitudinal angulation of the central ray with the long axis of the body part; projection that refers to images obtained with central ray angled 10 degrees or more along long axis of part

Orbitomeatal line (OML) line from outer canthus of the eye to the auricular point; also called the *radiographic baseline*

Infraorbitomeatal line (IOML) line from just below the eye to the auricular point; also called *Reid's baseline*

Glabellomeatal line line from the glabella to the auricular point

Acanthiomeatal line (AML) line from the acanthion to the auricular point

Median sagittal plane (MSP) plane that passes vertically through the midline of the body from front to back; also called *midsagittal plane*

Sagittal plane any plane parallel to the MSP

Midcoronal plane plane that passes vertically through midaxillary region of the body and coronal suture of the cranium at right angles to the MSP

Coronal plane any plane passing vertically through the body from side to side

Transverse plane passes crosswise through the body at right angles to its longitudinal axis and the MSP and coronal planes; also called *axial plane*

Related medical terminology prefixes, roots, and suffixes

Prefixes

a-, an- without

ab- away from

ante- front

anti- against

bi- two

co- together
contra- against
decub- side
dors- back
dys- difficult
ect- outside
en- in
endo- within
epi- on
ex- out
hemi- half
hydro- water
hyper- above or greater
hypo- below or lesser
infero- below
megal- large
peri- around
poly- many
post- after
pre- before
pseudo- false
retro- backward
scler- hard
sub- below
super- above
trans- across
vent- front

Roots

angio vessel
arth joint
cardi heart
cephal brain
cerebro head
cerv neck
chole bile
chondr cartilage
cost rib
crani skull
cysto bladder
derm skin
encephal brain
enter intestine
gastr stomach
hem blood
hepat liver
leuk white
lith stone
nephr kidney
osteo bone
phren diaphragm
pneum air
pyel pelvis (renal)
viscer organ

Suffixes

-algia pain
-centesis puncture
-ectasis expansion
-ectomy excision
-emia blood
-genic origin
-iasis condition
-itis inflammation
-megaly enlargement
-myel spinal cord
-oid like
-oma tumor
-osis condition
-pathy disease
-plasty surgical correction
-pulm lung
-pyel pelvis (renal)
-rhaphy suture
-scopy inspection
-tomy incision

📱 KEY REVIEW POINTS
Basic Procedures and Positioning Terminology

- Be able to define and understand the use of each of the terms presented.
- Be able to contrast the various recumbent, oblique, and decubitus positions.
- Locate and understand the use of the various body lines and planes.

BASIC PRINCIPLES OF POSITIONING AND PROCEDURES*

A. Body part placement
   1. Body part should be placed on the image receptor in a position that allows imaging of all anatomical features required for the procedure
   2. Allow for tight collimation
B. *Alignment:* The long axis of the body part should correspond to the long axis of the image receptor except when the image receptor must be rotated to fit the entire part on the image receptor

C. Two or more projections on the same image receptor
   1. Lead strip should always be used to mask unexposed portion of image receptor
   2. Using only collimation may cause overlap of images; the radiograph is not as easy to view
   3. Long axis of the bone should be oriented in the same direction for both projections
D. Precise visualization
   1. Positioning must be absolutely accurate
   2. No rotation of image present
E. Patient identification
   1. Identification marker on image receptor should not obstruct view of relevant anatomy
   2. Patient information should include patient's name and date of examination
F. Anatomical markers
   1. Right or left markers must always appear on the radiograph; use a radiopaque marker placed on the image receptor
   2. Stickers, grease pencil writing, and felt-tip writing on the radiograph after processing are not considered legal markings; these should be used only in rare circumstances
   3. Radiopaque markers must be placed just inside the collimation field and should not obstruct relevant anatomy

---

*Positioning routines vary from text to text and from department to department. The following is a general review of common routines. Questions on the certification exam could include any of these routines or combinations and variations of specific positions.

G. Other markers
   1. *Time:* Time indicators should always be used when radiographs are taken at specifically timed intervals
   2. *Direction:* If the radiograph was taken with the patient in an erect position, the lead marker indicating *erect* or *upright* must appear on the radiograph
   3. *Inspiration/expiration:* Must be used for comparison studies of the chest
   4. *Internal/external:* Must be used when both forms of rotation constitute part of an examination
   5. *Numeric markers:* Must be used when taking a series of radiographs in sequence (e.g., during trauma or surgical cases when follow-up is required in a short time)
H. Routines
   1. Minimum of two projections per examination except for certain cases in which a single survey radiograph suffices (e.g., KUB)
   2. A minimum of two projections, 90 degrees from one another, must always be taken
      a. Superimposition of structures may prevent visualization of some pathological conditions
      b. Lesions or foreign bodies require precise localization
      c. Fractures must be seen from two points precisely 90 degrees from each other
      d. Minimum of three projections (AP or PA, lateral, and oblique) required for proper visualization of joints

> **KEY REVIEW POINTS**
> *Basic Principles of Positioning and Procedures*
>
> These are basic points you learned early in positioning class. They are simple concepts that may be used as straightforward questions or to form the basis of more complex questions. Master them.

TOPOGRAPHY

A. Cervical region
   1. *C1:* Mastoid tip
   2. *C2, C3:* Gonion
   3. *C5:* Thyroid cartilage
   4. *C7:* Vertebra prominens
B. Thoracic region
   1. *T1:* 2 inches above sternal notch
   2. *T2, T3:* Level of manubrial notch and superior margin of scapula
   3. *T4, T5:* Level of sternal angle
   4. *T7:* Level of inferior angle of scapula
   5. *T10:* Level of xiphoid tip
C. Lumbar region
   1. *L3:* Costal margin
   2. *L3, L4:* Level of umbilicus
   3. *L4:* Level of superiormost aspect of iliac crest

D. Sacrum and pelvic region
   1. *S1:* Level of anterior superior iliac spine (ASIS)
   2. *Coccyx:* Level of pubic symphysis and greater trochanters
E. Lines
   1. Orbitomeatal line (OML)
      a. Line from outer canthus of the eye to the auricular point
      b. 7-degree angle with infraorbitomeatal line (IOML)
      c. 8-degree angle with glabellomeatal line
      d. Also called the *radiographic baseline*
   2. Infraorbitomeatal line (also called *Reid's baseline*)
      a. Line from just below the eye to the auricular point
      b. 7-degree angle with OML
   3. Glabellomeatal line
      a. Line from the glabella to the auricular point
      b. 8-degree angle with OML
   4. Acanthiomeatal line (AML)
      a. Line from acanthion to the auricular point

> **KEY REVIEW POINTS**
> *Topography*
>
> Positioning in the clinical setting and answering test questions on the certification exam are predicated on your knowledge of topography. Be certain you can identify these baselines.

MOTION CONTROL

A. Involuntary motion (controlled with short exposure time and high-speed image receptor)
   1. Cardiac motion
   2. Peristalsis
   3. Muscular spasm
   4. Chills
   5. Pain
B. Voluntary motion
   1. Belligerence
   2. Excitement
   3. Fear
   4. Nervousness
   5. Painful discomfort
   6. Age (children, elderly)
   7. Controlled by use of the following
      a. Clear communications
      b. Sandbags
      c. Sponges
      d. Tape
      e. Short exposure time
      f. Patient comfort
      g. Compression bands
      h. Pediatric immobilizer (Pigg-O-Stat) (for infants)
      i. Sheets for mummification techniques (for children)

j. Instructions—clearly explain the examination to the patient

k. Obtain signature on consent form if required

l. Ask patient if he or she has any questions, ensuring informed consent

m. Describe examination in terminology the patient understands

n. Describe exactly what will be done to the patient, including the approximate number of radiographs to be taken and the duration of the examination

o. Explain the reasons for removal of clothing and the extent of gowning

p. Explain the reason for removal of all radiopaque objects in the area of interest

q. Describe the required breathing pattern and the reasons for its use

KEY REVIEW POINTS
Motion Control

Be sure you can compare and contrast involuntary with voluntary motion. Understand all the factors that control each.

EXPOSURE MODIFICATION

A. Use of optimal radiographic technique ensures proper visualization of body parts

B. Exposure technique may require modification because of some factors
1. Pathological conditions
2. Age
3. Conditions under which the radiographs are being taken (e.g., mobile radiography, cross-table projections)
4. Body habitus

KEY REVIEW POINTS
Exposure Modification

Using this knowledge and the information in Chapter 4, be able to identify the various factors that affect exposure technique. Have a working knowledge of the changes needed and how to perform them.

GONADAL SHIELDING

A. Used when gonads are within the primary beam or within 5 cm of the primary beam

B. Used if the shielding does not interfere with the purpose of the examination

C. Used on patients of reproductive age and younger

KEY REVIEW POINTS
Gonadal Shielding

Understand the process of gonadal shielding and its role in radiation protection. Review the material in Chapter 2.

BODY HABITUS

A. Hypersthenic
1. Massive build
2. Represents 5% of population
3. Thorax is broad and deep
4. Ribs are almost horizontal
5. Thoracic cavity is shallow
6. Lungs are short; narrow above and broad at the base
7. Heart is short and wide
8. Diaphragm is high
9. Upper abdominal cavity is broad; lower part is small
10. Stomach and gallbladder are high and horizontal
11. Colon is high

B. Sthenic
1. Slight modification of hypersthenic
2. Most common body habitus
3. Present in 50% of population

C. Hyposthenic
1. Between asthenic and sthenic
2. Present in 35% of population

D. Asthenic
1. Slender build
2. Present in 10% of population
3. Thorax is narrow and shallow
4. Ribs slope sharply downward
5. Thoracic cavity is long
6. Lungs are long; broader above than at the base
7. Heart is long and narrow
8. Diaphragm is low, and abdominal cavity is short
9. Stomach and gallbladder are low, vertical, and near the midline
10. Colon is low; median position

KEY REVIEW POINTS
Body Habitus

Every patient is unique, but each fits into a certain category. Be able to identify each body habitus and the anatomy of each.

PEDIATRIC RADIOGRAPHY: GENERAL PRINCIPLES

A. Appropriately introduce radiographer to child and parent

B. Radiographer should show a positive attitude toward the child

C. Maintain clear communication with child and parent

D. Determine extent of parental involvement

E. Report suspected child abuse (nonaccidental trauma) to the appropriate radiologist, attending physician, radiology supervisor, or nurse

F. Determine type of immobilization to be used for the examination
1. Immobilization board
2. Pediatric immobilizer (Pigg-O-Stat)

3. Sandbags
4. Tape
5. Compression bands
6. Sheets and towels
G. Practice *as low as reasonably achievable* (ALARA) principle
   1. Gonadal shielding of children
   2. Tight collimation
   3. Pieces of lead used as contact shields
   4. Low mAs techniques
   5. No repeat radiographs
   6. High-speed image receptors
H. Determine whether patient preparation was adequately carried out
I. Interview the parent and write down the appropriate history
J. Briefly discuss case with radiologist to determine specifically which projections are needed and the extent of gonadal shielding that should be used if this is in doubt

KEY REVIEW POINTS
Pediatric Radiography: General Principles

Pediatric radiography requires specific skills, attention to detail, and attention to radiation protection. Be aware of all of the points in this section.

TRAUMA: GENERAL PRINCIPLES

A. Do no additional harm to the patient
B. Work quickly and confidently, observing standard precautions
C. Be prepared to modify conventional positions in response to patient's condition
D. If patient is immobilized, transfer to the x-ray table with as much help as possible, using a slide board or similar device when available
E. Skull and cervical spine injuries
   1. Cross-table lateral cervical spine radiograph must be obtained before the patient is moved in any way
   2. Radiograph must be approved by a physician before patient is moved or a cervical collar or sandbags are removed
F. Each body part requires at least two radiographs taken at 90-degree angles to one another
G. Projections should approach routine positioning (as patient's condition permits), with the image receptor placed as close to the body part as possible
H. Central ray entrance and exit points should be as close to routine as possible
I. Long bone radiography
   1. Always include joint nearest the trauma
   2. Joint farthest from the trauma should also be included if possible; otherwise, separate radiographs should be taken of that joint
J. Splints or bandages
   1. Should not be removed unless permission has been obtained from the physician

2. Modification of exposure technique may be necessary to compensate for splints and bandages
K. Allow patient as much control over movement as possible
L. Whether patient is conscious or unconscious, explain your movements clearly to encourage possible cooperation
M. Be prepared to perform several examinations at once
   1. *Example:* All AP projections should be taken in an uninterrupted sequence, then all lateral projections, and so on
   2. Reduces the number of times the patient or x-ray tube must be moved
   3. Allows overall procedure to be completed more quickly
N. Provide lead aprons for anyone who may need to be in the room caring for a critically injured patient
O. Move patient's extremities carefully to avoid displacing fractures further or causing internal hemorrhage
P. Maintain a cooperative spirit
   1. Cooperate with other health care professionals, such as phlebotomists, respiratory therapists, physicians, and nurses, who may need to be caring for the patient simultaneously during the radiographic examination in cases of severe trauma
   2. The radiographer is a vital part of a trauma team and needs to work in harmony with the other health care professionals present for the proper care of the patient
Q. Inability of the patient to move and difficulty obtaining routine projections must never be used as an excuse to submit poor-quality radiographs
   1. Patients with severe trauma need fully diagnostic radiographs to receive optimal care
   2. The radiographer must be proficient in radiographic exposure and positioning so that high-quality radiographs may be obtained under difficult conditions

KEY REVIEW POINTS
Trauma: General Principles

Trauma radiography requires fast, accurate work on the part of the radiographer. Be sure you understand each concept presented here.

REVIEW OF ANATOMY RELEVANT TO RADIOGRAPHY

PLANES OF THE BODY

A. Median sagittal plane (MSP); also called *midsagittal plane*
   1. Passes vertically through the midline of the body from front to back
   2. Divides body into equal right and left portions
   3. Any plane parallel to MSP is called a *sagittal plane*

B. Midcoronal plane
  1. Passes vertically through the midaxillary region of the body and the coronal suture of the cranium at right angles to the MSP
  2. Divides body into anterior and posterior portions
  3. Any plane passing vertically through the body from side to side is called a *coronal plane*
C. Transverse plane (axial plane)
  1. Passes crosswise through the body at right angles to its longitudinal axis and the MSP and coronal planes
  2. Divides body into superior and inferior portions

CLINICAL DIVISIONS OF THE ABDOMEN

A. Divided into four quadrants by a transverse plane and MSP intersecting at the umbilicus
B. Quadrants
  1. Right upper quadrant
  2. Right lower quadrant
  3. Left upper quadrant
  4. Left lower quadrant

ANATOMICAL DIVISIONS OF THE ABDOMEN

A. Abdomen is divided into nine regions using four planes
  1. Two transverse planes
  2. Two sagittal planes
B. Planes are called *Addison's planes*
C. Transverse planes are drawn
  1. At the levels of the tip of the ninth costal cartilage
  2. At the superior margin of the iliac crest
D. Two sagittal planes are drawn
  1. Each midway between ASIS of the pelvis and MSP of the body
E. Nine regions of the body
  1. Superior
    a. Right hypochondrium
    b. Epigastrium
    c. Left hypochondrium
  2. Middle
    a. Right lumbar
    b. Umbilical
    c. Left lumbar
  3. Inferior
    a. Right iliac
    b. Hypogastrium
    c. Left iliac

SKELETAL SYSTEM

Functions

A. Provides rigid support system
B. Protects delicate structures
C. Bones supply calcium to the blood and are involved in formation of blood cells
D. Bones provide attachment of muscles and form levers in the joint spaces, allowing movement

Ossification

A. Cartilage is covered with perichondrium that is converted to periosteum
B. *Diaphysis:* Central shaft
C. *Epiphysis:* Located at both ends of diaphysis
D. Growth in bone length is provided by the metaphyseal plate, located between the epiphyseal cartilage and the diaphysis
E. An osseous matrix is formed in the cartilage
F. Bone appears at the site where cartilage existed
G. Ossification is completed as the proximal epiphysis joins with the diaphysis between 20 and 25 years of age

Marrow

A. Fills spaces of spongy bone
B. Contains blood vessels and blood cells in various stages of development
C. Red bone marrow
  1. Site of formation of red blood cells and some white blood cells
  2. Found in spongy bone of adults
    a. Sternum
    b. Ribs
    c. Vertebrae
    d. Proximal epiphysis of long bones
D. Yellow bone marrow
E. *Fatty marrow:* Replaces red bone marrow in adults except in areas previously mentioned

Types of Bones

A. Long bones (e.g., femur, humerus)
B. Short bones (e.g., wrist, ankle bones)
C. Flat bones (e.g., ribs, scapulae)
D. Irregular bones (e.g., vertebrae, sesamoids [patella])

Descriptive Terminology for Bones

A. Projections
  1. *Process:* Prominence
  2. *Spine:* Sharp prominence
  3. *Tubercle:* Rounded projection
  4. *Tuberosity:* Larger rounded projection
  5. *Trochanter:* Very large bony prominence
  6. *Crest:* Ridge
  7. *Condyle:* Round process of an articulating bone
  8. *Head:* Enlargement at end of bone
B. Depressions
  1. *Fossa:* Pit
  2. *Groove:* Furrow
  3. *Sulcus:* Synonymous with groove
  4. *Sinus:* Cavity within a bone
  5. *Foramen:* Opening
  6. *Meatus:* Tubelike

Division of the Skeleton

A. Axial skeleton
  1. Composed of 74 bones
  2. Upright axis of the skeleton
  3. Components
    a. Skull
    b. Hyoid bone
    c. Vertebral column
    d. Sternum
    e. Ribs
B. Appendicular skeleton
  1. Composed of 126 bones
  2. Bones attached to the axial skeleton
    a. Upper and lower extremities
    b. Auditory ossicles—6 bones

Articulations

A. Classification basis
  1. Structure
  2. Composition
  3. Mobility
B. Fibrous joints (synarthroses)
  1. Surfaces of bones almost in direct contact, with limited movement
  2. Generally immovable
  3. No joint cavity or capsule
  4. *Examples:* Skull sutures
C. Cartilaginous joints (amphiarthroses)
  1. No joint cavity; contiguous bones united by cartilage and ligaments
  2. Slightly movable
  3. *Examples:* Intervertebral disks, pubic symphysis
D. Synovial joints (diarthroses)
  1. Approximating bone surfaces covered with cartilage
  2. Freely movable
  3. Bones held together by a fibrous capsule lined with synovial membrane and ligaments
  4. Examples of movement
    a. *Hinge:* Permits motion in one plane only (elbow)
    b. *Pivot:* Permits rotary movement in which a ring rotates around a central axis (proximal radioulnar articulation)
    c. *Saddle:* Opposing surfaces are concavoconvex, allowing flexion, extension, adduction, and abduction (carpometacarpal joint of thumb)
    d. *Ball and socket:* Capable of movement in an infinite number of axes; rounded head of one bone moves in a cuplike cavity of the approximating base (hip)
    e. *Gliding:* Articulation of contiguous bones allows only gliding movements (wrist, ankle)
    f. *Condyloid:* Permits movement in two directions at right angles to one another; circumduction occurs, rotation does not (radiocarpal joints)
E. Bursae
  1. Sacs filled with synovial fluid; located where tendons or muscles slide over underlying parts
  2. Some bursae communicate with a joint cavity
  3. Prominent bursae found at the elbow, shoulder, hip, and knee
F. Movements
  1. Gliding
    a. Simplest kind of motion in a joint
    b. Motion of a joint that does not involve any angular or rotary movements
  2. *Flexion:* Decreases angle formed by the union of two bones
  3. *Extension:* Increases the angle formed by the union of two bones
  4. *Abduction:* Occurs by moving part of the appendicular skeleton away from the median plane of the body
  5. *Adduction:* Occurs by moving part of the appendicular skeleton toward the median plane of the body
  6. Circumduction
    a. Occurs in ball-and-socket joints
    b. Circumscribes the conic space of one bone by the other bone
  7. *Rotation:* Turning on an axis without being displaced from that axis

Skull Morphology

A. Mesocephalic skull
  1. Considered "typical" skull
  2. Petrous ridge forms 47-degree angle with MSP
B. Brachycephalic skull
  1. Petrous ridge forms 54-degree angle with MSP
  2. Short from front to back
  3. Broad side to side
  4. Shallow from vertex to base
C. Dolichocephalic
  1. Petrous ridge forms 40-degree angle with MSP
  2. Long from front to back
  3. Narrow side to side
  4. Deep from vertex to base

Axial Skeleton

Skull

A. Cranium (Figures 5-1 and 5-2)
  1. Superior portion formed by frontal parietal and occipital bones
  2. Lateral portions formed by temporal and sphenoid bones
  3. Cranial base formed by temporal, sphenoid, and ethmoid bones
  4. *Fontanelles:* Soft spots at birth in which ossification is incomplete
B. Frontal bone
  1. Forms the forehead
  2. Contains the frontal sinuses

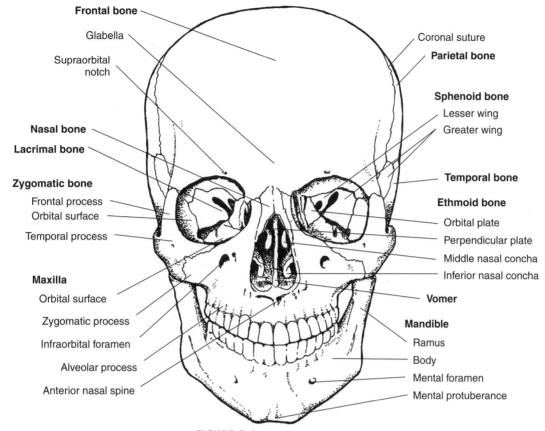

Frontal bone
Glabella
Supraorbital notch
Nasal bone
Lacrimal bone
Zygomatic bone
Frontal process
Orbital surface
Temporal process
Maxilla
Orbital surface
Zygomatic process
Infraorbital foramen
Alveolar process
Anterior nasal spine

Coronal suture
Parietal bone
Sphenoid bone
Lesser wing
Greater wing
Temporal bone
Ethmoid bone
Orbital plate
Perpendicular plate
Middle nasal concha
Inferior nasal concha
Vomer
Mandible
Ramus
Body
Mental foramen
Mental protuberance

FIGURE 5-1 Skull (anterior view).

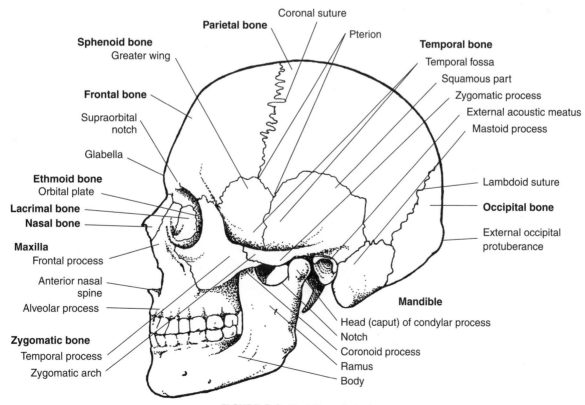

Sphenoid bone
Greater wing
Frontal bone
Supraorbital notch
Glabella
Ethmoid bone
Orbital plate
Lacrimal bone
Nasal bone
Maxilla
Frontal process
Anterior nasal spine
Alveolar process
Zygomatic bone
Temporal process
Zygomatic arch

Parietal bone
Coronal suture
Pterion
Temporal bone
Temporal fossa
Squamous part
Zygomatic process
External acoustic meatus
Mastoid process
Lambdoid suture
Occipital bone
External occipital protuberance
Mandible
Head (caput) of condylar process
Notch
Coronoid process
Ramus
Body

FIGURE 5-2 Skull (lateral view)

3. Forms the roof of the orbits
4. Union with the parietal bones forms the coronal suture

C. Parietal bones
   1. Union with occipital bone forms the lambdoid suture
   2. Union with temporal bone forms the squamous suture
   3. Union with sphenoid bone forms the coronal suture

D. Temporal bones
   1. Contain the external auditory meatus and middle and inner ear structures
   2. *Squamous portion:* Above the meatus; zygomatic process articulates with the zygoma to form the zygomatic arch
   3. Petrous portion
      a. Contains organs used for hearing and equilibrium
      b. Prominent elevation on the floor of the cranium
   4. Mastoid portion
      a. Protuberance behind the ear
      b. Mastoid process
   5. *Mandibular fossa:* Articulates with the condyle on the mandible
   6. *Styloid process:* Anterior to the mastoid process; several neck muscles attach here
   7. *Jugular foramen:* Located between the petrous portion and the occipital bones; opening from which CN IX, CN X, and CN XI exit

E. Sphenoid bone
   1. Bounded by ethmoid and frontal bones anteriorly and temporal and occipital bones posteriorly
   2. *Greater wings:* Lateral projections (Figure 5-3)
      a. Form outer wall and floor of the orbits
      b. *Foramen rotundum:* Round; located horizontally in anteromedial portion of the greater wing adjacent to lateral wall of the sphenoid sinus; maxillary division of CN V exits
      c. *Foramen ovale:* Oval; located laterally and posteriorly to foramen rotundum; mandibular division of CN V exits

d. *Foramen spinosum:* Located near posterior angle of the greater wing; lateral and posterior to foramen ovale; transmits an artery to the meninges
      e. *Foramen lacerum:* Contains internal carotid artery
      f. *Superior orbital fissure:* Transmits CN III and CN IV and part of CN V
   3. Lesser wings
      a. Posterior part of the roof of the orbits
      b. *Optic foramen:* CN II exits
   4. Body
      a. *Sella turcica:* Holds the pituitary gland (hypophysis)
      b. Contains the sphenoid sinuses
      c. Medial and lateral pterygoid processes located here

F. Ethmoid bone
   1. Contributes to formation of the base of the cranium, orbits, and roof of the nose
   2. *Perpendicular plate:* Forms superior part of the nasal septum
   3. Horizontal plate (cribriform plate)
      a. Located at right angles to perpendicular plate
      b. Olfactory nerves pass through
      c. Contains the crista galli; meninges of the brain attached to this process
   4. Lateral masses
      a. Form the orbital plates
      b. Contain superior and middle conchae (lateral walls of the nose)
      c. Contain ethmoid sinuses

G. Occipital bone
   1. Forms the posterior part of the cranium
   2. *Foramen magnum:* Spinal cord enters to attach to brainstem
   3. Condyles (two)
      a. On both sides of the foramen magnum
      b. Articulate with depressions on C1 vertebrae
   4. *External occipital protuberance:* Located on the posterior surface

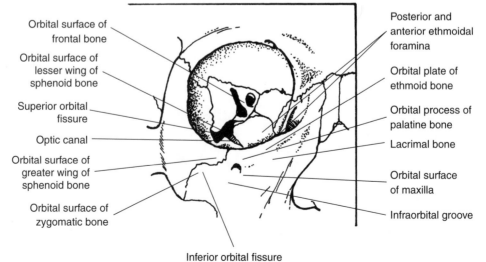

FIGURE 5-3 Right orbit.

Facial Bones

A. Appear suspended from middle and anterior parts of the cranium

B. Ethmoid and frontal bones also contribute to the framework of the face

C. Maxilla
  1. All facial bones except the mandible touch the maxilla
  2. *Alveolar process:* Forms upper jaw containing the maxillary teeth
  3. Forms the floor of the orbits; infraorbital foramen is inferior from the orbit
  4. Forms the walls of the nasal cavities and the hard palate (palatine process)
  5. *Maxillary sinus:* Large air space

D. Mandible (Figure 5-4)
  1. *Body:* Central horizontal portion
    a. *Chin:* Symphysis in midline
    b. *Alveolar process:* Contains the mandibular teeth
    c. Mental foramen
      (1) Below the first bicuspid on the outer surface
      (2) Transmits nerves and blood vessels
  2. *Ramus:* Upward process on both sides of the posterior body of the mandible
    a. *Condyle:* Articulates with the mandibular fossa
    b. *Coronoid process:* Attachment site for the temporalis muscle
    c. *Mandibular foramen:* Located on the inner surface

E. Zygomatic bone
  1. *Prominence of cheek:* Attaches to zygomatic process of the temporal bone to form the zygomatic arch
  2. Other margin of the orbit

F. *Lacrimal:* Medial part of the wall of the orbit

G. *Nasal bones:* Upper bridge of the nose

H. Inferior nasal concha
  1. Horizontally placed along the lateral wall of the nasal fossa
  2. Inferior to the middle and superior conchae of the ethmoid

I. Palatine bones
  1. Horizontal plates form the posterior part of the hard palate
  2. Perpendicular plates form the sphenoid palatine foramen

J. Vomer
  1. Plowshare-shaped bone
  2. Forms the lower part of the nasal septum

K. Hyoid
  1. U-shaped bone
  2. Body
  3. Greater horn
  4. Lesser horn
  5. Suspended by ligaments from the styloid process

Vertebral Column

A. Part of the axial skeleton
  1. Supports the head
  2. Gives base to the ribs
  3. Encloses the spinal cord

B. Vertebrae
  1. Consist of 34 bones that make up the spinal column
    a. *Cervical:* 7 bones
    b. *Thoracic:* 12 bones
    c. *Lumbar:* 5 bones
    d. *Sacral:* 5 bones
    e. *Coccygeal:* 4 or 5 bones
  2. In adults, the vertebrae of the sacral and coccygeal regions are united into two bones, the sacrum and the coccyx

C. *Curvatures:* From a lateral view, there are four curves, alternately convex and concave ventrally
  1. The two convex curves are the cervical and lumbar
  2. The two concave curves are the thoracic and sacral

D. Vertebral morphology
  1. Each vertebra differs in size and shape but has similar components
  2. *Body:* Central mass of bone
    a. Weight bearing
    b. Forms anterior part of vertebrae
  3. *Pedicles of the arch:* Two thick columns that extend backward from the body to meet the laminae of the neural arch
  4. *Processes:* Seven (one spinous [except C1], two transverse, two superior articular, and two inferior articular)
    a. Spinous process extends backward from the point of the union of the two laminae
    b. Transverse processes project laterally on both sides from the junction of the laminae and the pedicle
    c. Articular processes arise near the junction of the pedicle and the laminae; superior processes project upward, inferior processes project downward
    d. Surfaces of the processes are smooth

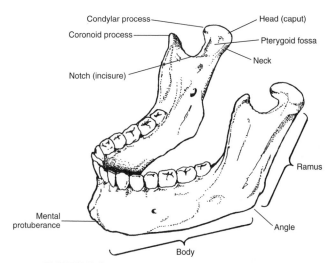

FIGURE 5-4 Mandible (anterolateral superior view).

e. Inferior articular processes of the vertebrae fit into the superior articular processes below

f. Form true joints, but the contacts established serve to restrict movement

E. Distinguishing features
1. *Cervical region:* Triangular shape
   a. All have foramina in the transverse processes (upper six transmit the vertebral artery)
   b. Spinous processes are short
      (1) C3 to C5 are bifurcated
      (2) C7 is a long prominence felt at the back of the neck
   c. Have small bodies (except for C1 vertebra)
   d. C1 vertebra (atlas) (Figure 5-5)
      (1) No body
      (2) Anterior and posterior arches and two lateral masses
      (3) Superior articular processes join with the condyles of the occipital bone

   e. *C2 vertebra (axis):* Process on the upper surface of the body (dens or odontoid) forms a pivot about which the axis rotates
2. Thoracic region (Figure 5-6)
   a. Presence of facets for articulation with the ribs
   b. Processes are larger and heavier than processes of the cervical region
   c. Spinous process is projected downward at a sharp angle
   d. Circular vertebral foramen
3. Lumbar region (Figure 5-7)
   a. Large and heavy bodies
   b. Four transverse lines separate the bodies of the vertebrae on the pelvic surface
   c. Triangular shape: Fitted between the halves of the pelvis
   d. Four pairs of dorsal sacral foramina communicate with four pairs of pelvic sacral foramina

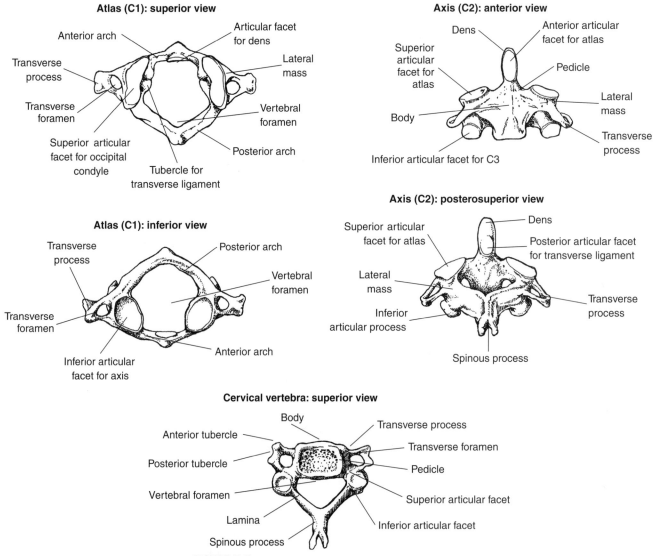

FIGURE 5-5 Distinguishing features of cervical vertebrae.

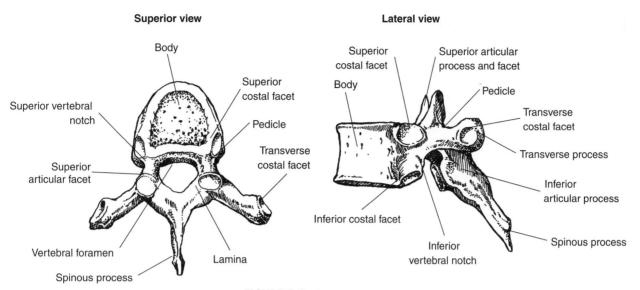

Superior view

Body
Superior costal facet
Superior vertebral notch
Pedicle
Superior articular facet
Transverse costal facet
Vertebral foramen
Spinous process
Lamina

Lateral view

Superior costal facet
Body
Superior articular process and facet
Pedicle
Transverse costal facet
Transverse process
Inferior articular process
Inferior costal facet
Inferior vertebral notch
Spinous process

FIGURE 5-6 Thoracic vertebra.

4. Sacral vertebrae
   a. Formed by fusion of five sacral segments in curved, triangular bone
   b. Base directed obliquely, superiorly, anteriorly
   c. Apex directed posteriorly, inferiorly
   d. Longer, narrower, more vertical in males than in females
   e. Body of sacrum has sacral promontory, a prominent ridge at upper anterior margin
5. Coccygeal vertebrae
   a. Four to five modular pieces fused together
   b. Triangular, with the base above and apex below
F. Defects
   a. *Lordosis:* Exaggerated lumbar concavity
   b. *Scoliosis:* Lateral curvature of any region
   c. *Kyphosis:* Exaggerated convexity in thoracic region

Bones of the Thorax

A. Sternum
   1. Forms medial part of the anterior chest wall

2. *Manubrium (upper part):* Clavicle and first rib articulate with the manubrium; contains notch on superior border called *jugular (manubrial) notch*
3. *Body (middle blade):* Ribs articulate with the body via the costal cartilages
4. Xiphoid (blunt cartilaginous tip)
B. Ribs—12 pairs (Figure 5-8)
   1. Each rib articulates with both the body and the transverse process of its corresponding thoracic vertebra

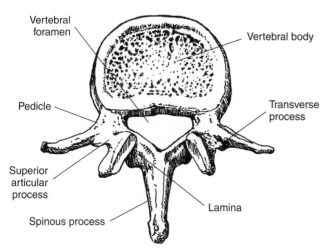

Vertebral foramen
Vertebral body
Pedicle
Transverse process
Superior articular process
Lamina
Spinous process

FIGURE 5-7 Lumbar vertebra (superior view).

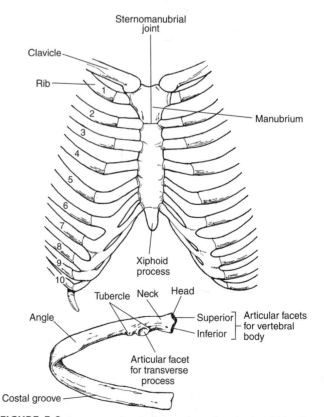

Sternomanubrial joint
Clavicle
Rib
1
2
3
4
5
6
7
8
9
10
Manubrium
Xiphoid process
Tubercle   Neck   Head
Angle
Superior
Inferior
Articular facets for vertebral body
Articular facet for transverse process
Costal groove

FIGURE 5-8 Sternocostal articulations (anterior view); middle rib (posterior view).

2. Second to ninth ribs articulate with the body of the vertebra above
3. Ribs curve outward, forward, and then downward
4. Anteriorly, each of the first seven ribs joins a costal cartilage that attaches to the sternum
5. Next three ribs (eighth to tenth) join the cartilage of the rib above
6. Eleventh and twelfth ribs do not attach to the sternum and are called *floating ribs*

Appendicular Skeleton

Upper Extremity

A. *Shoulder:* Clavicle and scapula (Figure 5-9)
  1. Clavicle
     a. Articulates with the manubrium at the sternal end
     b. Articulates with the scapula at the lateral end
     c. Slender S-shaped bone that extends horizontally across the upper part of the thorax
  2. Scapula (see Figure 5-9)
     a. Triangular bone with the base upward and the apex downward
     b. Lateral aspect contains the glenoid cavity (fossa), which articulates with the head of the humerus
     c. Spine extends across the upper part of the posterior surface; expands laterally and forms the acromion (point of shoulder)
     d. Coracoid process projects anteriorly from the upper part of the neck of the scapula
B. Humerus
  1. Consists of a shaft (diaphysis) and two ends (epiphyses)
  2. Proximal end has a head that articulates with the glenoid cavity (fossa) of the scapula
  3. Greater and lesser tubercles lie below the head
     a. Intertubercular groove (bicipital groove) is between them; long tendon of the biceps attaches here
     b. Surgical neck is below the tubercles
  4. Radial groove runs obliquely on the posterior surface; radial nerve is here
  5. Deltoid muscles attach in a V-shaped area in the middle of the shaft called the *deltoid tuberosity*
  6. Distal end has two projections
     a. *Capitulum:* Lateral, articulates with the radius; expanded area just superior is called the *lateral epicondyle*
     b. *Trochlea:* Medial, articulates with the ulna; expanded area just superior is called the *medial epicondyle*

C. Forearm (Figure 5-10)
  1. Radius
     a. Lateral bone of the forearm
     b. Radial tubercle (tuberosity) located below the head on the medial side
     c. Proximal end has disklike head
     d. Neck just inferior to head
     e. Distal end broad for articulation with the wrist
     f. Has styloid process on its lateral side
  2. Ulna
     a. Medial bone of the forearm
     b. Conspicuous part of the elbow joint (olecranon)
     c. Curved surface that articulates with the trochlea of the humerus is the trochlear notch
     d. Lateral side concave (radial notch); articulates with the head of the radius
     e. Distal end contains the styloid process
D. Hand and wrist (Figure 5-11)
  1. Carpal bones—8
     a. Arranged in two rows of four
     b. From lateral to medial, proximal row—scaphoid, lunate, triquetrum, and pisiform
     c. From lateral to medial, distal row—trapezium, trapezoid, capitate, and hamate
  2. Metacarpal bones—5
     a. Framework of the hand
     b. Numbered 1 through 5, beginning on the lateral side
  3. Phalanges—14
     a. Form the fingers
     b. Three phalanges in each finger; two phalanges in the thumb

Lower Extremity

A. Hip (os coxae or innominate) (Figure 5-12)
  1. Constitutes pelvic girdle
  2. United with the vertebral column
  3. Union of three parts that is marked by a cup-shaped cavity (acetabulum)
  4. Ilium
     a. Prominence of the hip
     b. Superior border is the crest
     c. *ASIS:* Projection at the anterior tip of the crest; just inferior to the ASIS is the anterior inferior iliac spine
     d. Corresponding projections on the posterior part are the posterior superior and posterior inferior iliac spines
     e. *Greater sciatic notch:* Located beneath the articular surface
     f. Most is a smooth concavity (iliac fossa)
     g. Posteriorly, it is rough and articulates with the sacrum in the formation of the sacroiliac joint

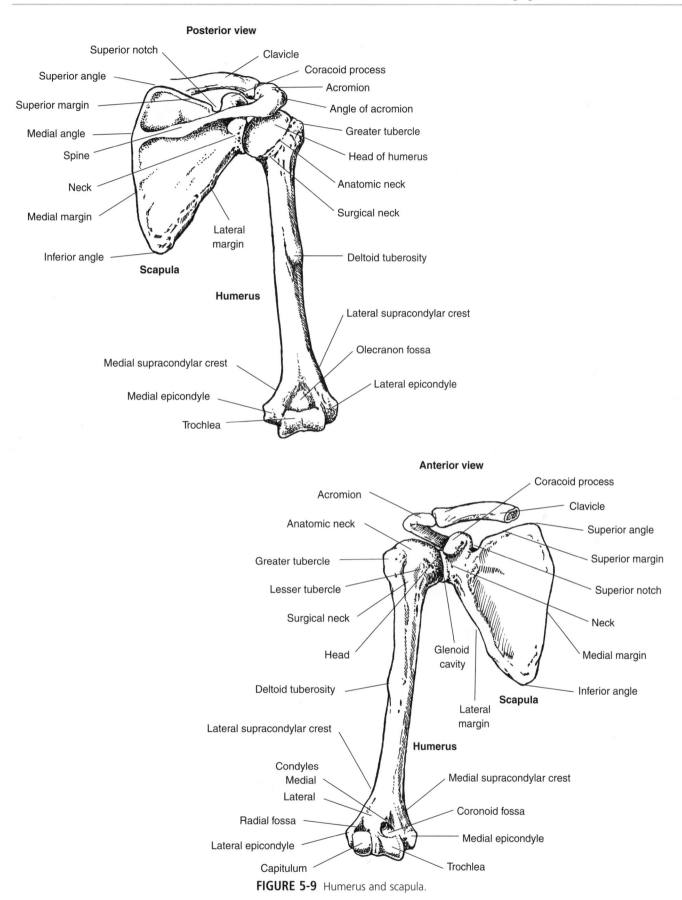

Posterior view

Superior notch
Clavicle
Superior angle
Coracoid process
Superior margin
Acromion
Medial angle
Angle of acromion
Spine
Greater tubercle
Neck
Head of humerus
Medial margin
Anatomic neck
Surgical neck
Inferior angle
Lateral margin
Scapula
Deltoid tuberosity
Humerus
Lateral supracondylar crest
Olecranon fossa
Medial supracondylar crest
Medial epicondyle
Lateral epicondyle
Trochlea

Anterior view

Acromion
Coracoid process
Anatomic neck
Clavicle
Greater tubercle
Superior angle
Lesser tubercle
Superior margin
Surgical neck
Superior notch
Head
Neck
Deltoid tuberosity
Glenoid cavity
Medial margin
Lateral supracondylar crest
Inferior angle
Scapula
Lateral margin
Condyles
Humerus
Medial
Medial supracondylar crest
Lateral
Coronoid fossa
Radial fossa
Medial epicondyle
Lateral epicondyle
Trochlea
Capitulum

FIGURE 5-9 Humerus and scapula.

5. Pubic bone
   a. Anterior part of the innominate bone
   b. *Symphysis pubis:* Joining of the right and left pubic bones at the midline
   c. Body and two rami
      (1) Body forms one-fifth of acetabulum
      (2) Superior ramus extends from the body to the median plane; superior border forms the pubic crest
      (3) Inferior ramus extends downward and meets with the ischium
      (4) Pubic arch is formed by the inferior rami of both pubic bones
6. Ischium
   a. Forms the lower and back part of the innominate bone
   b. Body
      (1) Forms two-fifths of the acetabulum
      (2) Ischial tuberosity supports the body in a sitting position
   c. *Ramus:* Passes upward to join the inferior ramus of the pubis
   d. Opening created by this ring is known as the *obturator foramen*
B. Pelvis
   1. Formed by the right and left hip bones, sacrum, and coccyx
   2. Greater pelvis
      a. Bounded by the ilia and lower lumbar vertebrae
      b. Gives support to the abdominal viscera

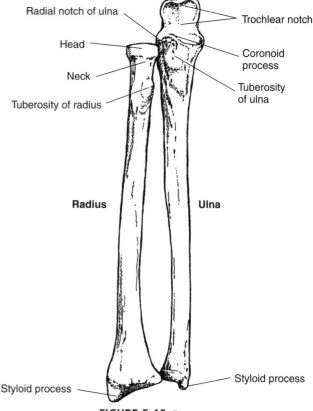

Radius and ulna in supination: anterior view

FIGURE 5-10 Forearm.

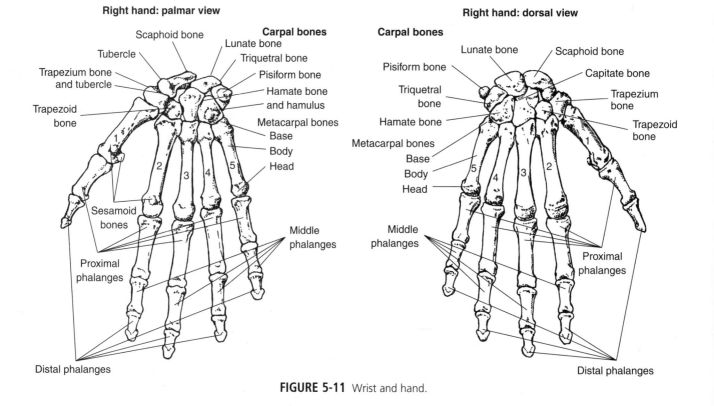

FIGURE 5-11 Wrist and hand.

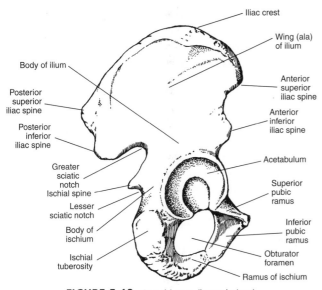

FIGURE 5-12 Coxal bone (lateral view).

3. Lesser pelvis
   a. Brim of the pelvis corresponds to the sacral promontory
   b. Inferior outlet is bounded by the tip of the coccyx, ischial tuberosities, and inferior rami of the pubic bones
4. Female pelvis
   a. Shows adaptations related to functions as a birth canal
   b. Wide outlet
   c. Angle of the pubic arch is obtuse
5. Male pelvis
   a. Shows adaptations that contribute to power and speed
   b. Heart-shaped outlet
   c. Angle of the pubic arch is acute
C. Femur (Figure 5-13)
   1. Longest and strongest bone of the body
   2. Proximal end has a rounded head that articulates with the acetabulum
   3. Constricted portion is neck
   4. Greater and lesser trochanters connected by inter-trochanteric crest
   5. Slightly arched shaft concave posteriorly
   6. Distal end has two condyles separated on the posterior side by the intercondyloid fossa
D. Patella
   1. Sesamoid bone
   2. Embedded in the tendon of the quadriceps muscle
   3. Articulates with the femur
E. Leg (Figure 5-14)
   1. *Tibia:* Medial bone
      a. Proximal end has two condyles that articulate with the femur
      b. Triangular shaft
         (1) *Anterior:* Shin
         (2) *Posterior:* Soleal line

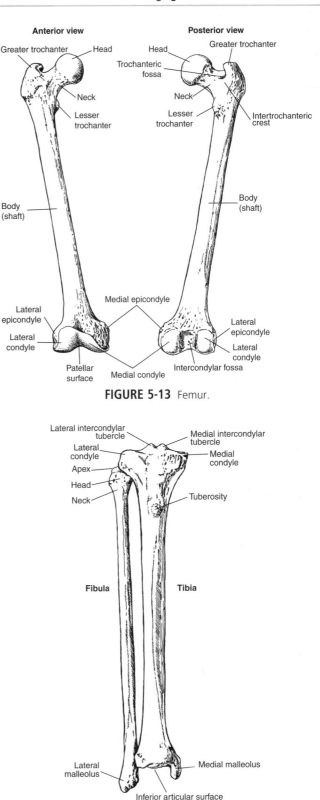

FIGURE 5-13 Femur.

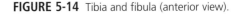

FIGURE 5-14 Tibia and fibula (anterior view).

      (3) *Distal:* Medial malleolus articulates with the lattice that forms the ankle joint
   2. *Fibula:* Lateral bone
      a. Articulates with lateral condyle of the tibia but does not enter the knee joint
      b. Distal end projects as the lateral malleolus

F. Ankle, foot, and toes (Figure 5-15)
   1. Adapted for supporting weight but similar in structure to the hand
   2. Talus
      a. Occupies the uppermost and central portion of the tarsus
      b. Distributes the body weight from the tibia above to the other tarsal bones
   3. *Calcaneus (os calcis, heel):* Located beneath the talus
   4. *Navicular:* Located in front of the talus on the medial side; articulates with three cuneiform bones distally
   5. *Cuboid:* Lies along the lateral border of the navicular bone
   6. Metatarsals
      a. First, second, and third metatarsals lie in front of the three cuneiform bones
      b. Fourth and fifth metatarsals lie in front of the cuboid bone
   7. Phalanges
      a. Distal to the metatarsals
      b. Two in the great toe; three in each of the other four toes
   8. Longitudinal arches of the foot—two
      a. *Lateral:* Formed by the calcaneus, talus, cuboid, and fourth and fifth metatarsal bones
      b. *Medial:* Formed by the calcaneus; talus; navicular; cuneiform; and first, second, and third metatarsal bones
   9. *Transverse arches:* Formed by the tarsal and metatarsal bones

NERVOUS SYSTEM

A. Adapts to environmental influences
   1. By stimulating skeletal, cardiac, and smooth muscles
   2. Adaptation by the muscular system is almost immediate
B. Organized into different systems
   1. Central nervous system (CNS)
      a. Consists of the brain and spinal cord
   2. Peripheral nervous system (PNS)
      a. Contains the nerves to and from the body wall that connect to the CNS
      b. Also known as the *somatic division* because it is under voluntary control
   3. Autonomic nervous system (ANS)
      a. Not under conscious control (involuntary)
      b. Provides stimulus for the viscera and smooth and cardiac muscles
      c. Sympathetic division includes motor (afferent) nerves from the ANS
      d. Parasympathetic division involves motor (efferent) nerves from the ANS
C. *Nerve cell:* Neuron
   1. Dendrite carries impulse toward the cell body under normal conditions

   2. Axon carries impulse away from the cell body and makes contact with the next cell; release of chemicals starts impulse in the next neuron
   3. *Myelin sheath:* Fatty substance around some cell axons provides insulation
   4. Neurons can carry impulses in different directions
      a. Afferent neurons carry the sensory information to the CNS
      b. Efferent neurons carry the motor information away from the CNS
   5. Central neurons are found entirely within the CNS; relay information within the system
      a. Spinal cord is approximately 45.8 cm long; occupies the upper two-thirds of the vertebral canal
      b. There are 31 pairs of spinal nerves; each has a dorsal (afferent) route and a ventral (efferent) route
D. Brain consists of four regions
   1. Cerebrum
      a. Seat of conscious activities
      b. Largest portion of the brain
      c. Superiormost location
      d. *Cerebral cortex:* Thin outside layer; gray color; consists of several layers of cells; convoluted surface
      e. *Longitudinal fissure:* Divides cerebrum into two hemispheres
      f. *Corpus callosum:* Heavy band of white fibers; forms the floor of the longitudinal fissure
      g. *Central fissure:* Posterior to midline
      h. *Frontal lobe:* Anterior to the central fissure
      i. *Parietal lobe:* Posterior to the central fissure
      j. *Temporal lobe:* Below the lateral fissure
      k. *Occipital lobe:* Posterior part of the brain
      l. *Broca's area:* Controls the muscular part of speech
      m. *Somesthetic area:* Interprets body sensations
      n. *Visual area:* Fibers from the medial part of the retina cross to opposite sides in the brain; fibers from the lateral portion do not cross
      o. *Auditory area:* Superior central portion of the temporal lobe
      p. *Prefrontal area:* Personality characteristics
   2. *Cerebellum:* Coordinates balance and equilibrium
   3. Medulla oblongata
      a. Bulb of the spinal cord located inside the foramen magnum
      b. White on the outside, gray on the inside
      c. Controls three vital functions—cardiac, respiratory, and basal motor
      d. Also controls chewing, salivation, swallowing, emesis, lacrimation, blinking, coughing, and sneezing
      e. *Pons:* Ropelike mass of white fibers; connects the halves of the cerebellum

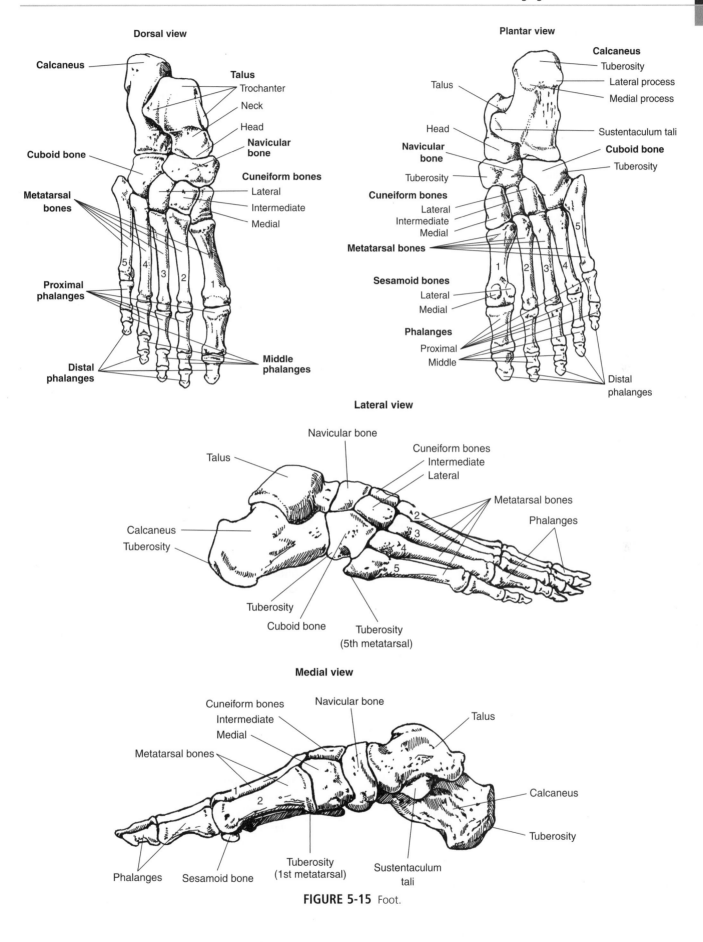

Dorsal view

Calcaneus

Talus
Trochanter
Neck
Head
Navicular bone

Cuboid bone

Cuneiform bones
Lateral
Intermediate
Medial

Metatarsal bones

5 4 3 2 1

Proximal phalanges

Distal phalanges

Middle phalanges

Plantar view

Calcaneus
Tuberosity
Lateral process
Medial process

Talus

Head

Sustentaculum tali

Navicular bone
Tuberosity

Cuboid bone
Tuberosity

Cuneiform bones
Lateral
Intermediate
Medial

Metatarsal bones

5

1 2 3 4

Sesamoid bones
Lateral
Medial

Phalanges
Proximal
Middle

Distal phalanges

Lateral view

Navicular bone

Talus

Cuneiform bones
Intermediate
Lateral

Metatarsal bones

Phalanges

Calcaneus
Tuberosity

2
3
4
5

Tuberosity
Cuboid bone
Tuberosity (5th metatarsal)

Medial view

Cuneiform bones
Intermediate
Medial

Navicular bone

Talus

Metatarsal bones

1
2

Calcaneus

Tuberosity

Phalanges Sesamoid bone Tuberosity (1st metatarsal) Sustentaculum tali

FIGURE 5-15 Foot.

4. Mesencephalon
   a. Short part of the brainstem
   b. Above the pons
   c. Mostly white matter
E. *Meninges:* Membranous coverings of the brain and spinal cord
   1. Dura mater
      a. Double layer around the brain
      b. Single layer around the spinal cord, including the cauda equina
   2. Arachnoid
      a. Membrane just inside the dura mater
      b. Relatively thin
   3. Pia mater
      a. Soft covering that fits against the brain and spinal cord
      b. Contains an enormous amount of blood
   4. Subarachnoid space
      a. Threadlike structure through which cerebrospinal fluid circulates
      b. Located between the pia mater and arachnoid
F. Cranial nerves
   1. Part of PNS
   2. Originate at the base of the brain
   3. 12 pairs of cranial nerves
   4. Referred to by name or Roman numerals
   5. Provide motor impulses, sensory impulses, or mixed impulses

HEART*

A. Composed of cardiac muscle; pumps the blood through the circulatory system
B. Located behind the sternum
C. The size of a human fist
D. The apex of the heart points down and to the left
E. Located in a space between the lungs and the thoracic cavity, known as the *mediastinum*
F. Consists of four chambers—two atria and two ventricles
   1. Blood from the superior and inferior venae cavae fills the right atrium and passes into the right ventricle through the tricuspid valve
   2. The unoxygenated blood moves from the right ventricle to the lungs through the semilunar valve and the pulmonary artery
   3. Oxygenated blood is sent from the lungs to the left atrium through the pulmonary veins; left semilunar valve separates the left atrium from the pulmonary veins

---

*The cardiovascular and lymphatic systems are not included in the content specifications for the certification exam. Their inclusion here supports the goal of this text as a study guide for use throughout the radiography program.

4. From the left atrium, blood flows through the mitral valve into the left ventricle
5. Blood enters circulation by passing through the left semilunar valve into the aorta
G. Heart wall consists of three layers
   1. Visceral pericardium or epicardium
   2. *Myocardium:* Heaviest covering
   3. *Endocardium:* Smooth continuous covering
   4. All valves and chambers are lined by endothelium
H. Heartbeat
   1. Averages 70 to 72 beats per minute
   2. Heart cannot contract without nerve impulses
   3. Nerves regulate the rate of the beat
I. Cardiac cycle
   1. Consists of a relaxation-contraction cycle
   2. Lasts for approximately 0.8 second
J. Electrocardiogram is a record of the action current as it travels across the heart

Circulatory System

A. Overview
   1. The connection of the heart to the arteries, arterioles, capillaries, venules, and veins
   2. The lymphatic system also interacts with the circulatory system
B. Arteries
   1. Thick-walled elastic vessels
   2. End in arterioles
C. Arterioles
   1. Smallest branch of an artery
   2. Connected to venules by capillaries
D. Capillaries
   1. Connect arterioles to venules
   2. Are lined by a thin layer of endothelium
   3. Capillaries can dilate or constrict, depending on the needs of the tissue
   4. Red blood cells go through capillaries one cell at a time
E. Venules
   1. Connected to veins that carry blood toward the heart and carry unoxygenated blood (except in the pulmonary vein)
F. Veins
   1. Have the same layers as arteries but are thinner
   2. Veins collapse without blood
   3. Valves in the veins help resist forces of gravity
G. Arteriovenous shunt (anastomosis)
   1. A large blood vessel that connects an artery and vein directly
   2. Skin color is caused by blood in the capillaries and anastomosis; anastomosis is important for heat distribution
   3. Found only in the hands, face, and toes, where the body is exposed to weather

Arterial Systemic Circulation

A. Aorta
1. Arises from the left ventricle of the heart
2. First 5 cm is called the *ascending aorta*
3. Two left and right coronary arteries branch off directly above the left semilunar valve and supply blood to the cardiac muscle

B. Aortic arch
1. Loops back over the top of the heart and left of the trachea
2. Continues down in back of the heart
3. Three arteries come off the arch
   a. Brachiocephalic
      (1) Only a few centimeters in length
      (2) Right subclavian artery arises from the brachiocephalic artery and supplies blood to the right shoulder
      (3) Right common carotid artery arises from the brachiocephalic artery and supplies blood to the right side of the head
   b. Left common carotid artery supplies blood to the left side of the head
   c. Left subclavian artery supplies branches to the upper chest and scapula

C. Carotid arteries
1. Supply the head
2. Right carotid artery originates from the brachiocephalic artery
3. Left carotid artery originates from the aortic arch

D. Subclavian arteries
1. Provide blood to the shoulder and arm
2. Left subclavian artery comes from the aortic arch
3. Right subclavian artery comes from the brachiocephalic artery
4. Pass over the first rib and under the clavicle
5. Become the axillary arteries as they pass through the shoulder region
6. First branch off the subclavian artery is the vertebral artery

E. Vertebral artery
1. Passes up the neck through the transverse foramen of the cervical vertebrae
2. Enters the skull through the foramen magnum
3. The two paired arteries join on the ventral side of the medulla and become the basilar artery; this artery joins branches from the internal carotid artery to form the circle of Willis, also called the *cerebral arterial circle*

F. Axillary artery
1. Becomes the brachial artery at the humerus
2. Moves along the medial surface across the elbow region and divides into radial and ulnar arteries

G. Radial artery
1. Moves along the radius and crosses it at the distal end
2. A pulse can be felt at the distal end
3. Moves across the metacarpals and deep into the palm
4. Forms a loop that connects with the ulnar artery

H. Ulnar artery
1. Travels down the medial surface of the forearm
2. Becomes the superficial palmar artery, which joins with the radial artery
3. Digital arteries supply the fingers and branch off from the palmar loop

I. *Descending aorta:* Consists of the thoracic and abdominal sections of the aorta
1. Thoracic aorta
   a. Starts after the left subclavian artery branches off the aortic arch
   b. Extends from T4-5 to T12-L1
   c. Passes down and in front of the vertebral column and through the diaphragm
   d. Gives off several branches supplying the ribs, lungs, and diaphragm
   e. After it passes through the diaphragm, it is called the *abdominal aorta*
2. Abdominal aorta
   a. Extends to the L4 vertebra
   b. Gives rise to the visceral and parietal arteries
   c. *Celiac artery:* Visceral artery that is 1.5 cm long; it divides into several branches
      (1) *Left gastric artery:* Smallest branch to the stomach
      (2) *Hepatic artery:* Supplies most of the blood to the liver; divides at the liver
         (a) *Cystic artery:* Serves the gallbladder
         (b) *Gastric duodenal artery:* Divides to serve the stomach, pancreas, and duodenum
      (3) *Splenic artery:* Largest branch to the spleen
   d. *Superior mesenteric artery:* Supplies all of the small intestine except the duodenum and superior ascending and transverse portion of the colon; comes off the front of the aorta below the celiac artery
   e. *Inferior mesenteric artery:* Supplies blood for part of the transverse colon and all of the descending and sigmoid colon, rectum, and bladder
   f. *Renal artery:* Supplies the kidneys; located below the superior mesenteric artery
      (1) Right renal artery slightly longer and lower because the aorta is slightly left of the midline
      (2) Enters the kidney at the hilus
   g. *Suprarenal artery:* Branches off the aorta above the renal artery (may be branches of the renal arteries)
   h. Aorta bifurcates and becomes the right and left common iliac arteries

J. Common iliac arteries bifurcate
1. Internal iliac artery supplies the pelvic wall and viscera
2. External iliac artery goes into the thigh
   a. Passes over the pelvic brim and under the inguinal ligament
   b. Becomes the femoral artery

K. Femoral artery
   1. Supplies thigh
   2. Becomes the popliteal artery just above the knee and goes behind the knee to bifurcate
      a. Anterior tibial artery
      b. Posterior tibial artery
      c. Anterior and posterior tibial arteries spread out at the ankle and become the dorsal artery of the foot

Venous Systemic Circulation

A. Consists of one set of superficial veins and one set of deep veins
B. Veins have a higher blood capacity than arteries but have lower blood pressure and velocity
C. Three sets of veins connect to the heart
   1. *Vena cava:* Superior and inferior
      a. Serve the body
      b. Return unoxygenated blood
   2. Coronary sinus
      a. Serves the heart
      b. Returns unoxygenated blood
   3. Pulmonary veins
      a. Serve the lungs (two per lung)
      b. Return oxygenated blood to the left atrium
D. Superior vena cava
   1. Begins at the level of the first rib
   2. Is formed by two veins
      a. Left and right brachiocephalic veins (return blood from the head, shoulders, and arms)
      b. Each brachiocephalic vein is a union of the internal jugular vein with the subclavian vein
E. Jugular veins drain blood from the head
   1. External jugular vein
      a. Drains the face and the scalp
      b. Is the union of three main veins that unite just below the ear and empty into the subclavian vein
   2. Internal jugular vein
      a. Returns from the internal carotid vein
      b. Originates in the skull
F. Vertebral veins
   1. Arise outside of the skull at the level of the atlas
   2. Pass through the transverse foramen to the subclavian artery
G. Arms and shoulders are drained by the deep veins that run alongside the arteries
H. Inferior vena cava
   1. Formed by two common iliac veins at the L5 vertebra in front of the vertebral column
I. Azygos vein
   1. Branches off the inferior vena cava at the level of the renal veins
   2. Goes through the aortic hiatus of the diaphragm just below the heart
   3. Empties into the superior vena cava
   4. Picks up veins from the esophagus and bronchi

J. Other veins serving the abdomen and thorax are named for the region or organs that they serve
K. Veins of the lower extremities
   1. Deep veins have the same names as the arteries
   2. Superficial veins
      a. *Great saphenous vein:* Drains the dorsalis pedis of the foot
      b. *Small saphenous vein:* Drains the lateral side of the foot
      c. *Popliteal vein:* Drains the lateral side of the leg

LYMPHATIC SYSTEM

A. Carries lymph
B. Involved in the maintenance of fluid pressure
C. Contains lymph glands that filter foreign particles
   1. Tissue fluid is located in the intracellular spaces and is derived from the blood
   2. Is constantly moving
   3. Similar to plasma without large proteins
D. Lymph is tissue fluid that has been reabsorbed into lymphatic vessels
E. Valves are necessary in the lymphatic system
   1. To keep fluid flowing in the right direction
   2. Most valves are located in the arms and legs, where gravity is a problem
F. Lymph nodes
   1. Spongy masses of tissue through which lymph filters
   2. Have more afferent vessels coming to the node than efferent vessels leaving the node
G. Lymphocytes are small white blood cells that originate from stem cells
H. Right lymphatic duct
   1. Drains the upper right quadrant of the thorax, right arm, and right side of the head
   2. Empties into the right subclavian vein
I. Thoracic duct
   1. Drains the rest of the body
   2. Begins at the cisterna chyli
   3. Passes up the left side of the vertebral column, through the aortic hiatus of the diaphragm, and into the left subclavian vein
J. Lymphoid tissue is found in various anatomical structures
   1. *Spleen:* The graveyard of red blood cells
   2. *Thymus:* Atrophies after puberty but is involved in the cell-mediated immune system
   3. *Tonsils:* Located in the oral cavity

RESPIRATORY SYSTEM

A. *Respiratory tract:* Begins at the nostril opening and extends to the alveoli of the lungs
B. Air is drawn in through the nose, where it is warmed, humidified, and cleansed

C. Nasal cavity is lined with olfactory epithelium in the sphenoethmoid recess and by respiratory epithelium in the lower part

D. Superior, middle, and inferior turbinates are located on the lateral surface of the nasal cavity

E. Frontal, ethmoidal, maxillary, and sphenoidal sinuses empty into the nasal cavity

F. Pharynx
   1. Second part of the respiratory tract
   2. Starts at the base of the skull and extends to the esophagus
   3. Divided into three parts
      a. *Nasopharynx:* Behind the nasal cavity
         (1) *Eustachian tube (auditory tube):* Connects the middle ear with the pharynx; open only during swallowing; equalizes pressure
         (2) *Pharyngeal tonsils (adenoids):* A mass of lymphoid tissue on the upper back wall of the nasopharynx
      b. *Oropharynx:* Extends from the soft palate to the base of the tongue; separated from the oral cavity by the palatine arches
      c. *Laryngopharynx:* Extends from the hyoid bone to the larynx

G. Larynx
   1. Located at the base of the tongue
   2. Comprises nine cartilages

H. Vocal chords
   1. Folds of mucous membranes
   2. Elastic connective tissue at the edges

I. Trachea
   1. Approximately 12 cm long
   2. In front of esophagus
   3. Composed of 16 to 20 C-shaped rings that prevent its collapse
   4. At the end of T4 vertebra, the trachea divides into left and right branches known as the *primary bronchi*

J. Primary bronchi
   1. Left primary bronchus is longer than the right and forms a sharp angle
   2. Right primary bronchus has a larger diameter than the left and comes off forming an almost straight line

K. Secondary bronchi branch off the primary bronchi
   1. Three secondary bronchi for the right lung, one per lobe
   2. Two secondary bronchi for the left lung, one per lobe

L. Tertiary bronchi
   1. Branch off the secondary bronchi
   2. Each lung has 10 tertiary bronchi because there are 10 segments per lung

M. *Bronchioles:* Smaller branches of the tertiary bronchi
   1. *Terminal bronchiole:* Not involved in gaseous exchange
      2. *Respiratory bronchiole:* Branch off terminal bronchiole; first site of diffusion of oxygen into the blood

N. Alveolar ducts
   1. Branch off respiratory bronchiole
   2. Alveolar sacs attach to the alveolar ducts

O. Two cone-shaped lungs in the thoracic cavity
   1. Base rests on the diaphragm
   2. Apex is located at the level of the clavicle
   3. Right lung
      a. Has three lobes—superior, middle, and inferior
      b. Larger than the left lung
   4. Left lung
      a. Smaller than the right lung because two-thirds of the heart is located on the left side
      b. Contains only two lobes
   5. 10 bronchopulmonary segments per lung
      a. Each has a branch from the tertiary bronchi
      b. Used as points of reference for surgery

P. *Cardiac notch:* Depression on the medial surface of the left lung
   1. Hilus
      a. Point of attachment to a lung
      b. Blood vessels, bronchial tree, and nerves enter at the hilus

Q. *Pleura:* Serous membrane surrounding the visceral and parietal layers of each lung
   1. Space between the two layers is the pleural cavity
   2. Lungs are not located in the pleural cavity

R. Mechanics of respiration
   1. Involve changing the pressure in the lungs to cause inspiration or expiration
   2. Inspiration
      a. Occurs when the air pressure in the lungs is decreased
      b. Causes the volume of the lungs to increase
      c. External intercostal muscles cause the ribs to elevate and increase the size of the chest cavity
      d. Dome-shaped diaphragm between the thoracic and abdominal cavities pulls downward when contracted
      e. Also increases the size of the chest cavity
   3. Expiration
      a. Basically a passive movement
      b. Ribs fall down
      c. Diaphragm is pushed up by the abdominal viscera
      d. Abdominal muscles force the abdominal contents up
      e. Internal intercostal muscles pull the ribs down

DIGESTIVE SYSTEM

A. Digestive or alimentary tract
   1. Consists of a tube 6 m long from the mouth to the anus
   2. Selectively absorbs nutrients and water for the body

B. Mouth
   1. Site where food processing and digestion begin
   2. Secondary teeth tear and grind the food
C. Tongue
   1. Fibromuscular organ
   2. Contains the taste buds
   3. Transmits the sensation of taste to the brain
   4. Rolls the food into a bolus for swallowing
D. Saliva
   1. Added to help food become a bolus for easier passage down the esophagus
   2. Produced by three major paired glands and many minor glands
E. Salivary glands
   1. Parotid glands
      a. Located in the preauricular region
      b. Saliva travels down Stensen's (parotid) duct, which opens opposite the second maxillary molar
   2. Sublingual glands
      a. Lie under the tongue and rest against the mandible
      b. Saliva travels down Bartholin's duct and enters the oral cavity through Rivinus' (lesser sublingual) ducts on the sublingual fold
   3. Submandibular glands
      a. Lie on the medial surface of the mandible
      b. Saliva travels down Wharton's (submandibular) duct and is released into the mouth at the sublingual caruncles
F. Swallowing
   1. Bolus of food moves from the mouth and pharynx to the esophagus
   2. During swallowing, the soft palate is pushed back against the posterior pharyngeal wall, closing the passage to the nasopharynx
   3. Larynx is elevated; superior opening is protected by the epiglottis
   4. Bolus moves into esophagus
   5. *Esophagus:* Muscular tube located posterior to the trachea and connected to the stomach
   6. Bolus moved through esophagus by peristalsis and gravity
G. *Stomach:* Dilated portion of the alimentary canal lying in the upper abdomen just under the diaphragm (Figures 5-16 and 5-17)
   1. Functions
      a. Stores food
      b. *Digests:* Secretes pepsin, renin, and gastric lipase
      c. Produces hydrochloric acid
   2. Shaped like the letter "J"; internal surface is wrinkled (rugae)
      a. *Cardiac portion:* Esophagus entrance
      b. *Body:* Main part
      c. *Fundus:* Bulge at the upper end, left of the esophageal area

      d. *Pyloric portion:* Narrow distal end that connects with the small intestine
H. *Small intestine:* Thin-walled muscular tube
   1. Three portions
      a. *Duodenum (horseshoe-shaped):* Bile and pancreatic secretions are added to the small intestine
      b. *Jejunum (1.5 m long):* Greatest amount of absorption
      c. *Ileum (2.5 m long):* Connects with the large intestine
   2. Secretes several enzymes and substances
I. *Large intestine:* Approximately 1.5 m long and in several divisions
   1. Cecum
      a. Blind pouch in the lower right quadrant
      b. Appendix attaches to cecum
      c. Ileocecal sphincter separates the ileum from the cecum
   2. Colon
      a. *Ascending:* From cecum to the hepatic flexure
      b. *Transverse:* From hepatic flexure to the splenic flexure
      c. *Descending:* From splenic flexure to the level of the pelvic bone on the left side of the body
   3. *Sigmoid:* S-shaped curve
   4. *Rectum:* From sigmoid colon down to the pelvic diaphragm
   5. *Anus:* 3 cm in length
J. *Pancreas:* Exocrine and endocrine gland
   1. Exocrine
      a. Produces pancreatic juice that is collected by the pancreatic (Wirsung's) duct and carried away
      b. Joins the common bile duct to form Vater's (hepatopancreatic) ampulla, which penetrates the walls of the abdomen
   2. *Endocrine:* Releases insulin that controls blood glucose levels; also releases glucagon and somatostatin
K. Liver
   1. Largest and most active gland in the body
   2. Two main lobes and several lobules
   3. Lobules produce bile that is carried away and stored in the gallbladder
   4. Stores glycogen
   5. Detoxifies waste
   6. Plays major role in metabolism
L. Bile ducts
   1. Two main hepatic ducts join to form common hepatic duct
   2. Common hepatic duct unites with cystic duct (attached to the gallbladder) to form common bile duct
   3. In some cases, common bile duct joins pancreatic duct to enter hepatopancreatic ampulla
   4. Hepatopancreatic ampulla opens into descending duodenum
   5. In other cases, common bile duct and pancreatic duct enter duodenum directly and separately

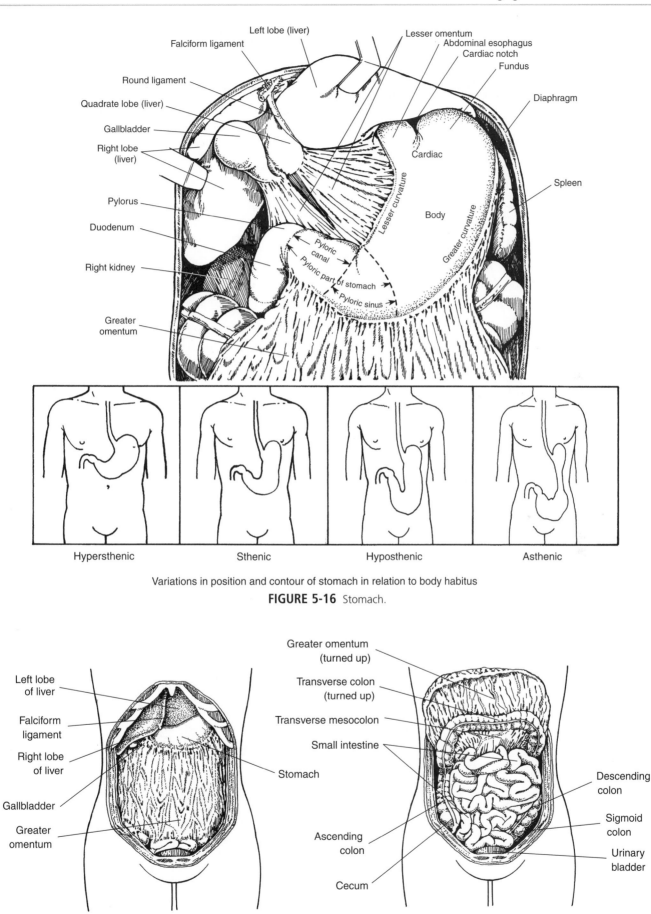

Left lobe (liver)

Falciform ligament

Round ligament

Quadrate lobe (liver)

Gallbladder

Right lobe (liver)

Pylorus

Duodenum

Right kidney

Greater omentum

Lesser omentum

Abdominal esophagus

Cardiac notch

Fundus

Diaphragm

Cardiac

Spleen

Lesser curvature

Body

Greater curvature

Pyloric canal

Pyloric part of stomach

Pyloric sinus

Hypersthenic   Sthenic   Hyposthenic   Asthenic

Variations in position and contour of stomach in relation to body habitus

FIGURE 5-16 Stomach.

Left lobe of liver

Falciform ligament

Right lobe of liver

Gallbladder

Greater omentum

Stomach

Greater omentum (turned up)

Transverse colon (turned up)

Transverse mesocolon

Small intestine

Ascending colon

Cecum

Descending colon

Sigmoid colon

Urinary bladder

FIGURE 5-17 Abdominal viscera.

6. Distal end of common bile duct controlled by hepatopancreatic sphincter (sphincter of Oddi)
M. Gallbladder
   1. Thin-walled sac with capacity of approximately 2 oz
   2. Concentrates and stores bile and evacuates bile during digestion
   3. Contraction of gallbladder is controlled by hormone cholecystokinin

URINARY SYSTEM

A. Kidneys (Figure 5-18)
   1. Paired bean-shaped organs on both sides of the vertebral column
   2. Renal artery and vein and ureter (which leads to the bladder) are attached to the center of the kidney at the hilus

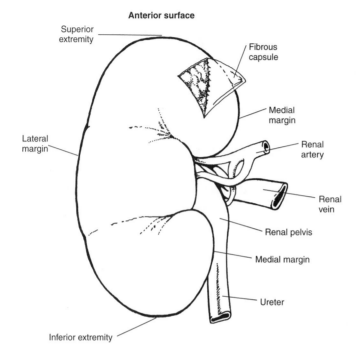

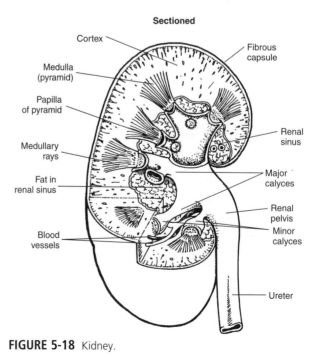

FIGURE 5-18 Kidney.

3. Outer part of the kidney is called the *cortex*, and inner part is called the *medulla*
   a. Medulla consists of several pyramids
   b. Apices of the pyramids project into the calyces
   c. Nephron is the functional unit of the kidney
4. Kidney connected to the bladder by the ureters

B. Ureters
   1. Approximately 27 cm long
   2. Urine flows down the ureters via peristalsis

C. Bladder
   1. Lies behind the symphysis pubis
   2. Serves as a reservoir for the urine

D. Urethra
   1. Connects the bladder to the exterior
   2. Female urethra is approximately 4 cm long
   3. Male urethra is approximately 20 cm long

E. Blood is filtered first in the glomeruli
   1. Passed through the glomerular membrane into Bowman's capsule and then into the proximal tubules
   2. Filtration rate determined by the filtration pressure
   3. Modified as it passes through the tubules by means of reabsorption and secretion
      a. Proximal convoluted tubule
      b. Loop of Henle
      c. Distal collecting tubule
   4. Waste products are not reabsorbed

📱 **KEY REVIEW POINTS**
Review of Anatomy Relevant to Radiography

- Identify, in words or on drawings, the various planes and divisions of the body.
- As you review the systems of the body, focus on the skeletal, respiratory, digestive, and urinary systems. These are the systems most often radiographed.
- The drawings in the chapter are invaluable. Be certain you can identify the labeled anatomy.

REVIEW OF RADIOGRAPHIC POSITIONING, PROCEDURES, AND PATHOLOGY

SKELETAL SYSTEM

*Pathological Conditions Imaged**

A. Acromegaly
   1. Endocrine disorder that causes bones to become thick and coarse
   2. Harder to penetrate

---

*Designation of "harder to penetrate" or "easier to penetrate" does not signify that alteration of exposure technique is required.

B. Ankylosing spondylitis
   1. Inflammatory disease of the spine and adjacent structures that causes severe pain and fusion of joints involved

C. Bony cyst
   1. Fluid-filled sacs in fibrous tissue
   2. Easier to penetrate

D. Bursitis
   1. Inflammation of bursa; causes severe pain
   2. Harder to penetrate if calcium has deposited

E. Callus
   1. New bony deposit surrounding healing fractures
   2. Harder to penetrate

F. Clubfoot (talipes)
   1. Congenital malformation of the foot that causes the foot to turn in at the ankle

G. Congenital hip anomaly
   1. Caused by malformation of the acetabulum in which the femoral head displaces superiorly and posteriorly

H. Disk herniation
   1. Protrusion of an intervertebral disk

I. Ewing's sarcoma
   1. Malignant destructive tumor of bone marrow
   2. Easier to penetrate

J. *Fractures:* Disruption of bone tissue
   1. *Complete fracture:* Discontinuity between two or more fragments
   2. *Incomplete fracture:* Partial discontinuity; portion of the cortex is intact
   3. *Closed fracture:* Overlying skin is intact
   4. *Compound fracture:* Overlying skin is broken; bony fragments
   5. *Transverse fracture:* Runs at right angle to the long axis of the bone
   6. *Oblique fracture:* Runs at approximately 45-degree angle to the long axis of the bone
   7. *Spiral fracture:* Encircles the shaft of the bone
   8. *Avulsion fracture:* Small fragments of bone torn off bony prominences
   9. *Comminuted fracture:* Produces more than two fragments
   10. *Compression fracture:* Causes compaction of the bone, resulting in decreased length or width
   11. *Stress fracture:* Results from repeated stresses placed on the bone
   12. *Pathological fracture:* Occurs as a result of bone disease
   13. *Greenstick fracture:* Incomplete fracture with cortex intact on opposite side of the bone from the fracture
   14. *Bowing fracture:* Occurs when stress applied to the bone causes the bone to bow but not fracture completely
   15. *Undisplaced fracture:* Lack of angulation or separation of fractured bone
   16. *Displacement:* Separation of bone fragments

17. *Angulation:* Deformity of the axes of major fragments of bone
18. *Dislocation:* Displacement of a bone from its normal site of articulation
19. *Subluxation:* Partial loss of continuity in a joint
20. *Fracture healing:* Characterized radiographically by calcium deposits across the fracture line that unite the fracture fragments
21. *Battered child syndrome:* Multiple fractures at various stages of healing located in long bones and the skull; also characterized by fractures at unusual sites (e.g., ribs, scapula, sternum, spine, clavicles)
22. *Colles' fracture:* Transverse fracture through the distal radius with posterior angulation and overriding of the distal fracture fragment
23. *Boxer's fracture:* Transverse fracture of neck of the fifth metacarpal with palmar angulation of the distal fragment
24. *Elbow fractures:* In addition to bony involvement, radiograph shows dislocation of elbow fat pads; this necessitates the use of appropriate radiographic exposure
25. *Pott's fracture:* Fracture of medial and lateral malleoli of the ankle with ankle joint dislocation
26. *Bimalleolar fracture:* Fracture of both medial and lateral malleoli
27. *Trimalleolar fracture:* Fracture of the posterior portion of the tibia and the medial and lateral malleoli
28. *Jefferson's fracture:* Comminuted fracture of the ring of the atlas involving both anterior and posterior arches and causing displacement of the fragments
29. *Hangman's fracture:* Caused by acute hyperextension of the head on the neck; characterized by fracture of the arch of C2 and anterior subluxation of C2 onto C3; caused primarily by motor vehicle accidents
30. *Seat belt fracture:* Transverse fracture of lumbar vertebrae in addition to substantial abdominal injuries

K. Hydrocephalus
   1. Abnormal accumulation of cerebrospinal fluid in the brain
   2. Harder to penetrate
L. Giant cell myeloma
   1. Benign or malignant tumor arising on bone with large bubble appearance
   2. Easier to penetrate
M. Gout
   1. Metabolic disorder in which urate crystals are deposited in the joints, most commonly the great toe, and cause extreme swelling
   2. Harder to penetrate

N. Multiple myeloma
   1. Malignancy of plasma cells resulting in destruction of bone, failure of bone marrow, and impairment of renal function
   2. Easier to penetrate
O. Osteoarthritis
   1. Form of arthritis characterized by degeneration of one or several joints
   2. Easier to penetrate
P. Osteoblastic metastases
   1. Dense, sclerotic tumors in bone
   2. Harder to penetrate
Q. Osteochondroma
   1. Benign projection of bone in the young
   2. Harder to penetrate
R. Osteogenic sarcoma
   1. Destructive cancer at the end of long bones
   2. Easier to penetrate (except for sclerotic area)
S. Osteoma
   1. Benign, small, round tumor
   2. Harder to penetrate
T. Osteogenesis imperfecta
   1. Inherited condition causing poor development of connective tissue and brittle, easily fractured bones
   2. Easier to penetrate
U. Osteomyelitis
   1. Bacterial infection of bone and bone marrow
   2. Easier to penetrate
V. Osteolytic metastases
   1. Arise in medullary canal to destroy bone
   2. Easier to penetrate
W. Osteomalacia
   1. Abnormal softening of bone
   2. Easier to penetrate
X. Osteopetrosis
   1. Inherited condition causing increased bone density
   2. Harder to penetrate
Y. Osteoporosis
   1. Abnormal demineralization of bone
   2. Easier to penetrate
Z. Paget's disease (osteitis deformans)
   1. Nonmetabolic bone disease causing bone destruction and unorganized bone repair
   2. Difficult to image properly because some areas that are easier to penetrate are adjacent to structures that are harder to penetrate
AA. Rheumatoid arthritis
   1. Destructive collagen disease with inflammation and joint swelling
   2. Harder to penetrate
BB. Rickets
   1. Soft, pliable bones resulting from deficiency of vitamin D and sunlight
   2. Easier to penetrate
CC. Scoliosis
   1. Abnormal lateral curvature of the spine

DD. Spina bifida
    1. Defect of posterior aspect of spinal canal caused by failure of vertebral arch to form properly
  EE. Spondylolysis
    1. Defect in pars articularis, which is between the superior and inferior articular processes of a vertebra
    2. No displacement present
  FF. Spondylolisthesis
    1. Spondylolysis with displacement

Digits (Fingers)

A. PA
    1. *Patient position:* Seated
    2. *Part position:* Separate and center extended digit of interest with palmar surface of hand firmly against image receptor
    3. *Central ray:* Perpendicular, entering proximal interphalangeal joint
B. Lateral
    1. *Patient position:* Seated
    2. Part position
      a. Extend digit of interest
      b. Close rest of digits into a fist
      c. Adjust digit of interest parallel to image receptor plane
      d. Immobilize extended digit
    3. *Central ray:* Perpendicular, entering proximal interphalangeal joint
C. Oblique
    1. *Patient position:* Seated
    2. Part position
      a. Place patient's hand in lateral position, ulnar side down
      b. Center to image receptor
      c. Rotate palm 45 degrees toward image receptor until digits are resting on support
      d. Immobilize separated digits
    3. *Central ray:* Perpendicular, entering proximal interphalangeal joint

Thumb

A. AP, lateral, oblique
    1. *Patient position:* Seated
    2. Part position
      a. *AP:* Patient's hand is turned in extreme internal rotation, thumb resting on image receptor and other fingers held out of the way
      b. *Lateral:* Hand in natural arched position, palm down; adjust hand to put thumb in true lateral
      c. *Oblique:* Abduct thumb, palm down
    3. *Central ray (all projections):* Perpendicular to metacarpophalangeal joint

Hand

A. PA
    1. *Patient position:* Seated
    2. Part position
      a. Patient rests forearm on table, with palmar surface firmly against image receptor
      b. Spread digits slightly
    3. *Central ray:* Perpendicular to third metacarpophalangeal joint
B. Oblique
    1. *Patient position:* Seated, forearm resting on table with hand on image receptor in lateral position, ulnar side down
    2. Part position
      a. Rotate hand medially
      b. Place digits on 45-degree radiolucent support to show interphalangeal joints
      c. Adjust digits parallel to image receptor
    3. *Central ray:* Perpendicular to third metacarpophalangeal joint
C. Lateral
    1. *Patient position:* Seated, resting ulnar surface of forearm on table with hand in true lateral position
    2. Part position
      a. Extend digits with first digit (thumb) placed at a right angle to palm of hand
      b. As an option, patient may "fan" fingers and place on positioning sponge to reduce superimposition of phalanges
      c. Center metacarpophalangeal joints to image receptor
      d. Adjust palmar surface of hand perpendicular to image receptor
    3. *Central ray:* Perpendicular to second metacarpophalangeal joint

Wrist

A. PA
    1. *Patient position:* Seated, forearm resting on table
    2. Part position
      a. Center carpus to image receptor area
      b. Digits are flexed slightly to place wrist in contact with image receptor
    3. *Central ray:* Perpendicular to midcarpal area (Figure 5-19)
B. Lateral
    1. *Patient position:* Elbow is flexed 90 degrees, with forearm and arm in contact with table
    2. *Part position:* Center carpals and adjust hand so wrist is lateral
    3. *Central ray:* Perpendicular to wrist joint (Figure 5-20)
C. Oblique
    1. *Patient position:* Seated, ulnar surface of wrist on image receptor

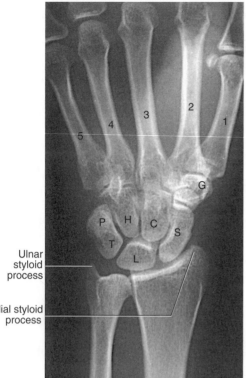

FIGURE 5-19 PA wrist. *C,* Capitate; *G,* trapezium; *H,* hamate; *L,* lunate; *P,* pisiform; *S,* scaphoid; *T,* triquetrum.

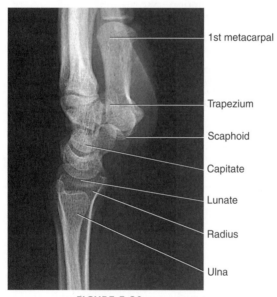

FIGURE 5-20 Lateral wrist.

2. Part position
   a. Center carpus to image receptor area
   b. From true lateral, rotate part approximately 45 degrees medially and support on sponge
3. *Central ray:* Perpendicular to image receptor, entering midcarpal area just distal to radius (Figure 5-21)

D. Scaphoid (navicular)
   1. *Patient position:* Elbow is flexed 90 degrees, with forearm and arm in contact with table

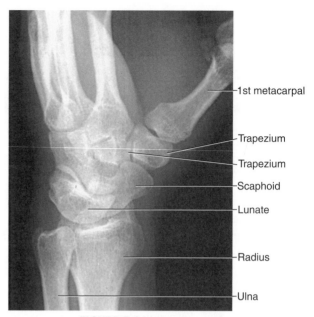

FIGURE 5-21 PA oblique wrist.

2. Part position
   a. Center carpals to image receptor area
   b. Place patient's wrist in extreme ulnar flexion
3. *Central ray:* Perpendicular to scaphoid; option to delineate fracture may require angulation of 10 to 15 degrees proximally (toward elbow) or distally; another approach is to elevate distal end of image receptor approximately 20 degrees

Forearm

A. AP
   1. *Patient position:* Seated
   2. *Part position:* Supinate hand and center forearm to image receptor to include joints of interest
   3. *Central ray:* Perpendicular to midpoint of forearm (Figure 5-22)
B. Lateral
   1. *Patient position:* Seated, with humerus and forearm in contact with table; elbow flexed
   2. Part position
      a. Elbow is flexed 90 degrees
      b. Adjust hand to lateral position (thumb up)
      c. Center forearm to image receptor to include joints of interest
   3. *Central ray:* Perpendicular to midpoint of forearm (Figure 5-23)

Elbow

A. AP
   1. *Patient position:* Seated, with arm extended
   2. Part position
      a. Extend patient's elbow
      b. Supinate hand

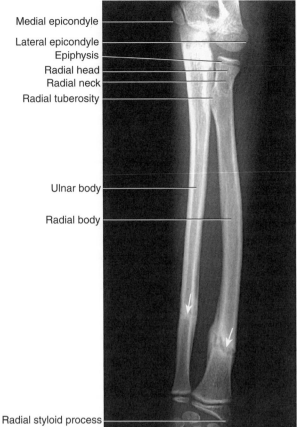

Medial epicondyle
Lateral epicondyle
Epiphysis
Radial head
Radial neck
Radial tuberosity

Ulnar body

Radial body

Radial styloid process

FIGURE 5-22 AP forearm with fractured radius and ulna.

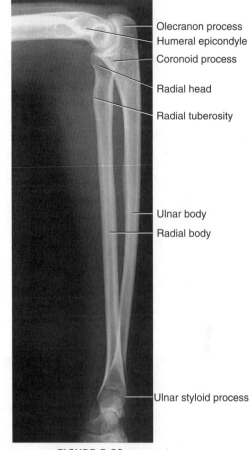

Olecranon process
Humeral epicondyle
Coronoid process

Radial head

Radial tuberosity

Ulnar body
Radial body

Ulnar styloid process

FIGURE 5-23 Lateral forearm.

c. Center elbow joint to image receptor
d. Patient may have to lean slightly laterally to ensure AP alignment
3. *Central ray:* Perpendicular to elbow joint (Figure 5-24)

B. Lateral
1. *Patient position:* Seated, with elbow flexed 90 degrees; humerus and forearm resting on table
2. Part position
a. Center 90-degree flexed elbow joint to image receptor
b. Adjust wrist and hand in lateral position
3. *Central ray:* Perpendicular to elbow joint (Figure 5-25)

C. Medial oblique
1. *Patient position:* Seated, with arm extended
2. Part position
a. Pronate hand
b. Medially rotate arm
c. Adjust anterior surface of elbow (epicondyles) at angle of 40 to 45 degrees
3. *Central ray:* Perpendicular to elbow joint (Figure 5-26)

D. Lateral oblique
1. *Patient position:* Seated, with arm extended

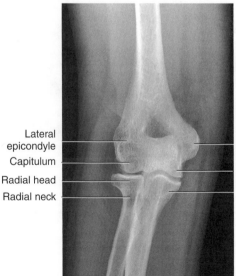

Lateral epicondyle
Capitulum
Radial head
Radial neck
Medial epicondyle
Trochlea
Proximal ulna

FIGURE 5-24 AP elbow.

2. Part position
a. Rotate patient's hand laterally
b. Adjust posterior surface of elbow at a 40-degree angle to image receptor
3. *Central ray:* Perpendicular to elbow joint

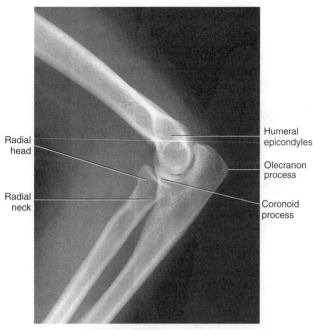

Radial head

Radial neck

Humeral epicondyles

Olecranon process

Coronoid process

FIGURE 5-25 Lateral elbow.

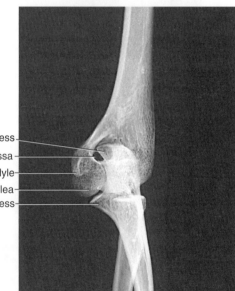

Olecranon process
Olecranon fossa
Medial epicondyle
Trochlea
Coronoid process

FIGURE 5-26 AP oblique elbow.

Humerus

A. AP
　1. *Patient position:* Erect or supine
　2. Part position
　　a. Unless it is contraindicated, supinate patient's hand and adjust humerus with epicondyles parallel to image receptor; keep humerus in neutral position if fracture is suspected or if reexamining healing fracture with a hanging cast
　　b. If patient is recumbent, elevate and support opposite shoulder
　　c. Center humerus to image receptor
　3. *Central ray:* Perpendicular to midpoint of humerus

B. Lateral
　1. *Patient position:* Erect or supine
　2. Part position
　　a. Unless it is contraindicated, slightly abduct the arm and center arm to image receptor
　　b. Medially rotate forearm until epicondyles are perpendicular to image receptor
　3. *Central ray:* Perpendicular to midpoint of humerus

Shoulder

A. AP
　1. *Patient position:* Erect or supine
　2. Part position
　　a. Center area of coracoid process to image receptor
　　b. Rotate patient slightly to place affected scapula parallel to image receptor
　　c. Adjust hand in (1) external rotation to obtain AP projection of humerus or (2) internal rotation for lateral position of humerus
　　d. *Respiration:* Suspended
　3. *Central ray:* Perpendicular to coracoid process (Figure 5-27)

B. Transthoracic lateral
　1. *Patient position:* Erect or supine
　2. Part position
　　a. Raise uninjured arm and rest on head
　　b. Elevate uninjured shoulder as much as possible
　　c. *Respiration:* Full inspiration or slow breathing
　3. *Central ray:* Adjust patient to project humerus between vertebral column and sternum; unless it is contraindicated, adjust humeral epicondyles perpendicular to image receptor; central ray perpendicular to median coronal plane, exiting surgical neck of affected humerus; if patient cannot elevate unaffected shoulder, the central ray may be angled 10 to 15 degrees cephalad

C. PA oblique (scapular Y)
　1. *Patient position:* Erect or prone oblique

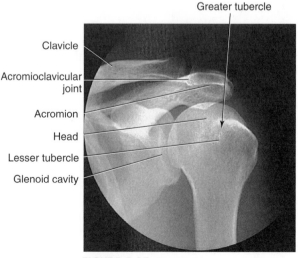

Greater tubercle

Clavicle

Acromioclavicular joint

Acromion

Head

Lesser tubercle

Glenoid cavity

FIGURE 5-27 AP shoulder.

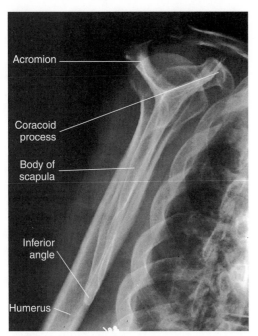

FIGURE 5-28 PA oblique shoulder (scapular Y).

2. Part position
   a. Center anterior surface of affected shoulder to image receptor
   b. Rotate patient so that midcoronal plane forms 60-degree angle from image receptor
   c. *Respiration:* Suspended
3. *Central ray:* Perpendicular to shoulder joint at level of scapulohumeral joint (Figure 5-28)

Acromioclavicular Articulations

A. AP
   1. *Patient position:* Upright if condition permits
   2. Part position
      a. Adjust midpoint of image receptor to level of acromioclavicular (AC) joints
      b. Center MSP of patient's body to midline of image receptor, if both AC joints can be shown on one radiograph
      c. Otherwise, center to each individual AC joint for two separate exposures
      d. To show AC separation, sandbags of equal weight should be attached to each wrist, and a second radiograph should be obtained without weights
      e. *Respiration:* Suspended
   3. *Central ray:* Perpendicular to image receptor, midway between AC joints or perpendicular to each AC joint

Clavicle

A. PA
   1. *Patient position:* Erect or prone; may be AP for patient comfort

2. Part position
   a. Center clavicle to center of image receptor midway between midline of body and coracoid process
   b. Head may be turned away from affected side
   c. *Respiration:* Suspended
3. *Central ray:* Perpendicular to midshaft of clavicle
B. PA axial
   1. *Patient position:* Erect or prone; may be supine (AP axial) for patient comfort
   2. Part position
      a. Center clavicle to midline of table with image receptor midway between MSP and coracoid process
      b. Head may be turned away from affected side
      c. *Respiration:* Suspended
   3. *Central ray:* Angle 25 to 30 degrees caudad, centered to the midshaft of the clavicle (25 to 30 degrees cephalad if performed AP)

Scapula

A. AP
   1. *Patient position:* Supine or upright (upright preferred when shoulder is tender)
   2. Part position
      a. Abduct arm
      b. Flex elbow
      c. Support hand near head
      d. Center palpated scapular area to image receptor approximately 2 inches inferior to coracoid process
      e. *Respiration:* Quiet breathing
   3. *Central ray:* Perpendicular to image receptor at midscapular area approximately 2 inches inferior to coracoid process (Figure 5-29)
B. Lateral
   1. *Patient position:* Prone oblique or upright (upright preferred when shoulder is tender)
   2. Part position
      a. Place patient in an oblique position with affected scapula centered to image receptor
      b. Extend affected arm across anterior thorax
      c. Palpate axillary and vertebral borders of scapula and adjust body rotation so that scapula is lateral and is projected free of rib cage
      d. *Respiration:* Suspended
   3. *Central ray:* Perpendicular to medial border of protruding scapula

Toes

A. AP axial
   1. *Patient position:* Supine or seated on table, knees flexed with feet separated

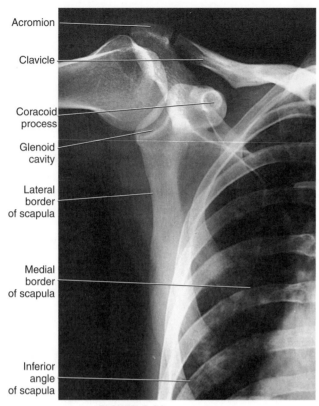

Acromion

Clavicle

Coracoid process

Glenoid cavity

Lateral border of scapula

Medial border of scapula

Inferior angle of scapula

FIGURE 5-29 AP scapula.

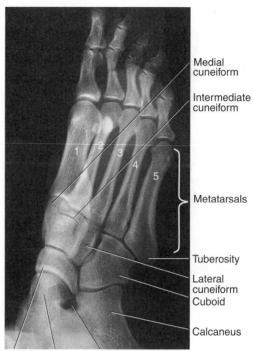

Medial cuneiform

Intermediate cuneiform

Metatarsals

Tuberosity

Lateral cuneiform

Cuboid

Calcaneus

Navicular   Talus   Sinus tarsi

FIGURE 5-30 AP oblique foot in medial rotation.

2. *Part position:* Center toes with plantar surface flat against image receptor
3. *Central ray:* 15 degrees cephalad, if positioning wedge is not used; enters the second metatarsophalangeal joint

B. Oblique
1. *Patient position:* Supine or seated on table, knees flexed with feet separated
2. *Part position:* Center patient's toes over image receptor area and medially rotate leg and foot until a 30- to 45-degree angle is formed from image receptor to plantar surface of foot
3. *Central ray:* Perpendicular, entering third metatarsophalangeal joint

Foot

A. AP axial
1. *Patient position:* Supine or seated on table, knees flexed with feet separated
2. Part position
   a. Plantar surface firmly resting on image receptor
   b. Center foot to image receptor
   c. Adjust midline of foot parallel to long axis of image receptor
3. *Central ray:* 10 degrees toward the heel, entering base of third metatarsal
B. Medial oblique
1. *Patient position:* Supine or seated on table, knees flexed with feet separated

2. Part position
   a. Center foot to image receptor
   b. Rotate leg medially until plantar surface forms angle of 30 degrees to image receptor
3. *Central ray:* Perpendicular to base of third metatarsal (Figure 5-30)
C. Lateral (mediolateral)
1. Patient position
   a. With the patient lying on the affected side, adjust leg and foot in lateral position
   b. Patella perpendicular to table
2. *Part position:* Center foot and adjust plantar surface perpendicular to image receptor
3. *Central ray:* Perpendicular to midpoint of image receptor, entering base of third metatarsal

Calcaneus

A. Axial (plantar dorsal)
1. *Patient position:* Supine or seated with leg fully extended
2. Part position
   a. Center image receptor to ankle
   b. Draw the plantar surface of foot perpendicular to image receptor
3. *Central ray:* 40 degrees cephalad to long axis of foot, entering midline at level of base of fifth metatarsal
B. Lateral
1. Patient position
   a. With the patient lying on the affected side, adjust leg and foot in lateral position
   b. Patella perpendicular to table

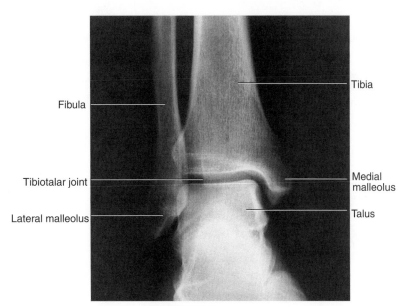

FIGURE 5-31 AP ankle.

2. *Part position:* Center calcaneus to image receptor, about 1 to 1½ inches distal to medial malleolus
C. *Central ray:* Perpendicular to midportion of calcaneus

Ankle

A. AP
  1. *Patient position:* Supine or seated on table with small support under knee
  2. Part position
    a. Center ankle to image receptor
    b. Dorsiflex foot
    c. Adjust ankle with toes pointing vertically
  3. *Central ray:* Perpendicular to ankle joint midway between malleoli (Figure 5-31)
B. Lateral
  1. *Patient position:* Supine; roll onto affected side
  2. Part position
    a. Rotate patient's ankle to lateral position
    b. Adjust foot in lateral position
    c. Center ankle to image receptor
  3. *Central ray:* Vertical through medial malleolus (Figure 5-32)
C. Medial oblique
  1. *Patient position:* Supine or seated on table
  2. Part position
    a. Rotate patient's leg and foot medially
    b. Adjust degree of medial rotation
      (1) *Mortise joint:* Until malleoli are parallel with image receptor (15 to 20 degrees)
      (2) *Bony structure:* To 45 degrees rotation
  3. *Central ray:* Vertical midway between malleoli

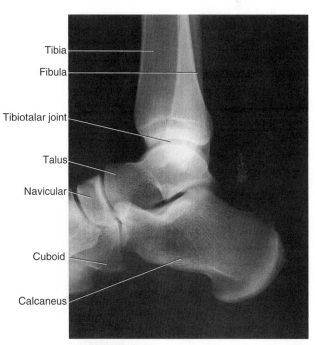

FIGURE 5-32 Lateral ankle.

Leg

A. AP
  1. *Patient position:* Supine with leg extended
  2. Part position
    a. Center leg to image receptor
    b. Adjust leg to AP position
    c. Both joints should be included
  3. *Central ray:* Vertical to midpoint of leg
B. Lateral
  1. *Patient position:* Supine and roll onto affected side

2. Part position
   a. Center leg to image receptor
   b. Adjust leg to lateral position
   c. Patella perpendicular
   d. Both joints should be included
3. *Central ray:* Perpendicular to midpoint of leg (Figure 5-33)

Knee

A. AP
   1. *Patient position:* Supine and with leg extended; adjust patient's body so that pelvis is not rotated
   2. Part position
      a. Center knee to image receptor
      b. Adjust leg to AP position
   3. *Central ray:* 5 to 7 degrees cephalad to a point ½ inch inferior to patellar apex (Figure 5-34)
B. Lateral
   1. *Patient position:* Turn patient onto affected side with knee flexed (usually 20 to 30 degrees)
   2. Part position
      a. Flex and center knee
      b. Center image receptor approximately 1 inch distal to medial epicondyle
      c. Patella perpendicular to image receptor
   3. *Central ray:* 5 degrees cephalad, entering knee joint inferior to medial condyle
C. Intercondylar fossa (tunnel)
   1. *Patient position:* Kneeling on radiographic table with affected knee flexed 70 degrees from full extension

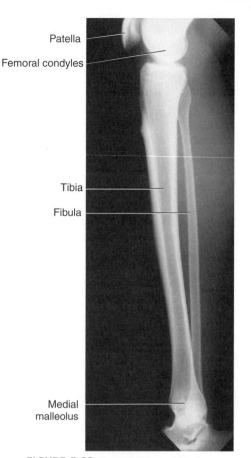

FIGURE 5-33 Lateral tibia and fibula.

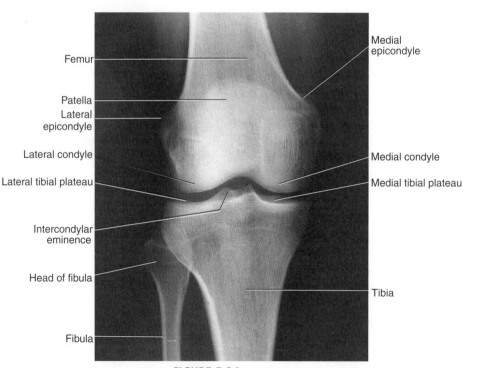

FIGURE 5-34 AP knee.

2. Part position
   a. Center knee to image receptor
   b. Place at level of patellar apex
   c. Flex knee 70 degrees from full extension
3. *Central ray:* Perpendicular to long axis of lower leg, entering midpopliteal area

Patella

A. PA
  1. *Patient position:* Prone with knee extended
  2. Part position
    a. Center patella
    b. Adjust to be parallel with image receptor plane
    c. Heel generally rotated 5 to 10 degrees laterally
  3. *Central ray:* Perpendicular to midpopliteal area
B. Tangential
  1. *Patient position:* Prone with foot resting on table
  2. *Part position:* Flex affected knee so that tibia and fibula form a 50- to 60-degree angle from table
  3. *Central ray:* 45 degrees cephalad through patellofemoral joint (Figure 5-35)
C. Lateral
  1. *Patient position:* Lying on affected side
  2. *Part position:* Flex knee 5 to 10 degrees, femoral epicondyles superimposed
  3. *Central ray:* Perpendicular to patella

Femur

A. AP
  1. *Patient position:* Supine with toes up
  2. Part position
    a. Center affected thigh to midline of table
    b. Internally rotate lower limb approximately 15 degrees

    c. Both joints should be included
    d. Apply gonadal shielding as appropriate
  3. *Central ray:* Perpendicular to midfemur
B. Lateral
  1. *Patient position:* Lying on affected side with knee slightly flexed
  2. Part position
    a. Rotate patient's unaffected hip (including hip joint) posteriorly to prevent superimposition of unaffected hip
    b. Center femur to midline of table
    c. Both joints should be included
    d. Apply gonadal shielding as appropriate
  3. *Central ray:* Perpendicular to midfemur

Pelvis

A. AP
  1. *Patient position:* Supine
  2. Part position
    a. Center MSP to table
    b. Adjust to AP position
    c. Internally rotate feet and lower limb 15 degrees
    d. Center image receptor approximately 2 inches superior to level of greater trochanter
    e. Use gonadal shielding as appropriate
    f. *Respiration:* Suspended
  3. *Central ray:* Perpendicular to midpoint of image receptor 2 inches superior to symphysis pubis

Hip

A. AP
  1. *Patient position:* Supine
  2. Part position
    a. Rotate lower limb 15 degrees medially
    b. Center hip to image receptor
    c. *Respiration:* Suspended

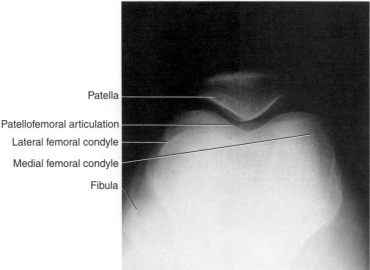

Patella
Patellofemoral articulation
Lateral femoral condyle
Medial femoral condyle
Fibula

FIGURE 5-35 Tangential patella (Settegast method).

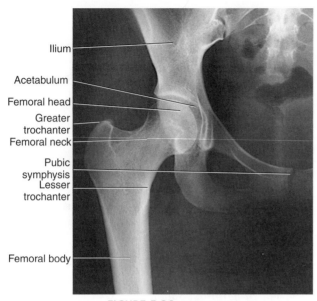

Ilium
Acetabulum
Femoral head
Greater trochanter
Femoral neck
Pubic symphysis
Lesser trochanter
Femoral body

FIGURE 5-36 AP hip.

3. *Central ray:* Perpendicular to a point 2 inches medial to ASIS and at level of superior margin of greater trochanter (Figure 5-36)

B. Lateral
1. *Patient position:* From supine position, turn patient toward affected side to posterior oblique body position
2. Part position
   a. Flex affected knee
   b. Center affected hip to midline of table
   c. Extend unaffected knee
   d. *Respiration:* Suspended
3. *Central ray:* Perpendicular to a point midway between ASIS and symphysis pubis

C. Axiolateral
1. *Patient position:* Supine with level of greater trochanter elevated to center of image receptor
2. Part position
   a. Flex knee and hip of unaffected side
   b. Elevate and rest on suitable support
   c. Adjust pelvis to supine position
   d. Unless it is contraindicated, rotate affected leg 15 to 20 degrees internally
   e. *Respiration:* Suspended
3. *Central ray:* Perpendicular to long axis of femoral neck and image receptor

Cervical Vertebrae

A. Atlas and axis
1. *Patient position:* Erect or supine
2. Part position
   a. MSP centered to image receptor at level of C2
   b. Arms by sides
   c. Shoulders in same plane
   d. Have patient open mouth wide

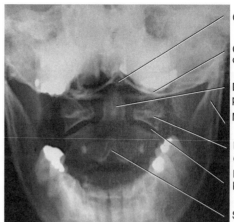

Occipital base
Occlusal surface of teeth
Dens (odontoid process)
Mandibular ramus
Lateral mass of atlas
Inferior articular process of atlas
Spinous process of axis

FIGURE 5-37 Open-mouth atlas and axis.

   e. Adjust head so that line from lower edge of upper incisors to mastoid process is perpendicular to image receptor
   f. *Respiration:* Phonate "ah" during exposure
3. *Central ray:* Perpendicular to image receptor, centered to open mouth (Figure 5-37)

B. AP axial
1. *Patient position:* Erect or supine
2. Part position
   a. MSP centered to image receptor
   b. Arms by sides
   c. Center image receptor at level of C4
   d. Adjust a line between upper occlusal plane and mastoid tip, perpendicular to image receptor
   e. *Respiration:* Suspended
3. *Central ray:* 15 to 20 degrees cephalad, entering slightly inferior to thyroid cartilage (Figure 5-38)

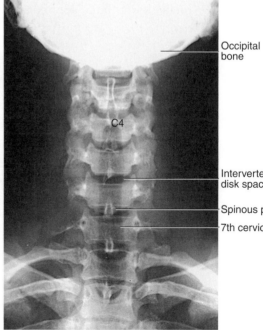

Occipital bone
C4
Intervertebral disk space
Spinous process
7th cervical

FIGURE 5-38 AP axial cervical vertebrae.

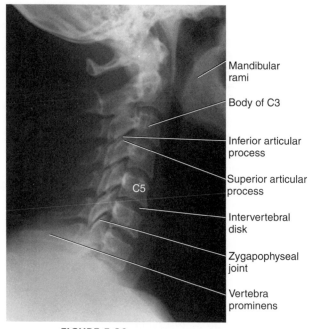

FIGURE 5-39 Lateral cervical vertebrae.

C. Lateral
1. *Patient position:* Seated or standing in lateral position
2. Part position
   a. Center coronal plane through mastoid tips to image receptor
   b. Adjust patient's shoulders to same horizontal level and body to true lateral position
   c. Elevate chin slightly
   d. Relax shoulders

   e. Weights may be attached to wrists to help lower shoulders
   f. Source-to-image receptor distance (SID) recommended—72 inches
   g. *Respiration:* Expiration
3. *Central ray:* Perpendicular to image receptor entering C4 (Figure 5-39)
D. LPO and RPO (AP axial oblique projections)
1. *Patient position:* Seated or standing
2. Part position
   a. Rotate body 45 degrees
   b. Place side of interest farther from image receptor
   c. Have patient slightly extend chin while looking forward
   d. Center spine to image receptor
   e. Obtain both oblique projections
   f. *Respiration:* Suspended
3. *Central ray:* 15 to 20 degrees cephalad, entering C4 (Figure 5-40)

Thoracic Vertebrae

A. AP
1. *Patient position:* Supine or upright
2. Part position
   a. MSP centered to image receptor
   b. Top of image receptor 1½ to 2 inches above shoulders
   c. Arms by sides
   d. Shoulders in same plane
   e. *Respiration:* Shallow or suspended expiration
3. *Central ray:* Perpendicular to T7, 3 to 4 inches distal to jugular (manubrial) notch

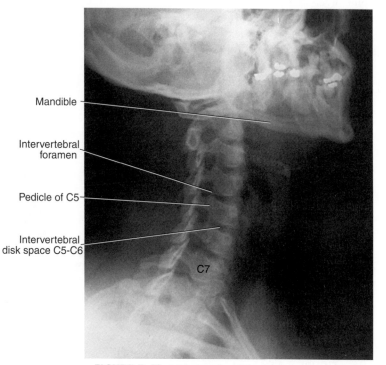

FIGURE 5-40 RAO showing right side.

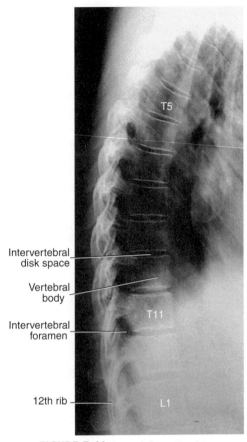

FIGURE 5-41 Lateral thoracic spine.

Labels on figure: T5; Intervertebral disk space; Vertebral body; Intervertebral foramen; 12th rib; T11; L1

B. Lateral
    1. *Patient position:* Lateral recumbent or erect
    2. Part position
        a. Elevate head to spine level
        b. Extend arms forward
        c. Place radiolucent support under lower thoracic region until spine is horizontal to top of table
        d. *Respiration:* Shallow or suspended expiration

    3. *Central ray:* Perpendicular to image receptor, entering level of T7, approximately 3 to 4 inches below sternal angle (Figure 5-41)
C. Cervicothoracic (Twining)
    1. *Patient position:* Lateral, seated or standing
    2. Part position
        a. Center midcoronal plane to grid
        b. Elevate arm adjacent to Bucky
        c. Center image receptor to level of T2
        d. Body in true lateral position
        e. *Respiration:* Suspended
    3. *Central ray:* Perpendicular to image receptor, entering at level of T2 (Figure 5-42)

Lumbar Vertebrae

A. AP
    1. *Patient position:* Supine
    2. Part position
        a. MSP centered to table
        b. Flex patient's knees and hips enough to place back in firm contact with table
        c. Center image receptor at level of iliac crest (L4)
        d. *Respiration:* Suspended
    3. *Central ray:* Perpendicular to midline, entering level of iliac crests (Figure 5-43)
B. Lateral
    1. *Patient position:* Lateral with hips and knees flexed
    2. Part position
        a. Center midaxillary line of body and L4 to table
        b. Extend arms forward
        c. Place radiolucent support under lower thorax, and adjust spine parallel to table
        d. Check for true lateral position
        e. *Respiration:* Suspended
    3. *Central ray:* Perpendicular to image receptor, entering midaxillary line at level of iliac crests (Figure 5-44)

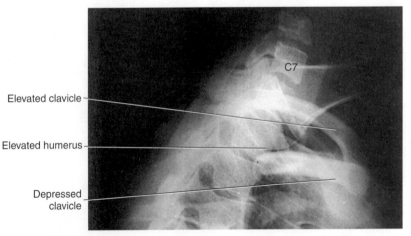

Labels on figure: Elevated clavicle; Elevated humerus; Depressed clavicle; C7

FIGURE 5-42 Lateral cervicothoracic region (twining method).

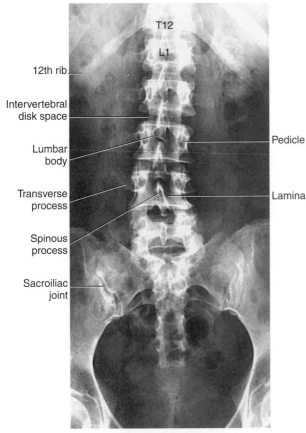

FIGURE 5-43 AP lumbar spine.

Labels: T12, L1, 12th rib, Intervertebral disk space, Lumbar body, Transverse process, Spinous process, Sacroiliac joint, Pedicle, Lamina

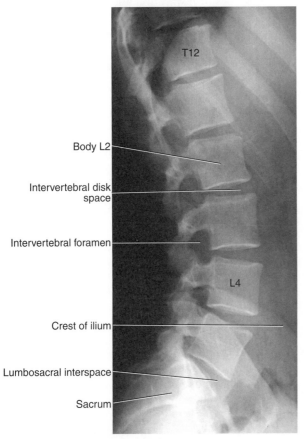

FIGURE 5-44 Lateral lumbar spine.

Labels: T12, Body L2, Intervertebral disk space, Intervertebral foramen, L4, Crest of ilium, Lumbosacral interspace, Sacrum

C. Lateral L5 to S1
  1. *Patient position:* Lateral with hips and knees flexed
  2. Part position
     a. Center 1½ inches posterior to midaxillary line and 1½ inches below iliac crest
     b. Extend arms forward
     c. Place radiolucent support under lower thorax, and adjust spine parallel to table
     d. Check for true lateral position
     e. Collimate tightly
     f. *Respiration:* Suspended
  3. *Central ray:* Perpendicular to a point 2 inches posterior to ASIS and 1½ inches inferior to iliac crest (if spine cannot be placed in true horizontal, may need to angle central ray caudally—5 degrees in male patients, 8 degrees in female patients)
D. LPO and RPO (AP oblique projections)
  1. *Patient position:* Posterior oblique; side closest to image receptor is side of interest
  2. Part position
     a. Adjust and support body obliquity to 45 degrees
     b. Adjust arms to a comfortable position
     c. Center spine to midline of table
     d. Center image receptor at level of L3
     e. Obtain oblique projections of both sides
     f. *Respiration:* Suspended
  3. *Central ray:* Perpendicular to L3, 1 to 2 inches above level of iliac crest, entering elevated side 2 inches laterally from patient's midline

Sacroiliac Joints

A. LPO and RPO (AP oblique)
  1. *Patient position:* Supine
  2. Part position
     a. Elevate and support side of interest 25 to 30 degrees from table
     b. Align sagittal plane passing 1 inch medial to ASIS of elevated side centered to image receptor
     c. Center to table
     d. Obtain both oblique projections
     e. *Respiration:* Suspended
  3. *Central ray:* Perpendicular to image receptor, 1 inch medial to elevated ASIS

Sacrum

A. AP axial
  1. *Patient position:* Supine
  2. Part position
     a. Center MSP to center of table
     b. *Respiration:* Suspended
  3. *Central ray:* 15 degrees cephalad, entering 2 inches superior to symphysis pubis

B. Lateral
1. *Patient position:* Lateral with hips and knees flexed
2. Part position
   a. Support body to place long axis of spine horizontally
   b. Align coronal plane, passing 3 inches posterior to median coronal plane
   c. Center to midline of table
   d. *Respiration:* Suspended
3. *Central ray:* Perpendicular to image receptor, entering 3 inches posterior to median coronal plane at level of ASIS

Coccyx

A. AP axial
1. *Patient position:* Supine
2. Part position
   a. Center MSP to center of table
   b. *Respiration:* Suspended
3. *Central ray:* 10 degrees caudad, entering 2 inches superior to symphysis pubis
B. Lateral
1. *Patient position:* Lateral with hips and knees flexed
2. Part position
   a. Support body to place long axis of spine horizontally
   b. Align coronal plane passing approximately 5 inches posterior to median coronal plane
   c. Center to midline of table
   d. *Respiration:* Suspended
3. *Central ray:* Perpendicular to image receptor, entering palpated coccyx located approximately 5 inches posterior to median coronal plane

Scoliosis Series

A. PA (to minimize exposure to breast tissue; AP may be performed with compensating filters)
1. *Patient position:* Seated or standing
2. Part position
   a. *First radiograph:* MSP centered to image receptor; image receptor adjusted to include 1 inch of the iliac crests; arms at sides
   b. *Second radiograph:* MSP centered to image receptor; elevate hip or foot of convex side of curve 3 or 4 inches on a block
3. *Central ray:* Perpendicular to the midpoint of the image receptor

THORAX

Pathological Conditions Imaged

A. Adult respiratory distress syndrome
1. Acute life-threatening respiratory distress
2. Large amount of fluid in interstitial and alveolar spaces
3. Harder to penetrate

B. Asthma
1. Pulmonary disorder with increased mucus production in bronchi, causing hyperventilation of the lungs
2. Bronchi harder to penetrate
3. Lungs easier to penetrate
C. Atelectasis
1. Collapse of lung tissue
2. Harder to penetrate
D. Bronchial adenoma
1. Neoplasm occurring in a bronchus, causing atelectasis and pneumonitis
2. Harder to penetrate
E. Bronchiectasis
1. Dilation and destruction of bronchial walls
2. Consolidation present
3. Harder to penetrate
F. Bronchogenic carcinoma
1. Lung cancer arising from the bronchial mucosa
2. Harder to penetrate
G. Chronic bronchitis
1. Debilitating pulmonary disease with substantial increase of mucus production in the trachea and bronchi
2. Harder to penetrate unless evolved into emphysema, which is easier to penetrate
H. Chronic obstructive pulmonary disease (COPD)
1. Progressive condition marked by diminished capabilities of inspiration and expiration
2. Harder to penetrate
I. Croup
1. Acute viral infection of respiratory system in infants
2. Lateral soft tissue neck radiograph taken to show subepiglottic narrowing
J. Cystic fibrosis
1. Inherited pathological condition of exocrine glands
2. Marked by increased mucus secretion in lungs and bronchi
3. Harder to penetrate
K. Emphysema
1. Overinflation of alveolar walls
2. Easier to penetrate
3. Should not be imaged with use of automatic exposure controls (AECs) because minimum reaction time of equipment usually results in overexposure, necessitating repeat exposures
L. Empyema
1. Pus in the pleural space
2. Harder to penetrate
M. Histoplasmosis
1. Infection caused by inhaling fungal spores
2. Harder to penetrate
N. Hyaline membrane disease
1. Respiratory distress syndrome of the newborn
2. Acute lung disease in newborn; characteristics include airless alveoli and rapid respirations
3. Harder to penetrate

O. Legionnaires' disease
   1. Form of acute bacterial pneumonia
   2. Harder to penetrate
 P. Pleural effusion
   1. Accumulation of fluid in intrapleural spaces
   2. Harder to penetrate
Q. Pneumoconiosis
   1. Lung disease caused by inhaling dust (usually mineral dust from the environment or workplace)
   2. *Silicosis:* Caused by prolonged inhalation of silicon dioxide (sand)
   3. *Anthracosis:* Caused by prolonged inhalation of anthracite (coal dust)
   4. *Asbestosis:* Caused by prolonged inhalation of asbestos
   5. *Siderosis:* Caused by prolonged inhalation of iron dust
   6. All are harder to penetrate
 R. Pneumonia
   1. Acute inflammation of the lungs
   2. Harder to penetrate
 S. Pneumothorax
   1. Air in the pleural space that causes the lung to collapse
   2. Easier to penetrate
 T. Pulmonary metastases
   1. Spread of cancer into the lungs from a primary site
   2. Harder to penetrate
U. Tuberculosis
   1. Chronic infection of the lungs caused by acid-fast bacillus
   2. More difficult to penetrate

Chest

A. PA
   1. Patient position
      a. Standing or seated erect
      b. Back of hands on hips
      c. Top of image receptor 1 to 2 inches above relaxed shoulders
   2. Part position
      a. MSP centered
      b. Chin extended and pointing straight ahead
      c. Roll shoulders forward
      d. SID recommended—72 inches
      e. *Respiration:* Full inspiration (expose at end of second inspiration)
   3. *Central ray:* Perpendicular to MSP at level of T7 (Figure 5-45)
B. Lateral
   1. Patient position
      a. Standing or seated erect
      b. Left side against image receptor unless otherwise specified
      c. Top of image receptor 1 to 2 inches above relaxed shoulder
   2. Part position
      a. MSP parallel to image receptor
      b. Adjacent shoulder resting against image receptor holder
      c. Arms raised and crossed over head
      d. Center thorax to image receptor
      e. SID recommended—72 inches
      f. *Respiration:* Full inspiration (expose at end of second inspiration)

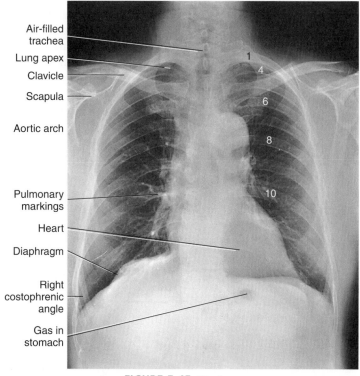

Air-filled trachea
Lung apex
Clavicle
Scapula
Aortic arch
Pulmonary markings
Heart
Diaphragm
Right costophrenic angle
Gas in stomach

FIGURE 5-45 PA chest.

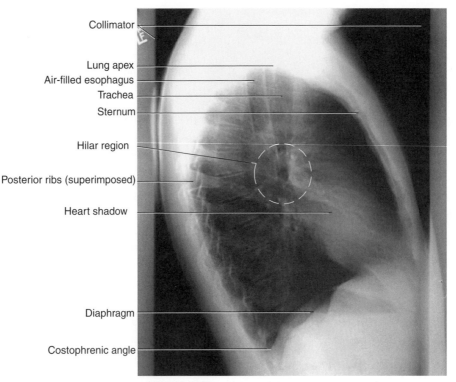

Collimator

Lung apex
Air-filled esophagus
Trachea
Sternum

Hilar region

Posterior ribs (superimposed)

Heart shadow

Diaphragm

Costophrenic angle

FIGURE 5-46 Left lateral chest.

3. *Central ray:* Perpendicular to image receptor, entering patient approximately 2 inches anterior to midaxillary plane at level of T7 (Figure 5-46)
C. LAO and RAO (PA oblique projections)
  1. Patient position
    a. Standing or seated
    b. Adjust coronal plane 45 degrees (or 60 degrees) from plane of image receptor
    c. Top of image receptor 2 inches above shoulders
    d. Side farther from image receptor is usually side of primary interest
  2. Part position
    a. Shoulder nearer image receptor rolled posteriorly
    b. Hand placed on hip
    c. Arm farther from image receptor placed on top of image receptor holder
    d. Thorax centered to image receptor
    e. SID recommended—72 inches
    f. Both 45-degree oblique projections (or 60-degree oblique projections) may be taken
    g. *Respiration:* Full inspiration
  3. *Central ray:* Perpendicular at level of T7
D. AP lordotic
  1. Patient position
    a. Standing approximately 1 foot in front of image receptor
    b. When patient is properly positioned, top of image receptor should be approximately 3 inches above shoulders

  2. Part position
    a. MSP centered with no rotation
    b. Elbows flexed
    c. Hands, with palms out, on hips
    d. Patient leans backward in extreme lordotic position
    e. SID recommended—72 inches
    f. *Respiration:* Full inspiration
  3. *Central ray:* Perpendicular to image receptor, entering midsternum
E. Lateral decubitus
  1. *Patient position:* Lateral recumbent
  2. Part position
    a. Lying on affected or unaffected side, depending on existing condition
    b. Elevate dependent side on firm pad
    c. Extend patient's arms above head
    d. Adjust thorax in true lateral position
    e. Place top of image receptor approximately 2 inches above shoulders
    f. *Respiration:* Full inspiration
  3. *Central ray:* Horizontal and perpendicular to image receptor, entering T7

Ribs

A. AP
  1. *Patient position:* Erect or recumbent
  2. Part position
    a. Center midsagittal plane to midline of grid

   b. *Above diaphragm:* Center to T7; top of image receptor should be 1 to 2 inches above shoulders; shoulders rotated anteriorly
      (1) *Respiration:* Full inspiration
   c. *Below diaphragm:* Center thorax with bottom of image receptor at level of iliac crests
      (1) *Respiration:* Full expiration
   3. *Central ray:* Perpendicular to T7 for upper ribs; perpendicular to T12 for lower ribs (bilateral)
B. LPO and RPO (AP oblique projections)
   1. *Patient position:* Erect or recumbent
   2. Part position
      a. Rotate body 45 degrees with affected side toward image receptor
      b. Center midway between MSP and lateral surface of body to center of grid
      c. Abduct arm nearer image receptor
      d. Place hand on head
      e. Abduct opposite limb
      f. Place hand on hip
      g. *Respiration:* Above diaphragm, full inspiration; below diaphragm, full expiration
   3. *Central ray:* Perpendicular to image receptor; above diaphragm, center at level of T7; below diaphragm, center at level of T10

Sternum

A. RAO (PA oblique)
   1. *Patient position:* Prone position for RAO (right PA oblique)
   2. Part position
      a. Center sternum to image receptor
      b. Rotate body 15 to 20 degrees to prevent superimposition of vertebral and sternal images
      c. *Respiration:* Shallow breathing or suspended expiration
   3. *Central ray:* Perpendicular, exiting midsternum (Figure 5-47)
B. Lateral
   1. *Patient position:* Lateral, seated or standing
   2. Part position
      a. Top of image receptor 1 to 2 inches above jugular notch
      b. Shoulders and arms rotated posteriorly
      c. Center sternum to image receptor
      d. Adjust to true lateral position
      e. *Respiration:* Full inspiration
   3. *Central ray:* Perpendicular to center of midsternum

Sternoclavicular Joints

A. PA
   1. *Patient position:* Prone or upright, MSP centered to table

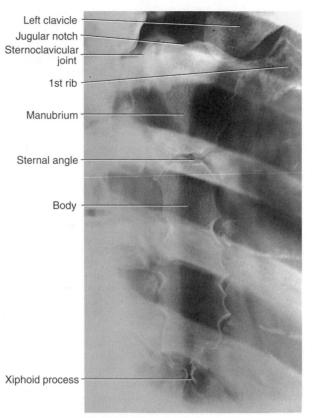

Left clavicle
Jugular notch
Sternoclavicular joint
1st rib
Manubrium
Sternal angle
Body
Xiphoid process

FIGURE 5-47 RAO of sternum.

   2. Part position
      a. Image receptor centered to T3
      b. Arms on side of body, palms up, shoulders in same plane
      c. *Bilateral examination:* Head rests on chin, MSP vertical to table
      d. *Unilateral examination:* Turn head toward affected side, rest cheek on table
   3. *Central ray:* Perpendicular to T3
B. RAO
   1. *Patient position:* Prone or upright
   2. Part position
      a. Rotate patient to an oblique position to place vertebral shadow behind sternoclavicular joint nearer image receptor (10 to 15 degrees)
      b. Center joint to midline of image receptor
   3. *Central ray:* Perpendicular to affected joint

Skull

Cranium

A. PA or Caldwell (PA axial) (Figures 5-48 and 5-49)
   1. *Patient position:* Prone or seated erect
   2. Part position
      a. Head resting on forehead and nose
      b. MSP perpendicular to midline of grid device
      c. OML perpendicular to image receptor
      d. *Respiration:* Suspended

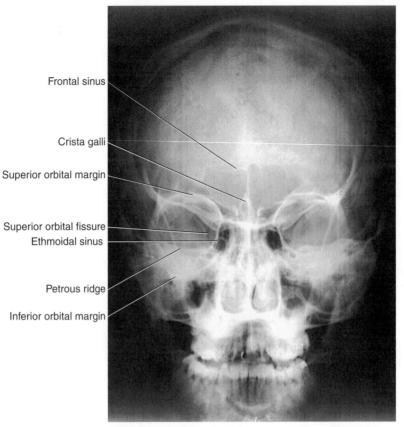

Frontal sinus

Crista galli

Superior orbital margin

Superior orbital fissure
Ethmoidal sinus

Petrous ridge

Inferior orbital margin

FIGURE 5-48 PA axial skull (Caldwell method).

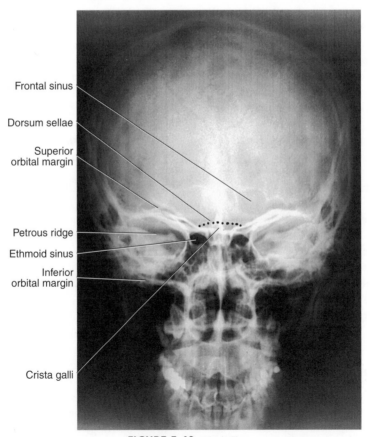

Frontal sinus

Dorsum sellae

Superior
orbital margin

Petrous ridge

Ethmoid sinus

Inferior
orbital margin

Crista galli

FIGURE 5-49 PA skull.

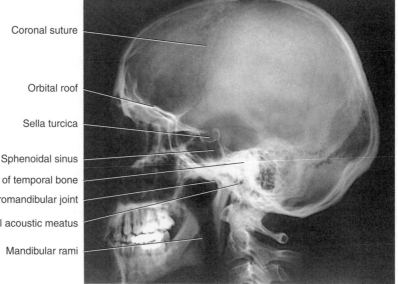

FIGURE 5-50 Lateral skull.

Labels (top to bottom): Coronal suture, Orbital roof, Sella turcica, Sphenoidal sinus, Petrous portion of temporal bone, Temporomandibular joint, External acoustic meatus, Mandibular rami

3. Central ray
   a. *Caldwell method (PA axial):* Direct central ray 15 degrees caudad to OML, exiting nasion, for survey examination
   b. *PA:* Perpendicular to image receptor, exiting nasion, to examine frontal bone
B. Lateral (Figure 5-50)
   1. *Patient position:* Seated erect or semiprone
   2. Part position
      a. Center a point to the image receptor that is 2 inches superior to the external auditory meatus (EAM)
      b. MSP parallel to image receptor

   c. IOML parallel to transverse axis of image receptor
   d. Interpupillary line (IPL) perpendicular to image receptor
   e. *Respiration:* Suspended
3. Central ray
   a. Perpendicular, entering 2 inches superior to EAM for survey examination
   b. When sella turcica is of primary interest, image receptor is centered, and central ray enters ¾ inch superior and ¾ inch anterior to EAM
C. AP axial (Towne) (Figure 5-51)

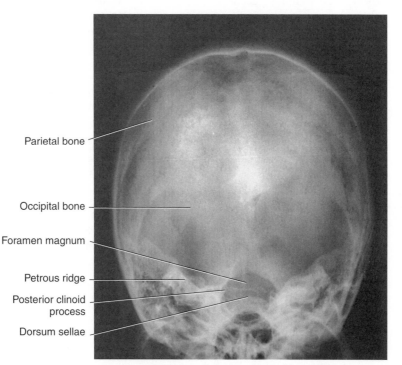

FIGURE 5-51 AP axial skull.

Labels (top to bottom): Parietal bone, Occipital bone, Foramen magnum, Petrous ridge, Posterior clinoid process, Dorsum sellae

1. *Patient position:* Supine or seated erect
2. Part position
   a. Center MSP to midline of grid device
   b. Adjust to be perpendicular
   c. Flex head and adjust OML perpendicular to image receptor
   d. Place top of image receptor at level of cranial vertex
   e. *Respiration:* Suspended
3. Central ray
   a. Direct through foramen magnum with caudal angle of 30 degrees to OML or 37 degrees to IOML, entering 2 to 2½ inches above glabella
D. Submentovertex (full basal)
   1. *Patient position:* Seated erect at head unit or supine on elevated table support
   2. Part position
      a. Extend neck
      b. Rest head on vertex
      c. Center and adjust MSP perpendicular to image receptor
      d. Adjust IOML parallel to plane of image receptor
      e. *Respiration:* Suspended
   3. *Central ray:* Direct perpendicular to IOML, entering between angles of mandible

Orbit

A. Parietoorbital oblique (Rhese) (Figure 5-52)
   1. *Patient position:* Prone or seated erect
   2. Part position
      a. Center affected orbit to image receptor
      b. Rest head on zygoma, nose, and chin
      c. Adjust AML perpendicular to image receptor
      d. Rotate MSP 53 degrees from image receptor
      e. *Respiration:* Suspended

3. *Central ray:* Perpendicular, entering 1 inch superior and posterior to top of ear attachment, exiting affected orbit

Facial Bones

A. Lateral (Figure 5-53)
   1. *Patient position:* Semiprone or seated erect
   2. Part position
      a. Center zygoma
      b. Adjust MSP parallel to image receptor
      c. IOML parallel to transverse axis of image receptor
      d. IPL perpendicular to image receptor
      e. *Respiration:* Suspended
   3. *Central ray:* Perpendicular, entering lateral surface of zygomatic bone
B. Parietoacanthial (Waters) (Figure 5-54)
   1. *Patient position:* Prone or seated erect
   2. Part position
      a. Center and adjust MSP perpendicular to image receptor
      b. Rest patient's head on extended chin
      c. Adjust OML to form 37-degree angle to image receptor plane
      d. *Respiration:* Suspended
   3. *Central ray:* Perpendicular, exiting acanthion

Nasal Bones

A. Lateral (performed as bilateral examination)
   1. *Patient position:* Semiprone or seated erect
   2. Part position
      a. Center nasion to image receptor
      b. Adjust MSP parallel to image receptor
      c. IOML parallel to transverse axis of image receptor

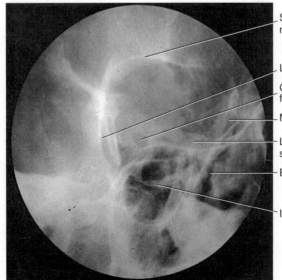

Superior orbital margin

Lateral orbital margin

Optic canal and foramen

Medial orbital margin

Lesser wing of sphenoid

Ethmoidal sinus

Inferior orbital margin

FIGURE 5-52 Parietoorbital oblique optic canal (Rhese method).

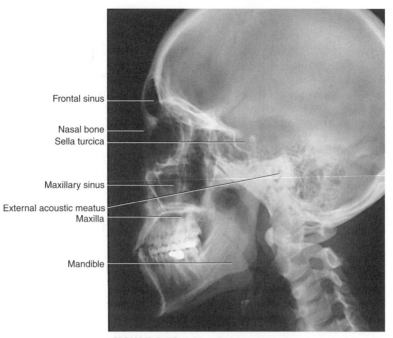

Frontal sinus

Nasal bone
Sella turcica

Maxillary sinus

External acoustic meatus
Maxilla

Mandible

FIGURE 5-53 Lateral facial bones.

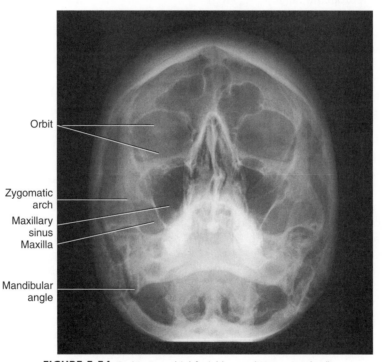

Orbit

Zygomatic
arch
Maxillary
sinus
Maxilla

Mandibular
angle

FIGURE 5-54 Parietoacanthial facial bones (Waters method).

d. IPL perpendicular to image receptor
e. *Respiration:* Suspended
3. *Central ray:* Perpendicular to the bridge of the nose, entering ¾ inch distal to nasion

Zygomatic Arches

A. Bilateral tangential (basal)
  1. *Patient position:* Seated erect or supine on elevated table support
  2. Part position

a. Have patient extend head and rest on vertex
b. Center and adjust MSP perpendicular to image receptor
c. Adjust IOML parallel to image receptor
d. *Respiration:* Suspended
3. *Central ray:* Perpendicular to IOML, entering midway between zygomatic arches, approximately 1 inch posterior to outer canthi

B. Unilateral tangential (May)
  1. *Patient position:* Prone or seated erect at vertical grid device

2. Part position
   a. Extend neck and rest chin on grid device
   b. Rotate MSP 15 degrees away from side being examined; if AP, rotate MSP 15 degrees toward side being examined
   c. Center image receptor 3 inches distal to most prominent point of zygoma
   d. IOML parallel to plane of image receptor
   e. *Respiration:* Suspended
3. Central ray
   a. Perpendicular to IOML
   b. Directed through zygomatic arch 1½ inches posterior to outer canthus

Mandible

A. PA
   1. *Patient position:* Prone or seated erect
   2. Part position
      a. Have patient rest head on nose and chin
      b. For mandibular body, center image receptor at level of lips
      c. For rami and temporomandibular joint (TMJ), center to tip of nose
      d. MSP perpendicular to image receptor
      e. *Respiration:* Suspended
   3. Central ray
      a. For mandibular body, direct perpendicular to image receptor at level of lips
      b. For rami and condylar processes, direct midway between TMJs at 30-degree cephalad angle
B. Axiolateral oblique (for mandibular body)
   1. *Patient position:* Semiprone or seated erect
   2. Part position
      a. Adjust image receptor under affected cheek
      b. Extend neck to place long axis of mandibular body parallel to image receptor
      c. Center to first molar region
      d. Adjust broad surface of mandibular body parallel to image receptor
      e. *Respiration:* Suspended
   3. *Central ray:* Direct slightly posteriorly to mandibular angle farthest from image receptor at a 25-degree cephalad angle
C. Axiolateral oblique (for mandibular ramus)
   1. *Patient position:* Semiprone or seated erect
   2. Part position
      a. Center image receptor ½ inch anterior and 1 inch inferior to affected side EAM
      b. Extend chin
      c. Adjust broad surface of ramus parallel to image receptor
      d. *Respiration:* Suspended
   3. *Central ray:* Direct 25 degrees cephalad, entering 2 inches distal to the mandibular angle on side farther from image receptor

D. Submentovertex (basal)
   1. *Patient position:* Seated erect or supine on elevated table support
   2. Part position
      a. Extend neck and rest head on vertex
      b. Center and adjust MSP perpendicular to image receptor
      c. Adjust IOML parallel to plane of image receptor
      d. *Respiration:* Suspended
   3. *Central ray:* Perpendicular to IOML, entering midway between mandibular angles

Temporomandibular Articulations

A. Open-mouth and closed-mouth laterals
   1. *Patient position:* Seated erect or semiprone
   2. Part position
      a. Center a point ½ inch anterior and 1 inch inferior to EAM to image receptor
      b. MSP angled 15 degrees (nose toward image receptor)
      c. AML adjusted parallel to transverse axis of image receptor
      d. IPL perpendicular to image receptor
      e. After first exposure (made with mouth closed and patient completely still), image receptor is changed, and second exposure is made with patient's mouth fully open
      f. *Respiration:* Suspended
   3. *Central ray:* Direct 15 degrees caudad, exiting TMJ against image receptor

Paranasal Sinuses

A. Lateral (Figure 5-55)
   1. *Patient position:* Seated erect
   2. Part position
      a. Center image receptor ½ to 1 inch posterior to outer canthus
      b. Adjust head to true lateral position
      c. MSP parallel and IPL perpendicular to image receptor
      d. IOML adjusted parallel to transverse axis of image receptor
      e. *Respiration:* Suspended
   3. *Central ray:* Perpendicular, entering ½ to 1 inch posterior to outer canthus
B. PA axial (Caldwell)
   1. *Patient position:* Seated erect at vertical grid device
   2. Part position
      a. Rest head on forehead and nose
      b. MSP perpendicular to midline of image receptor
      c. OML perpendicular to image receptor
      d. *Respiration:* Suspended
   3. *Central ray:* Direct to nasion at angle of 15 degrees caudal to the OML

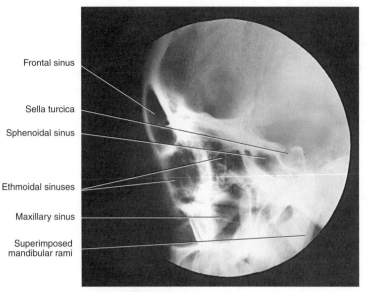

FIGURE 5-55 Lateral sinuses.

C. Parietoacanthial (Waters)
  1. *Patient position:* Seated erect; use horizontal central ray to demonstrate fluid level
  2. Part position
     a. Center and adjust MSP perpendicular to image receptor
     b. Rest head on extended chin
     c. Adjust OML to form 37-degree angle to image receptor
     d. *Respiration:* Suspended
  3. *Central ray:* Horizontal and perpendicular to image receptor, exiting acanthion

D. Submentovertex (basal) (Figure 5-56)
  1. *Patient position:* Seated erect at vertical grid device
  2. Part position
     a. Extend head and rest on vertex
     b. Center and adjust MSP perpendicular to image receptor
     c. Adjust IOML parallel to image receptor
     d. *Respiration:* Suspended
  3. *Central ray:* Perpendicular to IOML through sella turcica, approximately ¾ inch anterior to level of EAM

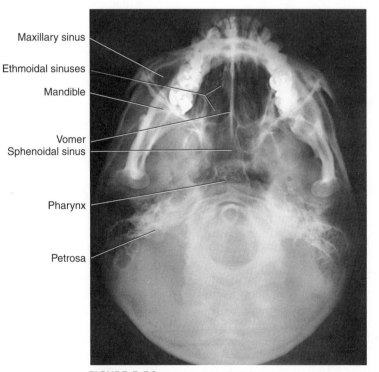

FIGURE 5-56 Submentovertical sinuses.

GASTROINTESTINAL SYSTEM

Pathological Conditions Imaged

A. *Acute cholecystitis:* Inflammation of gallbladder
B. Cancer of the colon and rectum
  1. Leading cause of death from cancer in the United States
  2. More typical form is annular carcinoma, with classic "apple-core" pattern when imaged using barium enema
C. Cancer of the esophagus
  1. Malignant neoplasm
  2. Imaged during barium study
D. Cancer of the stomach
  1. May appear as gross changes in the stomach wall or as a large mass
  2. Imaged during barium study
  3. Harder to penetrate
E. Cholelithiasis
  1. Gallstones
  2. Harder to penetrate
F. Crohn's disease
  1. Chronic inflammation of the bowel
  2. Sometimes separated by normal segments of bowel
G. Diverticulosis
  1. Presence of diverticula (pouchlike herniations through the wall of the colon)
H. Diverticulitis
  1. Inflammation of diverticula
I. Esophageal varices
  1. Varicose veins at distal end of esophagus
J. Esophagitis
  1. Inflammation of esophageal mucosal lining
K. Gastritis
  1. Inflammation of the stomach
L. Hiatal hernia
  1. Condition in which a portion of the stomach protrudes through the diaphragm
M. Ileus
  1. Intestinal obstruction
  2. *Adynamic ileus:* Ileus caused by immobility of the bowel
  3. *Mechanical ileus:* Ileus caused by mechanical obstruction
N. Intussusception
  1. Prolapse of one segment of bowel into another section of bowel
O. Irritable bowel syndrome
  1. Abnormal increase in small and large bowel motility
P. Large bowel obstruction
  1. Characterized by massive accumulation of gas proximal to obstruction
  2. Absence of gas distal to obstruction
  3. High risk of bowel perforation
  4. Extent of obstruction determines ease or difficulty of penetration

Q. Peptic ulcer disease
  1. Loss of mucous membrane in a portion of gastrointestinal (GI) system
  2. Imaged using barium study
  3. Has craterlike appearance
R. *Pyloric stenosis:* Narrowing of pyloric sphincter
S. Small bowel obstruction
  1. Seen as distended loops of bowel filled with gas
  2. Bowel proximal to obstruction may be filled with fluid
  3. Extent of obstruction determines ease or difficulty of penetration
T. Ulcerative colitis
  1. Severe inflammation of the colon and rectum characterized by ulceration
U. *Volvulus:* Twisting of bowel on itself, causing an obstruction

General Survey Examinations

Abdomen

A. AP (KUB)
  1. *Patient position:* Supine
  2. Part position
    a. Center MSP to table
    b. Shoulders in same transverse plane
    c. Support under knees
    d. Center image receptor at level of iliac crests
    e. Apply gonadal shielding as appropriate
    f. *Respiration:* Expiration
  3. *Central ray:* Perpendicular to midline at level of iliac crests
B. AP (upright)
  1. *Patient position:* Erect
  2. Part position
    a. Center MSP to table or upright grid device
    b. Shoulders in same transverse plane
    c. Center image receptor 2 to 3 inches above iliac crests to include diaphragm
    d. Apply gonadal shielding as appropriate
    e. *Respiration:* Expiration
  3. *Central ray:* Horizontal, entering MSP 2 to 3 inches superior to iliac crests
C. Lateral decubitus (Figure 5-57)
  1. Patient position
    a. Lateral recumbent (usually left side down), lying on pad
    b. Arms above level of diaphragm
    c. Knees slightly flexed
  2. Part position
    a. MSP centered to grid device
    b. Center image receptor at level of iliac crest
    c. Apply gonadal shielding as appropriate
    d. *Respiration:* Expiration
  3. *Central ray:* Horizontal and parallel to the MSP at level of iliac crest

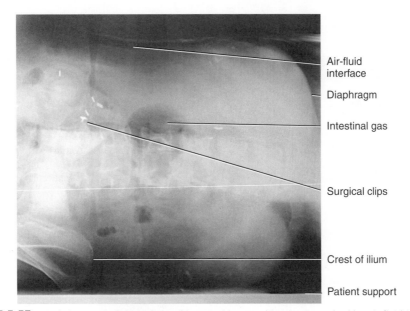

Air-fluid interface

Diaphragm

Intestinal gas

Surgical clips

Crest of ilium

Patient support

FIGURE 5-57 AP abdomen. Left lateral decubitus position resulting in air marked by air-fluid interface.

Upper Gastrointestinal System

Esophagus

A. RAO (PA oblique)
  1. *Patient position:* Recumbent with right arm posterior, left arm by head
  2. Part position
     a. Elevate left side to obliquity of 35 to 40 degrees
     b. Support patient on flexed knee and elbow
     c. Align esophagus and center at level of T5 or T6
     d. Feed barium to patient
     e. *Respiration:* Suspended
  3. *Central ray:* Perpendicular to image receptor, entering level of T5 or T6

Stomach

A. PA
  1. *Patient position:* Prone
  2. Part position
     a. Center at level of pylorus (approximately midway between xiphoid process and umbilicus)
     b. Center halfway between midline and lateral border of abdominal cavity for 10- × 12-inch image receptor or MSP for 14- × 17-inch image receptor
     c. *Respiration:* Expiration
  3. *Central ray:* Perpendicular to image receptor at level of pylorus (L2)
B. RAO (PA oblique) (Figure 5-58)
  1. *Patient position:* Recumbent with right arm posterior, left arm by head
  2. Part position

     a. Elevate left side and support patient to obliquity of 40 to 70 degrees
     b. Longitudinal plane midway between vertebrae and anterior surface of elevated side is centered to image receptor
     c. Center at level of duodenal bulb
     d. *Respiration:* Expiration
  3. *Central ray:* Perpendicular to center of image receptor midway between vertebral column and lateral border of abdominal cavity at level of L2
C. Lateral
  1. *Patient position:* Recumbent (right lateral) or erect (left lateral)
  2. Part position
     a. Center image receptor between midaxillary plane and anterior abdominal surface
     b. Center at level of pylorus
     c. Adjust to true lateral
     d. *Respiration:* Expiration
  3. *Central ray:* Perpendicular to center of image receptor midway between midaxillary line and anterior surface of abdomen at the level of L1 for recumbent position or L3 for upright position

Small Bowel

A. PA
  1. *Patient position:* Prone
  2. Part position
     a. MSP centered to table
     b. Center image receptor at level of iliac crest (may be slightly higher for early time exposures)
     c. *Respiration:* Suspended
  3. *Central ray:* Perpendicular to image receptor entering midline at level of iliac crest (or slightly above)

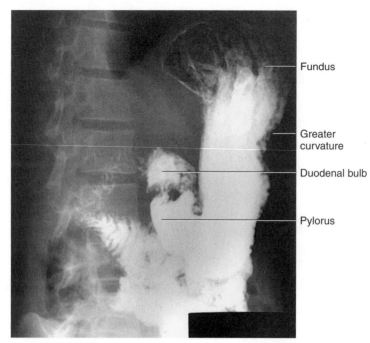

FIGURE 5-58 Single-contrast PA oblique stomach (RAO position).

Lower Gastrointestinal System

Colon

A. PA (Figure 5-59)
1. *Patient position:* Prone
2. Part position
a. MSP centered to table
b. Center image receptor at level of iliac crest
c. *Respiration:* Suspended
3. *Central ray:* Perpendicular to image receptor, entering level of iliac crest
B. PA axial
1. *Patient position:* Prone
2. Part position
a. MSP centered to table
b. Center image receptor at level of iliac crest
c. *Respiration:* Suspended
3. Central ray
a. From 30 to 40 degrees caudad
b. To show rectosigmoid area using smaller image receptor, central ray enters midline at level of ASIS
C. LAO and RAO (PA oblique) (Figure 5-60)
1. *Patient position:* PA oblique
2. Part position
a. Patient rotated 35 to 45 degrees
b. Either right or left side up
c. Center abdomen to table
d. Image receptor centered at level of iliac crest
e. *Respiration:* Suspended
3. *Central ray:* Perpendicular to image receptor, entering level of iliac crest

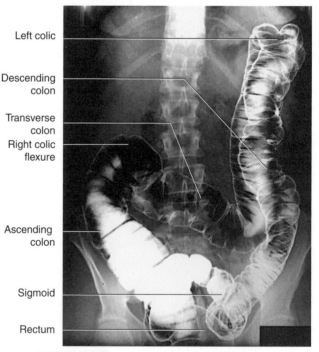

FIGURE 5-59 Double-contrast PA large intestine.

D. Lateral rectum
1. *Patient position:* Lying on side
2. Part position
a. Adjust patient's body to true lateral position (right or left side down)
b. Center midaxillary plane of abdomen to center of table
c. *Respiration:* Suspended
3. *Central ray:* Perpendicular to image receptor, entering midaxillary plane at level of ASIS

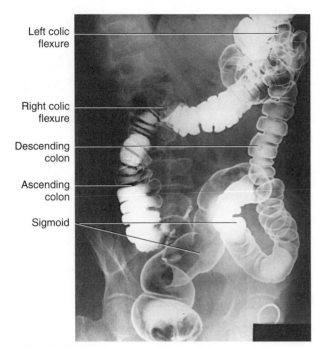

Left colic
flexure

Right colic
flexure

Descending
colon

Ascending
colon

Sigmoid

FIGURE 5-60 Double-contrast PA oblique large intestine.

E. AP
1. *Patient position:* Supine
2. Part position
   a. MSP centered to table
   b. Image receptor centered at level of iliac crest
   c. *Respiration:* Suspended
3. *Central ray:* Perpendicular to image receptor, entering level of iliac crest
F. AP axial
1. *Patient position:* Supine
2. Part position
   a. MSP centered to table
   b. Image receptor centered 2 inches above iliac crest
   c. *Respiration:* Suspended
3. Central ray
   a. Cephalad 30 to 40 degrees, entering approximately 2 inches below level of ASIS
   b. When rectosigmoid is of interest, central ray enters inferior margin of symphysis pubis
G. Lateral decubitus
1. *Patient position:* Lying on either right or left side, patient's MSP centered to midline of grid
2. Part position
   a. Arms above head
   b. Knees slightly flexed
   c. Image receptor centered to abdomen at level of iliac crest
   d. *Respiration:* Suspended
3. *Central ray:* Horizontal, entering midline at level of iliac crest
H. LPO and RPO (AP oblique)
1. *Patient position:* AP oblique

2. Part position
   a. Patient rotated 35 to 45 degrees from AP position; either right or left side up
   b. Center abdomen to table
   c. Image receptor centered at level of iliac crest
   d. *Respiration:* Suspended
3. *Central ray:* Perpendicular to image receptor at level of iliac crest

Surgical Cholangiogram

A. AP or AP oblique
1. *Patient position:* Supine on operating table
2. Part position
   a. Right upper quadrant centered to image receptor
   b. Left side of body may be elevated into a 15- to 20-degree oblique angle to prevent bile ducts from being superimposed over the spine
3. *Central ray:* Perpendicular to exposed biliary tract
4. Procedure notes
   a. Surgeon directs imaging sequence
   b. Equipment must be properly cleaned and ready to use
   c. Radiographer must be in proper operating room attire
   d. Appropriate radiation protection standards must be maintained for the radiographer and for the operating room staff, using distance and lead shielding
   e. Exposure times must be as short as possible, with patient respiration controlled by the anesthetist
5. *Examination evaluation:* Patency of the bile ducts, operation of the sphincter of the hepatopancreatic ampulla, and presence of calculi

Endoscopic Retrograde Cholangiopancreatography

A. Endoscopic retrograde cholangiopancreatography (ERCP) examination notes
1. Used to evaluate biliary and pancreatic pathological conditions
2. Endoscope is passed into duodenum under fluoroscopic control
3. Contrast medium is injected into the common bile duct or pancreatic duct through a cannula passed through the endoscope
4. Patient is placed prone for imaging
5. ERCP may be preceded by ultrasound

Urinary System

Pathological Conditions Imaged

A. Carcinoma of the bladder
1. Seen as solid mass arising from the bladder wall
2. Harder to penetrate

B. *Cystitis:* Inflammation of bladder and ureters
C. *Glomerulonephritis:* Inflammation of glomerulus of kidney
D. Polycystic kidney disease
   1. Enlarged kidneys containing numerous cysts
   2. Harder to penetrate
E. *Pyelonephritis:* Inflammation of renal pelvis and parenchyma
F. Renal calculus
   1. Kidney stone
   2. Harder to penetrate stone, but overall technique is not increased to compensate
G. Renal carcinoma
   1. Solid mass cancer that causes renal bulging or enlargement with impact on collecting system
   2. Harder to penetrate
H. Renal cysts
   1. Fluid-filled masses in kidney
   2. Harder to penetrate
I. Wilms' tumor
   1. Malignant cancer of kidney in children
   2. Harder to penetrate

Urinary System Procedures

Intravenous Urography

A. KUB (AP) (Figure 5-61)
   1. *Patient position:* Supine, centered to the table
   2. Part position
     a. Spine centered to table

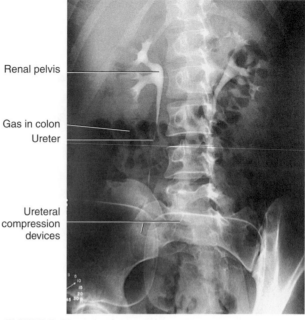

FIGURE 5-62 AP oblique urogram 10 minutes after injection.

     b. Include entire renal outlines, bladder, and symphysis pubis and prostatic region on older male patients
   3. *Central ray:* Perpendicular to image receptor, centered at level of iliac crest
B. Oblique (RPO, LPO) (Figure 5-62)
   1. *Patient position:* Supine
   2. *Part position:* Patient's body rotated to a 30-degree oblique angle; kidney farther from the image receptor is parallel to image receptor, and kidney nearer to the image receptor is perpendicular to image receptor
   3. *Central ray:* Perpendicular to image receptor at iliac crest
C. AP bladder
   1. *Patient position:* Supine
   2. *Part position:* Supine, centered to image receptor
   3. *Central ray:* Perpendicular to image receptor, centered at level of ASIS
D. Intravenous pyelogram (IVP) (intravenous urogram) procedure notes
   1. Patient should be properly prepared with a low-residue diet for 1 to 2 days before the examination and cleansing of GI tract
   2. NPO (nothing by mouth) after midnight the day of the examination but not dehydrated
   3. Preliminary KUB is performed before contrast agent injection to verify positioning, visualize renal anatomy, or detect the presence of lesions
   4. Based on patient weight, 30 to 100 mL of iodinated contrast medium is injected; pelvicalyceal system appears in 2 to 8 minutes, with greatest visualization occurring in 15 to 20 minutes

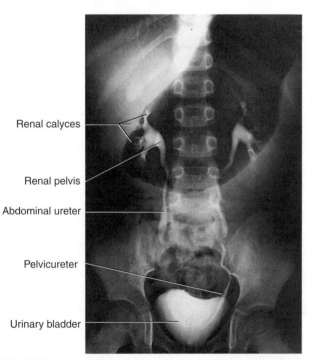

FIGURE 5-61 Urogram from supine position at 15-minute interval with gas-filled stomach.

5. AP and oblique radiographs are obtained at specific intervals after injection of contrast medium

6. All images must be carefully identified using right, left, upright, and "postvoid" markers and numbers indicating postinjection time; stickers, felt-tip markers, and grease pencils should not be used to place identification on a radiograph

7. All image receptor sizes needed for examination should be made readily available before beginning procedure

8. AP upright positions may be used to show kidney mobility and filled bladder

9. Oblique radiographs may be used to image kidney rotation or localize tumor masses

10. Postvoid radiographs may be taken to image tumor masses or prostatic enlargement

11. Tomography may be used during IVP to blur gas patterns and to image intrarenal lesions better; this is termed *nephrotomography*

Cystography and Cystourethrography

A. Positioning
 1. AP axial
   a. Angle 10 to 15 degrees caudal; only 5 degrees caudal for bladder neck
   b. Image receptor centered at level 2 to 3 inches above symphysis pubis
 2. Oblique (RPO, LPO)
   a. Patient rotated 40 to 60 degrees
   b. Pubic arch closest to table centered to midline of table
 3. PA of bladder
   a. Patient centered
   b. Central ray enters 1 inch distal to tip of coccyx with 10- to 15-degree cephalad angle
 4. Lateral
   a. Bladder centered to image receptor; image receptor 2 to 3 inches above symphysis pubis
   b. Central ray centered and perpendicular to image receptor
B. Procedure notes
 1. Bladder is drained with catheter that has been put in place
 2. Bladder is filled with contrast medium through urethral catheter
 3. After bladder is filled, clamp is closed to prevent contrast agent from draining
 4. Imaging follows filling of bladder
 5. Cystourethrography may follow cystogram
   a. Patient is instructed to void contrast material from bladder while on fluoroscopic table
   b. Radiologist takes spot images during urination to evaluate urethra and to image reflux

Retrograde Pyelography

A. Positioning
 1. AP
 2. RPO
 3. LPO
B. Procedure notes
 1. Ureters are catheterized to allow filling of the pelvicalyceal system
 2. Urologist performs procedure
 3. Image receptor is placed to include both kidneys and ureters
 4. After catheterization and introduction of contrast material, urologist directs imaging sequence

Table 5-1 lists common additive and destructive diseases and conditions.

Other Radiological Examinations

A. Myelography
 1. Pathological conditions imaged
   a. Herniated intervertebral disks
   b. Degenerative diseases of the CNS
   c. Space-occupying lesions

TABLE 5-1	Common Additive and Destructive Diseases and Conditions by Anatomical Area	
Additive Conditions	**Destructive Conditions**	
Abdomen		
Aortic aneurysm	Bowel obstruction	
Ascites	Free air	
Cirrhosis		
Hypertrophy of some organs (e.g., splenomegaly)		
Chest		
Atelectasis	Emphysema	
Congestive heart failure	Pneumothorax	
Malignancy		
Pleural effusion		
Pneumonia		
Skeleton		
Hydrocephalus	Gout	
Metastases (osteoblastic)	Metastases (osteolytic)	
Osteochondroma (exostoses)	Multiple myeloma	
Paget disease	Paget's disease	
Osteoporosis		
Nonspecific Sites		
Abscess	Atrophy	
Edema	Emaciation	
Sclerosis	Malnutrition	

From Fauber TL: *Radiographic imaging and exposure*, ed 4, St. Louis, 2012, Mosby.

2. Pathological changes are imaged by displacement of column of contrast material in the subarachnoid space
3. Lumbar puncture performed by physician at L3-4 interspace allows injection of water-soluble contrast agent into subarachnoid space
4. Small amount of spinal fluid is withdrawn for laboratory analysis
5. X-ray table is tilted up and down to distribute contrast medium
6. Contrast medium should not be allowed to enter cerebral ventricles; head must be kept hyperextended to compress cisterna magna when contrast medium is used in cervical region
7. Images are taken under fluoroscopic control in PA and oblique positions
8. Cross-table lateral radiographs are taken by radiographer to provide right-angle views
9. Contrast medium is absorbed by patient's body

B. Arthrography
1. Contrast examination of an encapsulated joint
   a. Knee
   b. Shoulder
   c. Hip
   d. Wrist
   e. TMJ
2. Pathological conditions imaged
   a. Joint trauma
   b. Meniscal tears
   c. Capsular damage
   d. Deformities caused by arthritis
   e. Rupture of articular ligaments
3. Performed under local anesthetic with use of asepsis
4. Physician injects contrast material
5. Joint is manipulated to distribute contrast agent
6. Fluoroscopic images may be taken
7. Arthrography is gradually being replaced by MRI

KEY REVIEW POINTS
Review of Radiography Positioning, Procedures, and Pathology

These three topics are collectively tested as part of one category on the certification exam. These topics constitute the heart of radiographic procedures. Use this review to reinforce what you have learned in class and clinical education. Make use of the labeled radiographs. Be able to define, in words, the pathological conditions presented.

REVIEW QUESTIONS

1. What body type is a slender build?
   a. Hypersthenic habitus
   b. Sthenic habitus
   c. Hyposthenic habitus
   d. Asthenic habitus

2. What body type is a massive build?
   a. Hypersthenic habitus
   b. Sthenic habitus
   c. Hyposthenic habitus
   d. Asthenic habitus
3. What body type has the stomach and gallbladder low, vertical, and near the midline?
   a. Hypersthenic habitus
   b. Sthenic habitus
   c. Hyposthenic habitus
   d. Asthenic habitus
4. What body type is average build, present in about 35% of the population?
   a. Hypersthenic habitus
   b. Sthenic habitus
   c. Hyposthenic habitus
   d. Asthenic habitus
5. What is the most common body habitus, present in about 50% of the population?
   a. Hypersthenic habitus
   b. Sthenic habitus
   c. Hyposthenic habitus
   d. Asthenic habitus
6. What body type has the stomach and gallbladder high and horizontal?
   a. Hypersthenic habitus
   b. Sthenic habitus
   c. Hyposthenic habitus
   d. Asthenic habitus
7. What body type has the thorax narrow and shallow?
   a. Hypersthenic habitus
   b. Sthenic habitus
   c. Hyposthenic habitus
   d. Asthenic habitus
8. What body type has the thorax broad and deep?
   a. Hypersthenic habitus
   b. Sthenic habitus
   c. Hyposthenic habitus
   d. Asthenic habitus
9. Key points in performing pediatric radiography are:
   a. Work quickly and impersonally, use gonadal shielding, report suspected child abuse, keep parents in waiting room
   b. Work quickly, communicate clearly with child and parents, use gonadal shielding, report suspected child abuse
   c. Work quickly and impersonally, report suspected child abuse, keep parents in waiting room, always use Pigg-O-Stat
   d. Work quickly and impersonally, use gonadal shielding only on abdominal examinations, report suspected child abuse, keep parents in waiting room
10. The most important point to remember when performing trauma radiography is:
   a. Use gonadal shielding because this patient will be having many follow-up examinations
   b. Work quickly because the injuries may be life-threatening

c. Do no additional harm to the patient

d. Perform only the projections ordered by the physician

11. When you are performing trauma radiography:

a. Splints, bandages, and cervical collars should be removed so that they do not obstruct the anatomy that must be imaged

b. Remove cervical collars only under the direction of a radiologist

c. Remove cervical collars only under the direction of an emergency department physician or radiologist

d. Splints, bandages, and cervical collars should be removed after preliminary images have been viewed by a physician so that they do not obstruct the anatomy that must be imaged

12. What plane passes transversely across the body?

a. Transverse plane

b. Midcoronal plane

c. Median sagittal plane

d. Sagittal plane

13. What plane passes vertically through the midline of the body from front to back?

a. Transverse plane

b. Midcoronal plane

c. Median sagittal plane

d. Sagittal plane

14. What plane divides the body into superior and inferior portions?

a. Transverse plane

b. Midcoronal plane

c. Median sagittal plane

d. Sagittal plane

15. What plane passes vertically through the midaxillary region of the body and through the coronal suture of the cranium at right angles to the midsagittal plane?

a. Transverse plane

b. Midcoronal plane

c. Median sagittal plane

d. Sagittal plane

16. What describes any plane parallel to the MSP?

a. Transverse plane

b. Midcoronal plane

c. Median sagittal plane

d. Sagittal plane

17. What type of joint is the hip?

a. Ball-and-socket joint

b. Pivot joint

c. Hinge joint

d. Saddle joint

18. What type of joint has a rounded head of one bone that moves in a cuplike cavity?

a. Ball-and-socket joint

b. Pivot joint

c. Hinge joint

d. Saddle joint

19. What type of joint permits motion in one plane only?

a. Ball-and-socket joint

b. Pivot joint

c. Hinge joint

d. Saddle joint

20. What type of joint has opposing surfaces that are convex-concave, allowing great freedom of motion?

a. Ball-and-socket joint

b. Pivot joint

c. Hinge joint

d. Saddle joint

21. What type of joint permits rotary movement in which a ring rotates around a central axis?

a. Ball-and-socket joint

b. Pivot joint

c. Hinge joint

d. Saddle joint

22. Which of the following conditions would not be an indication for performing hysterosalpingography?

a. Determination of the patency of the oviducts

b. Status of pregnancy

c. Abnormal uterine bleeding

d. Uterine polyps

23. Which of the following statements are true regarding venography?

1. Venography is performed to visualize thrombophlebitis, varicose veins, or vessel damage secondary to trauma

2. Venography requires AP and lateral projections

3. Use of this examination is limited because deep veins cannot be imaged

4. Injection is made into superficial veins

a. 1, 2, 3

b. 1, 4

c. 2, 3

d. 1, 2, 4

24. Which of the following statements are true regarding contrast arthrography?

1. Asepsis is required

2. The examination may be performed on knee, shoulder, TMJ, hip, and wrist

3. Indications include trauma, capsular damage, meniscal tears, rupture of ligaments, and arthritis

4. The joint is manipulated by hand to distribute contrast medium

a. 1, 2, 3, 4

b. 1, 2

c. 3, 4

d. 2, 3

25. Which of the following statements are true concerning myelography?

1. Injection is always performed at the L3-4 interspace

2. Oily, iodinated contrast agent is the medium of choice

3. Indications include herniated intervertebral disks, space-occupying lesions, and degenerative diseases of the CNS

4. Contrast medium is distributed by manual manipulation of the subarachnoid space

5. The head must be kept hyperflexed so that contrast medium does not enter the cerebral ventricles
6. Spinal fluid may be withdrawn for laboratory analysis
   a. 1, 2, 4
   b. 2, 4, 5
   c. 1, 2, 3, 5
   d. 3, 6

26. An examination that uses motion and blurring to view anatomy by setting the x-ray tube and image receptor in motion is:
   a. CT
   b. Autotomography
   c. Conventional tomography
   d. Fluoroscopy

27. The proper centering point for a PA projection of the hand is the:
   a. Third metatarsophalangeal joint
   b. Third metacarpophalangeal joint
   c. Midshaft of the third metacarpal
   d. First metacarpophalangeal joint

28. For a lateral projection of the wrist:
   a. The radius and ulna should be superimposed
   b. The radial surface must be in contact with the image receptor
   c. The central ray is parallel
   d. Use the fastest image receptor speed possible

29. For a lateral projection of the forearm, which of the following statements are true?
   1. The ulnar surface must be in contact with the image receptor
   2. The thumb should be in a relaxed position
   3. The humerus and forearm should be in contact with the table
   4. The elbow should be flexed 45 degrees
   5. The central ray is directed toward the injured joint
   a. All are true
   b. 1, 2, 5
   c. 1, 3
   d. 2, 4, 5

30. For an AP projection of the elbow, which of the following statements are true?
   1. The forearm and humerus should be at right angles
   2. The central ray is directed perpendicular to the joint
   3. The forearm and humerus should be parallel to the table
   4. The hand must be pronated
   5. The patient may have to lean laterally to ensure AP alignment
   a. 1, 2
   b. 2, 3, 5
   c. 1, 4
   d. 2, 3, 4, 5

31. For a lateral projection of the humerus, which of the following statements are true?
   1. The hand should be pronated
   2. The patient may be upright or supine
   3. The humeral epicondyles are placed perpendicular to the cassette
   4. The arm should be slightly adducted
   5. The central ray is directed perpendicular to the midshaft
   a. 2, 3, 5
   b. 1, 4
   c. 2, 4
   d. 1, 2, 3, 5

32. For a PA oblique (scapular Y) projection of the shoulder, which of the following statements are true?
   1. The central ray is directed to the shoulder at a 10-degree cephalad angle
   2. The anterior surface of the affected shoulder is centered to the cassette
   3. The patient is rotated so that the midcoronal plane forms a 60-degree angle with the cassette
   4. The patient continues shallow breathing during exposure
   a. 1, 2
   b. 2, 3, 4
   c. 2, 3
   d. 1, 2, 3

33. For an AP projection of the AC joints:
   a. To show AC separation properly, joints both with and without weights should be shown on one image receptor if possible
   b. To show AC separation properly, separate images must be acquired with equal weights attached to both wrists and without weights
   c. The central ray is always directed midway between the AC joints
   d. The patient should be seated upright and instructed to continue shallow breathing during the exposure

34. When the clavicle is being radiographed, which of the following statements are true?
   1. PA projection must always be used
   2. A central ray angle of 25 to 30 degrees cephalad is used for the PA axial projection
   3. The patient's head should be turned away from the affected side
   4. AP projection may be used for patient comfort
   5. An erect position may be used for patient comfort
   6. A central ray angle of 25 to 30 degrees caudad is used for the PA axial projection
   a. 1, 2, 3, 4, 5
   b. 1, 3, 4, 5
   c. 2, 3, 4, 5
   d. 3, 4, 5, 6

35. For the lateral projection of the scapula, which of the following statements are true?
   1. Patient should be upright to reduce pain

2. Patient is positioned obliquely with unaffected scapula centered to the cassette
3. The body is adjusted by palpating axillary and vertebral borders of the scapula so that the scapula is lateral
4. Scapula must be projected free of the rib cage
   a. 1, 3, 4
   b. 2, 3
   c. 3, 4
   d. 2, 3, 4

36. What is the name of a fracture of the medial and lateral malleoli of the ankle with ankle joint dislocation?
    a. Trimalleolar fracture
    b. Giant cell myeloma
    c. Osteoarthritis
    d. Pott fracture

37. What condition involves the posterior portion of the tibia and the medial and lateral malleoli?
    a. Trimalleolar fracture
    b. Giant cell myeloma
    c. Osteoarthritis
    d. Pott fracture

38. What condition is more commonly seen in elderly patients?
    a. Trimalleolar fracture
    b. Giant cell myeloma
    c. Osteoarthritis
    d. Pott fracture

39. What is a tumor that arises on bone with a large bubble appearance and may be benign or malignant?
    a. Trimalleolar fracture
    b. Giant cell myeloma
    c. Osteoarthritis
    d. Pott fracture

40. What condition is characterized by the degeneration of one or several joints?
    a. Trimalleolar fracture
    b. Giant cell myeloma
    c. Osteoarthritis
    d. Pott fracture

41. For AP radiography of the foot, which of the following statements are true?
    1. A trough-compensating filter may be used
    2. The dorsal surface rests on the cassette
    3. The central ray is directed 10 degrees anterior
    4. The central ray is directed at the head of the third metatarsal
       a. All are true
       b. 1, 3, 4
       c. 2, 4
       d. None are true

42. When an AP axial projection is performed for the os calcis, which of the following statements are true?
    1. The leg should be fully extended
    2. The plantar surface of the foot should be parallel to the cassette

3. The central ray is directed 40 degrees cephalad to the long axis of the foot
4. The central ray enters the foot at the head of the fifth metatarsal
5. A cylinder cone may be used for this projection
   a. 1, 3, 5
   b. 2, 4
   c. 2, 5
   d. 1, 3, 4, 5

43. For a medial oblique position of the ankle, which of the following statements are true?
    1. The leg and foot are rotated medially
    2. The ankle is adjusted to a 90-degree angle
    3. The medial rotation is adjusted to 45 degrees to show the mortise joint
    4. The medial rotation is adjusted to 15 to 20 degrees to show the bony structure
    5. The central ray is directed vertically midway between the malleoli
       a. 1, 4
       b. 1, 5
       c. 1, 3, 4, 5
       d. 1, 2, 3, 4

44. For a lateral lower leg projection, which of the following statements are true?
    1. The leg is centered to the cassette
    2. The examination may be performed with the patient on the tabletop or Bucky
    3. Roll the patient away from the affected side
    4. The patella should be perpendicular to the cassette
    5. Include both joints
    6. The tibia and fibula should be superimposed
    7. The central ray is directed to the midpoint of the leg
       a. 1, 2, 3
       b. 1, 2, 3, 4, 5, 7
       c. 1, 4, 5, 6, 7
       d. 1, 2, 4, 5, 7

45. When a lateral knee projection is performed, which of the following statements are true?
    1. The patient turns onto the affected side
    2. The knee is flexed 20 to 30 degrees
    3. The patella must be parallel to the image receptor
    4. The central ray is directed 5 degrees caudad
    5. The central ray enters the knee joint inferior to the medial condyle
       a. 1, 2, 3
       b. 1, 2, 3, 5
       c. 1, 2, 5
       d. 1, 2, 4, 5

46. For a tangential projection of the patella, which of the following statements are true?
    1. The patient is prone
    2. The affected knee is flexed so that the tibia and fibula form a 50- to 60-degree angle with the table

3. The central ray is directed 45 degrees cephalad through the patellofemoral joint
4. The tangential patella projection may also be performed with the patient supine
   a. 1, 2, 3, 4
   b. 2, 3, 4
   c. 1, 2, 3
   d. 1, 2, 4

47. For an AP projection of the femur:
    a. The lower leg should be rotated laterally 15 degrees
    b. The central ray is directed toward the affected joint
    c. The patient is prone
    d. The lower leg is rotated medially 15 degrees

48. The central ray for an AP projection of the hip is:
    a. Directed parallel to a point 2 inches medial to the ASIS and at the level of the superior margin of the greater trochanter
    b. Directed parallel to a point 2 inches lateral to the ASIS and at the level of the superior margin of the greater trochanter
    c. Directed parallel to a point 2 inches medial to the ASIS and at the level of the inferior margin of the greater trochanter
    d. Directed perpendicular to a point 2 inches medial to the ASIS and at the level of the superior margin of the greater trochanter

49. What condition is commonly caused by motor vehicle accidents?
    a. Jefferson's fracture
    b. Hangman's fracture
    c. Spondylolysis
    d. Spina bifida

50. What condition is caused by acute hyperextension of the head on the neck and a fracture of the arch of C2?
    a. Jefferson's fracture
    b. Hangman's fracture
    c. Spondylolysis
    d. Spina bifida

51. What is a defect of the posterior aspect of the spinal canal caused by failure of the vertebral arch to form properly?
    a. Jefferson's fracture
    b. Hangman's fracture
    c. Spondylolysis
    d. Spina bifida

52. What is a defect in the pars articularis?
    a. Jefferson's fracture
    b. Hangman's fracture
    c. Spondylolysis
    d. Spina bifida

53. What is a comminuted fracture of the ring of the atlas involving both anterior and posterior arches and causing displacement of the fragments?
    a. Jefferson's fracture

b. Hangman's fracture
c. Spondylolysis
d. Spina bifida

54. For a lateral projection of the cervical spine, which of the following statements are true?
    1. The patient may be upright, seated, or supine, depending on his or her condition
    2. SID of 72 inches should be used because of increased object-to-image receptor distance
    3. The shoulders should lie in the same plane
    4. The cervical collar should be removed so that it does not obstruct pertinent anatomy
    5. The chin should be in contact with the chest
       a. 1, 2, 4
       b. 1, 2, 3
       c. 1, 2, 3, 5
       d. 1, 2, 4, 5

55. For a lateral projection of the thoracic spine, which of the following statements are true?
    1. The head and spine should be in the same plane
    2. The central ray is directed to T7, at a cephalad angle of 10 degrees
    3. The patient should continue shallow breathing during exposure
    4. The examination should not be performed in a room with a falling load generator, if possible
       a. 1, 2
       b. 1, 3
       c. 1, 3, 4
       d. 1, 2, 3

56. For a lateral projection of L5-S1, which of the following statements are true?
    1. The patient is in lateral position
    2. The hips and knees are extended
    3. The cassette is centered at the level of the transverse plane that passes midway between the iliac crests and the ASIS
    4. A cylinder cone may be used to reduce greatly the production of scatter radiation
    5. The central ray is directed to a point 1½ inches anterior to the palpated spinous process of L5
       a. 1, 2, 3, 4, 5
       b. 1, 2
       c. 1, 2, 3, 5
       d. 1, 3, 4, 5

57. For RPO and LPO positions for sacroiliac joints:
    a. Image the joint nearest the image receptor
    b. The part must be angled at 10 to 15 degrees to coincide with the angle of the joints
    c. Image the joint farthest from the image receptor
    d. The central ray must be angled 25 degrees cephalad

58. For an AP projection of the coccyx:
    a. The central ray should be directed 10 degrees caudad, entering 2 inches superior to the symphysis pubis

b. The central ray should be directed 10 degrees cephalad, entering 2 inches superior to the symphysis pubis

c. The central ray should be directed 25 degrees caudad, entering 2 inches superior to the symphysis pubis

d. The central ray should be directed 25 degrees caudad, entering 4 inches superior to the symphysis pubis

59. Which pathological condition is easy to penetrate?
   a. Atelectasis
   b. Bronchogenic carcinoma
   c. COPD
   d. Emphysema

60. What condition is a collapse of lung tissue and is harder to penetrate?
   a. Atelectasis
   b. Bronchogenic carcinoma
   c. COPD
   d. Emphysema

61. What condition is characterized by air trapped in the alveoli, which makes the condition very easy to penetrate?
   a. Atelectasis
   b. Bronchogenic carcinoma
   c. COPD
   d. Emphysema

62. What condition should not be imaged with use of an AEC?
   a. Atelectasis
   b. Bronchogenic carcinoma
   c. COPD
   d. Emphysema

63. What is lung cancer arising from bronchial mucosa?
   a. Atelectasis
   b. Bronchogenic carcinoma
   c. COPD
   d. Emphysema

64. What progressive condition is marked by diminished capabilities of inspiration and expiration?
   a. Atelectasis
   b. Bronchogenic carcinoma
   c. COPD
   d. Emphysema

65. For an AP projection of the ribs above the diaphragm, which of the following statements is true?
   1. The top of the cassette is placed 1 to 2 inches above the shoulders
   2. The shoulders are relaxed, and the scapulae are flat against the table
   3. The central ray is directed to T7
   4. Exposure is performed on full expiration to depress the diaphragm
   a. 1, 3
   b. 1, 2, 3, 4
   c. 1, 2, 3
   d. 1, 3, 4

66. For RAO position of the sternum:
   a. The body should be rotated 45 to 60 degrees to prevent superimposition of the sternum and spine
   b. The patient is supine
   c. Breathing should be shallow during exposure; a falling load generator should not be used, if possible
   d. The best image is obtained with suspended breathing

67. For radiography of the sternoclavicular articulations:
   a. PA and lateral projections are required
   b. RAO or LAO positions are used to eliminate superimposition of joints onto vertebral shadow
   c. The patient should breathe during exposure; a falling load generator should be used if possible
   d. An AP projection is used to reduce magnification of joints

68. What condition is characterized by soft bones resulting from deficiency of vitamin D and sunlight?
   a. Hydrocephalus
   b. Paget's disease
   c. Osteoporosis
   d. Rickets

69. What condition is a bone disease causing bone destruction and unorganized bone repair and is generally difficult to penetrate?
   a. Hydrocephalus
   b. Paget's disease
   c. Osteoporosis
   d. Rickets

70. What condition is an abnormal demineralization of bone, seen more often in females?
   a. Hydrocephalus
   b. Paget's disease
   c. Osteoporosis
   d. Rickets

71. What condition is marked by abnormal accumulation of cerebrospinal fluid in the brain?
   a. Hydrocephalus
   b. Paget's disease
   c. Osteoporosis
   d. Rickets

72. What condition is most often seen in elderly patients?
   a. Hydrocephalus
   b. Paget's disease
   c. Osteoporosis
   d. Rickets

73. For a direct PA projection of the skull, the central ray is directed:
   a. 15 degrees caudad
   b. 25 degrees caudad
   c. Perpendicular to the image receptor
   d. Perpendicular to the image receptor, exiting the nasion when the OML is perpendicular to the IR

74. When the skull is radiographed in the lateral position:
    a. The MSP must be perpendicular to the IR, the IOML must be parallel to the IR, and the IPL must be parallel to the IR
    b. The MSP and IOML are parallel to the IR, and the IPL is perpendicular to the IR
    c. The MSP is perpendicular to the IR, and the IPL is parallel to the IR
    d. The MSP and IOML are perpendicular to the IR, and the IPL is parallel to the IR

75. For a parietoorbital (Rhese) projection of the optic foramen:
    a. The head is resting on the forehead, nose, and zygoma
    b. The MSP forms an angle of 53 degrees from the perpendicular
    c. The central ray exits the unaffected orbit
    d. The head rests on the zygoma, nose, and chin while the MSP is rotated 53 degrees from the IR

76. When a parietoacanthial (Waters) projection is performed for the facial bones:
    a. The MSP is parallel to the IR
    b. The MSP is perpendicular to the IR, the head rests on the chin, and the OML forms a 53-degree angle with the plane of the image receptor
    c. The MSP is perpendicular to the IR, the head rests on the chin, and the OML forms a 37-degree angle with the plane of the image receptor
    d. The MSP is perpendicular to the IR, the head rests on the nose, and the OML forms a 37-degree angle with the plane of the image receptor

77. For a unilateral tangential (May) projection of the zygomatic arches:
    a. The IOML is parallel to the plane of the image receptor, the MSP is rotated 15 degrees away from the affected side, the IR is centered 3 inches distal to the most prominent point of the zygoma, and the central ray is directed perpendicular to the IOML through the zygomatic arch 1½ inches posterior to the outer canthus
    b. The IOML is parallel to the plane of the image receptor, the MSP is rotated 15 degrees toward the affected side, the IR is centered 3 inches distal to the most prominent point of the zygoma, and the central ray is directed perpendicular to the IOML through the zygomatic arch 1½ inches posterior to the outer canthus
    c. The IOML is parallel to the plane of the image receptor, the MSP is rotated 15 degrees away from the affected side, the IR is centered 3 inches distal to the most prominent point of the zygoma, and the central ray is directed perpendicular to the zygomatic arch 1½ inches posterior to the outer canthus
    d. The IOML is parallel to the plane of the image receptor, the MSP is rotated 25 degrees away from the affected side, the IR is centered 3 inches distal to the most prominent point of the zygoma, and the central ray is directed perpendicular to the IOML through the zygomatic arch 1½ inches posterior to the outer canthus

78. When the mandibular body is radiographed with the patient in the SMV position:
    a. The head and neck are extended and resting on the chin
    b. The MSP is parallel with the IR
    c. The IOML is perpendicular with the plane of the image receptor, the head and neck are resting on the vertex, and the MSP is perpendicular to the IR
    d. The IOML is parallel with the plane of the image receptor, the head is resting on the vertex, and the MSP is perpendicular to the IR

79. The best survey study of the paranasal sinuses is obtained by use of what projection?
    a. Lateral
    b. Parietoacanthial (Waters)
    c. Upright lateral
    d. SMV

80. What is a condition in which a portion of the stomach protrudes through the diaphragm?
    a. Annular carcinoma
    b. Crohn's disease
    c. Hiatal hernia
    d. Ileus

81. What condition involves an intestinal obstruction?
    a. Annular carcinoma
    b. Crohn's disease
    c. Hiatal hernia
    d. Ileus

82. What condition involves chronic inflammation of portions of the bowel?
    a. Annular carcinoma
    b. Crohn's disease
    c. Hiatal hernia
    d. Ileus

83. What condition may be adynamic or mechanical?
    a. Annular carcinoma
    b. Crohn's disease
    c. Hiatal hernia
    d. Ileus

84. What condition appears in an "apple-core" pattern on barium enema examination?
    a. Annular carcinoma
    b. Crohn's disease
    c. Hiatal hernia
    d. Ileus

85. What condition is visualized by performing an upper GI series?
    a. Diverticula
    b. Ulcerative colitis
    c. Pyloric stenosis
    d. Adynamic ileus

86. What describes a bowel obstruction caused by immobility of bowel?
    a. Diverticula
    b. Ulcerative colitis
    c. Pyloric stenosis
    d. Adynamic ileus
87. What condition is characterized by pouchlike herniations of the colonic wall?
    a. Diverticula
    b. Ulcerative colitis
    c. Pyloric stenosis
    d. Adynamic ileus
88. What condition causes a narrowing of the sphincter at the distal end of the stomach?
    a. Diverticula
    b. Ulcerative colitis
    c. Pyloric stenosis
    d. Adynamic ileus
89. What condition is a severe inflammation of the colon and rectum with loss of mucosal lining?
    a. Diverticula
    b. Ulcerative colitis
    c. Pyloric stenosis
    d. Adynamic ileus
90. For RAO position of the esophagus:
    a. The patient is rotated obliquely by elevation of the right side 35 to 40 degrees, and the esophagus is centered to the image receptor at the level of T5 or T6
    b. The patient is rotated obliquely by elevation of the left side 35 to 40 degrees, and the esophagus is centered at the level of T5 or T6
    c. The patient is rotated obliquely by elevation of the right side 55 to 60 degrees, and the esophagus is centered to the image receptor at the level of T5 or T6
    d. The patient is rotated obliquely by elevation of the left side 55 to 60 degrees, and the esophagus is centered to the image receptor at the level of T5 or T6
91. For a PA projection of the stomach:
    a. Center midway between the xiphoid process and the umbilicus
    b. Center halfway between the midline and lateral border of abdominal cavity
    c. Center midway between the manubrium and the umbilicus and halfway between the midline and lateral border of abdominal cavity
    d. Center midway between the xiphoid process and the umbilicus and halfway between the midline and lateral border of the abdominal cavity
92. For the LPO or RPO positions for the colon:
    a. The patient is prone, rotated 35 to 45 degrees, with the central ray at the level of the iliac crest
    b. The patient is supine, rotated 55 to 60 degrees, with the central ray at the level of ASIS

c. The patient is supine, rotated 35 to 45 degrees from AP, with the central ray at the level of the iliac crest
    d. The patient is prone, rotated 55 to 60 degrees, with the central ray at the level of the iliac crest
93. For a lateral decubitus position of the colon:
    a. The patient is lying on one side, the cassette is centered to the iliac crest, and the central ray is horizontal to the midline at the level of the iliac crest
    b. The patient is prone, the cassette is centered to the iliac crest, and the central ray is horizontal to the midline at the level of the iliac crest
    c. The patient is lying on one side, the cassette is centered 3 inches above the iliac crest, and the central ray is horizontal 3 inches above the iliac crest
    d. The patient is prone, the cassette is centered to L1, and the central ray is horizontal to L1
94. A procedure used to evaluate biliary and pancreatic pathological conditions with an endoscope is:
    a. Ultrasound
    b. MRI
    c. ERCP
    d. IVP
95. What condition is characterized by fluid-filled masses in the kidney?
    a. Polycystic kidney disease
    b. Renal calculus
    c. Wilms' tumor
    d. Renal cysts
96. Which of the following is a malignant cancer of the kidney?
    a. Polycystic kidney disease
    b. Renal calculus
    c. Wilms' tumor
    d. Renal cysts
97. What condition includes enlarged kidneys containing numerous cysts?
    a. Polycystic kidney disease
    b. Renal calculus
    c. Wilms' tumor
    d. Renal cysts
98. Which of the following conditions is seen primarily in children?
    a. Polycystic kidney disease
    b. Renal calculus
    c. Wilms' tumor
    d. Renal cysts
99. What describes a kidney stone?
    a. Polycystic kidney disease
    b. Renal calculus
    c. Wilms' tumor
    d. Renal cysts
100. For RPO and LPO positions of the kidneys:
    a. The patient is prone, the body is rotated obliquely 30 degrees, the kidney farther from the image

receptor is imaged in profile and the kidney nearer the image receptor is imaged in its entirety, and the central ray is perpendicular

b. The patient is supine, the body is rotated obliquely 45 degrees, the kidney farther from the image receptor is imaged in profile and the kidney nearer the image receptor is imaged in its entirety, and the central ray is perpendicular

c. The patient is supine, the body is rotated obliquely 30 degrees, the kidney farther from the image receptor is imaged parallel to the image receptor and the kidney nearer the image receptor is imaged perpendicular to the image receptor, and the central ray is perpendicular to the image receptor

d. The patient is supine, the body is rotated obliquely 30 degrees, the kidney nearer the image receptor is imaged in profile and the kidney farther from the image receptor is imaged in its entirety, and the central ray is perpendicular

Review of Patient Care and Education

The difference between a successful person and others is not a lack of strength, not a lack of knowledge, but rather a lack of will.

BASIC PATIENT CARE TERMINOLOGY

Verbal communication speaking using clear, concise language understood by the patient

Nonverbal communication communicating with facial expressions, eye contact, or body motions

Diversity factors that distinguish humans from one another, including age, gender, race or ethnicity, sexual preference, traditional versus nontraditional families, nuclear versus extended families, marital status, socioeconomic background, political beliefs, religious beliefs, geographic origin or residence, generation, physical or mental disability

Patient education providing the patient with information regarding the procedure being performed, other imaging procedures, or other medical center services

Torts personal injury law

Assault action that causes fear or apprehension in the patient

Battery inappropriate touching or harm done to the patient

False imprisonment unjustified restraint

Invasion of privacy violation of any aspect of patient confidentiality

Libel written defamation of character

Slander spoken defamation of character

Negligence unintentionally omitting reasonable care

Respondeat superior an employer is responsible for the employee's actions

Res ipsa loquitur cause of the negligence is obvious

Implied consent assumes the patient would approve of care if conscious

Informed consent patient provides consent after being fully informed of need, risks, and alternatives

Patient bill of rights establishes rights for patients regarding diagnosis, treatment, privacy, prognosis, and alternatives

Health Insurance Portability and Accountability Act (HIPAA) establishes legal regulations regarding confidentiality of patient records

Do not resuscitate order (DNR) no code

Advance directive document used by patient to provide directives regarding medical care before becoming incapacitated

Durable power of attorney patient provides for another person (personal representative) to make decisions regarding medical care if the patient is unable to communicate

Patient history provides information for the radiographer about the extent of a patient's injury and the range of motion the patient can tolerate

Medical asepsis microorganisms have been eliminated as much as possible

Surgical asepsis complete removal of all organisms from equipment and environment

Standard precautions first tier of transmission-based isolation precautions; uses barriers to prevent contact with blood, all body fluids, nonintact skin, and mucous membranes when there is a chance infection could be transmitted

Airborne precautions respiratory protection required for individuals entering a patient's room

Droplet precautions masks required for persons coming in close contact with a patient

Contact precautions masks, gloves, and gowns required for individuals coming in contact with a patient

Direct contact transmission infected person touches susceptible host

Indirect contact transmission inanimate object containing pathogenic organisms is placed in contact with a susceptible person

Airborne transmission droplets and dust

Droplet transmission primarily transmission by coughs, sneezes, or other methods of spraying onto a nearby host

Common vehicle transmission primarily transmission by contaminated items such as food, water, medications, devices, and equipment

Vectorborne transmission an animal contains and transmits an infectious organism to humans

Handwashing most effective method to prevent the spread of infection

Infection control barriers gloves, protective clothing, masks, eye protection

Temperature normal adult oral temperature is 98° F to 99° F

Pulse normal adult pulse is 60 beats per minute

Tachycardia heart rate more than 100 beats per minute

Bradycardia heart rate less than 60 beats per minute

Respiration normal adult rate is 12 to 16 breaths per minute

Blood pressure normal adult blood pressure is 120/80 mm Hg

Sphygmomanometer device used to measure blood pressure

Systolic pressure measurement of the pumping action of the heart

Diastolic pressure measurement of the heart at rest

Oxygen administration usual oxygen flow rate is 3 to 5 L per minute

Suction unit used to maintain patient's airway

Cardiac arrest cessation of heart function

Crash cart used in cardiac arrest; contains medications, airways, sphygmomanometers, stethoscopes, defibrillators, cardiac monitors

Respiratory arrest cessation of breathing

Shock failure of circulation in which blood pressure is inadequate to oxygenate tissues and remove by-products of metabolism

Hypovolemic shock follows loss of a large amount of blood or plasma

Septic shock occurs when toxins produced during massive infection

cause a dramatic decrease in blood pressure

Neurogenic shock causes blood to pool in peripheral vessels

Cardiogenic shock secondary to cardiac failure or other interference with heart function

Allergic shock (anaphylaxis) allergic reaction to foreign proteins after injection of an iodinated contrast agent

Trauma serious and potentially life-threatening injuries

Ventilators mechanical respirators attached to tracheostomies

Nasogastric (NG) tubes tube inserted through the nose and down the esophagus into the stomach

Chest tube tube placed to remove fluid or air from the pleural space

Negative contrast agent most commonly used negative contrast agent is air

Positive contrast agent iodine or barium

Aqueous iodine compound water-soluble sterile contrast agent

Iodinated ionic contrast agents salts of organic iodine compounds; composed of positively and negatively charged ions

Iodinated nonionic contrast agents agents that do not ionize into separate positive and negative charges

Anaphylactic reactions flushing, hives, nausea

Cardiovascular reactions hypotension, tachycardia, cardiac arrest

Psychogenic factors may be caused by patient anxiety

Hypodermic needle gauge unit of measurement that indicates diameter; the larger the gauge, the smaller the diameter of the needle opening

Intravenous (IV) catheter combination unit with a needle inside a flexible plastic catheter

Biohazardous materials—possible routes of entry inhalation, swallowing, absorption through the skin or mucous membranes

Material safety data sheets (MSDS) provide direction for handling precautions, safe use of the product, cleanup and disposal of biohazardous materials

PPE personal protective equipment

OSHA Occupational Safety and Health Administration

COMMUNICATION WITH THE PATIENT

A. Importance of clear communication
1. Establishes a respectful and professional relationship with the patient
2. Provides an accurate explanation of the examination
3. Helps the patient feel more comfortable to ask questions
4. Shows respect for the patient
5. Demonstrates a professional demeanor on the part of the radiographer

B. Verbal communication
1. Verbal communication must be clear and distinct
2. Terms used must be in a language the patient can understand
3. Care must be taken that a "difficult day" for the radiographer does not enter the tone of verbal communication with the patient; that is, the radiographer should always be aware of the tone of voice being used to communicate
4. Verbal communication implies that the radiographer should also possess excellent listening skills to interpret properly what the patient is saying

C. Nonverbal communication
1. The radiographer must be continually aware of how facial expressions or other body motions may be interpreted
2. Words may be saying one thing, but nonverbal actions may be communicating an entirely different attitude toward the patient
3. The use of touch must be appropriate and never open to uncertainty or miscommunication
4. Nonverbal communication, including eye contact, must be respectful of the patient's age and ethnicity
5. The radiographer must be a good listener

D. Diversity in medical imaging
1. The radiographer must be aware of the extensive diversity of patients
2. Respect for diversity is vital in the performance of medical imaging
3. Diversity may include any of, or any combination of, the following factors
   a. Age
   b. Gender
   c. Race or ethnicity
   d. Sexual preference
   e. Traditional versus nontraditional families
   f. Nuclear versus extended families

g. Marital status

h. Socioeconomic background

i. Political beliefs

j. Religious beliefs

k. Geographic origin or residence

l. Generation

m. Physical or mental disability

n. Language

4. The radiographer must be fully aware that the patient population is composed of infinite diversity in infinite combinations

E. Patient education

1. Patient education is part of the radiographer's scope of practice

2. The radiographer must be able to explain to the patient, in words the patient understands, the imaging procedure being performed

3. Patient education includes answering questions from the patient regarding the procedure

4. The radiographer should also be able to answer basic questions regarding other imaging modalities, such as the following:

a. Mammography

b. Nuclear medicine

c. Angiography

d. CT

e. MRI

f. Bone densitometry

g. Ultrasound

h. Positron emission tomography (PET)

5. The radiographer should be able to answer basic questions, or provide directions to the patient, regarding other medical center services, such as the following

a. Social services

b. Discharge planning

c. Pastoral care

d. Rehabilitation

e. Business office

f. Other medical departments

KEY REVIEW POINTS

Communication with the Patient

- Clear and comfortable communication—establishing this with the patient is of paramount importance
- Verbal communication—must be clear and in a language the patient understands
- Nonverbal communication—conveys the radiographer's attitude and demeanor
- Diversity—the radiographer must be aware of age, gender, race or ethnicity, sexual preference, traditional versus nontraditional families, nuclear versus extended families, marital status, socioeconomic background, political beliefs, religious beliefs, geographic origin or residence, generation, physical or mental disability

---

- Patient education—the radiographer must understand the role of patient educator and be prepared to answer basic questions regarding mammography, nuclear medicine, angiography, CT, MRI, bone densitometry, ultrasound, social services, discharge planning, pastoral care, rehabilitation, business office, other medical departments

---

MEDICOLEGAL ASPECTS OF PRACTICE

A. Torts

1. Violations of civil law

2. Also known as *personal injury law*

3. Injured parties have a right to compensation for injury

B. Intentional misconduct

1. Assault

a. Patient is apprehensive about being injured

b. Imprudent conduct of radiographer that causes fear in patient is grounds for an allegation of civil assault

2. Battery

a. Unlawful touching or touching without consent

b. Harm resulting from physical contact with radiographer

c. May also include radiographing the wrong patient or the wrong body part or performing radiography against a patient's will

3. False imprisonment

a. Unjustified restraint of a person

b. Care must be taken when using restraint straps or having other individuals assist with holding a patient still

4. Invasion of privacy

a. Violation of confidentiality of information

b. Unnecessarily or improperly exposing the patient's body

c. Unnecessarily or improperly touching a patient's body

d. Photographing patients without their permission

5. *Libel:* Written information that results in defamation of character or loss of reputation

6. *Slander:* Orally spreading false information that results in defamation of character or loss of reputation

C. Unintentional misconduct (negligence)

1. Neglect or omission of reasonable care

2. Based on doctrine of the reasonably prudent person

3. *Reasonably prudent person doctrine:* Based on how a reasonable person with similar education and experience would perform under similar circumstances

4. *Gross negligence:* Acts that show reckless disregard for life or limb

5. *Contributory negligence:* Instance in which the injured person is a contributing party to the injury

D. Four conditions needed to establish malpractice
 1. Establishment of standard of care
 2. Demonstration that standard of care was violated by the radiographer
 3. Demonstration that loss or injury was caused by radiographer who is being sued
 4. Demonstration that loss or injury actually occurred and is a result of the negligence

E. *Respondeat superior*
 1. "Let the master answer"
 2. Legal doctrine stating that an employer is held liable for an employee's negligent act

F. *Rule of personal responsibility:* Individuals are responsible for their own actions

G. *Res ipsa loquitur*
 1. "The thing speaks for itself"
 2. Legal doctrine stating that cause of the negligence is obvious (e.g., forceps left inside a patient during surgery)

H. Charting
 1. Writing on the patient's chart by radiographer
 2. Varies by institution
 3. Radiographer's responsibilities in this regard must be carefully outlined during new employee orientation
 4. Write clear statements regarding patient's condition, reaction to contrast agents, and amount of contrast material injected
 5. Must be clearly stated on the chart
 6. Information must also include the date and time of the occurrence
 7. Radiographer must sign chart entries using full name and credentials
 8. In case of error, strike over once and rewrite correct entry; never erase or obscure erroneous information

I. Radiographs
 1. Radiographs are legal documents
 2. Radiographs must include the following information
   a. Patient identification
   b. Anatomical markings, including left and right markers
   c. Carefully placed markings on each radiograph using lead markers
   d. Date of exposure
   e. Other markings (e.g., with stickers, grease pencils) applied to the radiograph after processing may not be legally admissible
 3. Retention of radiographs
   a. Varies according to state law
   b. Normally maintained for 5 to 7 years after the date of the last radiographic examination (mammograms and black lung images are kept for the life span of the patient)
   c. Film folders on minors are normally retained for 5 to 7 years after the minor reaches age 18 or 21, depending on the state of residence

 4. Careful documentation must be maintained when radiographs are checked out for use by physicians, students, or other health care practitioners

J. Patient's rights
 1. Patient's bill of rights from the American Hospital Association provides for patient consent or refusal of any procedure; the patient has the right to the following:
   a. Respectful care
   b. Obtain up-to-date and understandable medical information regarding diagnosis, treatment, and likely outcomes
   c. Be involved in the decision-making process throughout diagnosis and treatment
   d. Have an advance directive (living will, health care proxy, durable power of attorney) on file
   e. Privacy in all aspects of diagnosis and treatment
   f. Complete confidentiality
   g. View medical records of the case
   h. Expect that a hospital will respond to a request for needed care and services
   i. Be informed of business or educational relationships that may affect treatment and care
   j. Consent to or decline participation in research studies
   k. Continuity of care and other options for care beyond the hospital
   l. Be informed of hospital policies and procedures related to diagnosis and treatment
   m. Be informed of all resources available for resolving disputes
   n. Be informed of charges for services and payment options
 2. Implied consent
   a. Provides for care when patient is unconscious
   b. Based on assumption that patient would approve care if conscious
 3. Valid consent
   a. Also called *informed consent*
   b. Patient must be mentally competent
   c. Consent must be offered voluntarily
   d. Patient must be adequately informed
   e. Patient must be of legal age
   f. Requires that radiographer or radiologist carefully explain all aspects of procedure and risks involved
   g. Requires that explanation be provided in lay terms the patient understands
 4. Health Insurance Portability and Accountability Act (HIPAA)
   a. Passed by U.S. Congress and enacted under rules and regulations of U.S. Department of Health and Human Services
   b. Hospitals must put in place policies and procedures regarding the release of patient information
   c. Patient must provide clear permission for release of any information to outside parties (e.g., medical, financial, employment)

d. Patient must be informed in writing of how the released information will be used

e. Patient must be allowed to view and copy records and amend records as needed

f. Any history of information sharing must be disclosed to the patient

g. Patient must freely provide consent for information to be shared

h. Patient has the right to restrict sharing of information

i. Patient may file a complaint regarding a violation of HIPAA

5. Do not resuscitate order (DNR)
   a. Also called *no code*
   b. May be placed on file when the quality of life has seriously declined or the patient's condition is terminal
   c. Agreement is between the physician and the patient (or the designated person holding power of attorney if the patient is incompetent)
   d. The agreement or appropriate notation is made on the patient's chart

6. Advance directive
   a. Patient provides directives regarding medical care before becoming incapacitated
   b. Patient may do this so that directions are in place should the patient be unable to communicate wishes regarding care
   c. Copies should be provided to physician, attorney, family member, and medical record

7. Durable power of attorney
   a. Patient provides for another person (personal representative) to make decisions regarding medical care if the patient is unable to communicate
   b. This personal representative may sign informed consent forms for the patient
   c. The patient and personal representative should communicate clearly ahead of time the patient's thoughts regarding extraordinary methods of treatment and end-of-life wishes

K. American Registry of Radiologic Technologists (ARRT) Mission and Standards of Ethics
   1. The accompanying box contains the ARRT Mission Statement and Standards of Ethics, including the preamble, code of ethics, and rules of ethics
   2. The Standards of Ethics promote the goals of the Mission Statement
   3. The Standards of Ethics comprise the Code of Ethics and the Rules of Ethics

---

AMERICAN REGISTRY OF RADIOLOGIC TECHNOLOGISTS (ARRT) MISSION STATEMENT AND RULES OF ETHICS (NOT INCLUDING CODE OF ETHICS)

Mission
The American Registry of Radiologic Technologists promotes high standards of patient care by recognizing qualified individuals in medical imaging, interventional procedures, and radiation therapy.

ARRT Standards of Ethics
Preamble
The Standards of Ethics of the ARRT shall apply solely to persons holding certificates from ARRT who either hold current registrations by ARRT or formerly held registrations by ARRT (collectively, "Registered Technologists" or "Registered Radiologist Assistants"), and to persons applying for examination and certification by ARRT in order to become Registered Technologists ("Candidates"). "Radiologic Technology" is an umbrella term that is inclusive of the disciplines of radiography, nuclear medicine technology, radiation therapy, cardiovascular-interventional radiography, mammography, computed tomography, magnetic resonance imaging, quality management, sonography, bone densitometry, vascular sonography, cardiac-interventional radiography, vascular-interventional radiography, breast sonography, and radiologist assistant. The Standards of Ethics are intended to be consistent with the Mission Statement of ARRT and to promote the goals set forth in the Mission Statement.

Rules of Ethics
The Rules of Ethics form the second part of the Standards of Ethics. They are mandatory standards of minimally acceptable professional conduct for all present Registered Technologists, Registered Radiologist Assistants, and Candidates. Certification is a method of assuring the medical community and the public that an individual is qualified to practice within the profession.

Because the public relies on certificates and registrations issued by ARRT, it is essential that Registered Technologists and Candidates act consistently with these Rules of Ethics. These Rules of Ethics are intended to promote the protection, safety, and comfort of patients. The Rules of Ethics are enforceable. Registered Technologists, Registered Radiologist Assistants, and Candidates engaging in any of the following conduct or activities, or who permit the occurrence of the following conduct or activities with respect to them, have violated the Rules of Ethics and are subject to sanctions as described hereunder:

1. Employing fraud or deceit in procuring or attempting to procure, maintain, renew, or obtain reinstatement of certification or registration as issued by ARRT; employment in radiologic technology; or a state permit, license, or registration certificate to practice radiologic technology. This includes altering in any respect any document issued by the ARRT or any state or federal agency, or by indicating in writing certification or registration with the ARRT when that is not the case.

2. Subverting or attempting to subvert ARRT's examination process. Conduct that subverts or attempts to subvert ARRT's examination process includes, but is not limited to:

(i) conduct that violates the security of ARRT examination materials, such as removing or attempting to remove examination materials from an examination room, or having unauthorized possession of any portion of or information concerning a future, current, or previously administered examination of ARRT; or disclosing information concerning any portion of a future, current, or previously administered examination of ARRT; or disclosing what purports to be, or under all circumstances is likely to be understood by the recipient as, any portion of or "inside" information concerning any portion of a future, current, or previously administered examination of ARRT;

Continued

(ii) conduct that in any way compromises ordinary standards of test administration, such as communicating with another Candidate during administration of the examination, copying another Candidate's answers, permitting another Candidate to copy one's answers, or possessing unauthorized materials; or

(iii) impersonating a Candidate or permitting an impersonator to take the examination on one's own behalf.

3. Convictions, criminal proceedings, or military court-martials as described below:

   (i) Conviction of a crime, including a felony, a gross misdemeanor, or a misdemeanor, with the sole exception of speeding and parking violations. All alcohol and/or drug related violations must be reported. Offenses that occurred while a juvenile and that are processed through the juvenile court system are not required to be reported to ARRT.

   (ii) Criminal proceeding where a finding or verdict of guilt is made or returned but the adjudication of guilt is either withheld, deferred, or not entered or the sentence is suspended or stayed; or a criminal proceeding where the individual enters a plea of guilty or *nolo contendere* (no contest).

   (iii) Military court-martials that involve substance abuse, any sex-related infractions, or patient-related infractions.

4. Failure to report to the ARRT that:

   (i) charges regarding the person's permit, license, or registration certificate to practice radiologic technology or any other medical or allied health profession are pending or have been resolved adversely to the individual in any state, territory, or country (including, but not limited to, imposed conditions, probation, suspension, or revocation); or

   (ii) the individual has been refused a permit, license, or registration certificate to practice radiologic technology or any other medical or allied health profession by another state, territory, or country.

5. Failure or inability to perform radiologic technology with reasonable skill and safety.

6. Engaging in unprofessional conduct, including, but not limited to:

   (i) a departure from or failure to conform to applicable federal, state, or local governmental rules regarding radiologic technology practice; or, if no such rule exists, to the minimal standards of acceptable and prevailing radiologic technology practice;

   (ii) any radiologic technology practice that may create unnecessary danger to a patient's life, health, or safety; or

   (iii) any practice that is contrary to the ethical conduct appropriate to the profession that results in the termination from employment. Actual injury to a patient or the public need not be established under this clause.

7. Delegating or accepting the delegation of a radiologic technology function or any other prescribed health care function when the delegation or acceptance could reasonably be expected to create an unnecessary danger to a patient's life, health, or safety. Actual injury to a patient need not be established under this clause.

8. Actual or potential inability to practice radiologic technology with reasonable skill and safety to patients by reason of illness; use of alcohol, drugs, chemicals, or any other material; or as a result of any mental or physical condition.

9. Adjudication as mentally incompetent, mentally ill, a chemically dependent person, or a person dangerous to the public, by a court of competent jurisdiction.

10. Engaging in any unethical conduct, including, but not limited to, conduct likely to deceive, defraud, or harm the public; or demonstrating a willful or careless disregard for the health, welfare, or safety of a patient. Actual injury need not be established under this clause.

11. Engaging in conduct with a patient that is sexual or may reasonably be interpreted by the patient as sexual, or in any verbal behavior that is seductive or sexually demeaning to a patient; or engaging in sexual exploitation of a patient or former patient. This also applies to any unwanted sexual behavior, verbal or otherwise, that results in the termination of employment. This rule does not apply to preexisting consensual relationships.

12. Revealing a privileged communication from or relating to a former or current patient except when otherwise required or permitted by law.

13. Knowingly engaging or assisting any person to engage in, or otherwise participating in, abusive or fraudulent billing practices, including violations of federal Medicare and Medicaid laws or state medical assistance laws.

14. Improper management of patient records, including failure to maintain adequate patient records or to furnish a patient record or report required by law; or making, causing, or permitting anyone to make false, deceptive, or misleading entry in any patient record.

15. Knowingly aiding, assisting, advising, or allowing a person without a current and appropriate state permit, license, or registration certificate or a current certificate of registration with ARRT to engage in the practice of radiologic technology, in a jurisdiction which requires a person to have such a current and appropriate state permit, license, or registration certificate or a current and appropriate registration of certification with ARRT in order to practice radiologic technology in such jurisdiction.

16. Violating a rule adopted by any state board with competent jurisdiction, an order of such board, or state or federal law relating to the practice of radiologic technology, or any other medical or allied health professions, or a state or federal narcotics or controlled-substance law.

17. Knowingly providing false or misleading information that is directly related to the care of a former or current patient.

18. Practicing outside the scope of practice authorized by the individual's current state permit, license, or registration certificate, or the individual's current certificate of registration with ARRT.

19. Making a false statement or knowingly providing false information to ARRT or failing to cooperate with any investigation by ARRT or the Ethics Committee.

20. Engaging in false, fraudulent, deceptive, or misleading communications to any person regarding the individual's education, training, credentials, experience, or qualifications, or the status of the individual's state permit, license, or registration certificate in radiologic technology or certificate of registration with ARRT.

21. Knowing of a violation or a probable violation of any Rule of Ethics by any Registered Technologist, Registered Radiologist Assistant, or Candidate and failing to promptly report in writing the same to the ARRT.

22. Failing to immediately report to his or her supervisor information concerning an error made in connection with imaging, treating, or caring for a patient. For purposes of this rule, errors include any departure from the standard of care that reasonably may be considered to be potentially harmful, unethical, or improper (commission). Errors also include behavior that is negligent or should have occurred in connection with a patient's care, but did not (omission). The duty to report under this rule exists whether or not the patient suffered any injury.

4. The Code of Ethics serves as a guide to professional conduct (not included here)
5. The Rules of Ethics are mandatory and enforceable and carry sanctions for violations
6. The Standards of Ethics also include a section addressing administrative procedures, not included here (for details, visit www.arrt.org)

▢ KEY REVIEW POINTS
Medicolegal Aspects of Practice

- *Torts:* Violations of civil law; personal injury law
- *Intentional misconduct:* Assault (patient is apprehensive about being injured)
- *Intentional misconduct:* Battery (unlawful touching or touching without consent); may also include radiographing the wrong patient or wrong body part or performing radiography against a patient's will
- *Intentional misconduct:* False imprisonment (unjustified restraint of a person)
- *Intentional misconduct:* Invasion of privacy (violation of confidentiality of information; unnecessary or improper exposure or touching of the patient's body)
- *Intentional misconduct:* Libel (written information that results in defamation of character or loss of reputation)
- *Intentional misconduct:* Slander (orally spreading false information that results in defamation of character or loss of reputation)
- *Unintentional misconduct:* Negligence (neglect or omission of reasonable care)
- *Unintentional misconduct:* Based on doctrine of the reasonably prudent person
- *Reasonably prudent person doctrine:* How a reasonable person with similar education and experience would perform under similar circumstances
- *Gross negligence:* Acts that demonstrate reckless disregard for life or limb
- *Four conditions needed to establish malpractice: (1)* Establishment of standard of care; *(2)* demonstration that standard of care was violated by the radiographer; *(3)* demonstration that loss or injury was caused by radiographer who is being sued; *(4)* demonstration that loss or injury actually occurred and is a result of the negligence
- *Respondeat superior ("Let the master answer"):* Legal doctrine stating that an employer is held liable for an employee's negligent act
- *Res ipsa loquitur ("The thing speaks for itself"):* Legal doctrine stating that cause of the negligence is obvious (e.g., forceps left inside a patient during surgery)
- *Charting:* Writing of clear statements regarding the patient's condition, reaction to contrast agents, and amount of contrast material injected
- *Radiographs:* Legal documents; must include patient identification, anatomical markings (including left and right markers), and date of exposure
- *Patient's rights:* Patient bill of rights provides for patient's consent to or refusal of any procedure and access to appropriate medical information; allows for advance directive

- *Implied consent:* Provides for care when patient is unconscious
- *Valid consent:* Patient must be mentally competent; consent must be offered voluntarily; patient must be adequately informed; patient must be of legal age; requires radiographer and radiologist to explain carefully, in lay terms the patient understands, all aspects of procedure and risks involved; also called *informed consent*
- *Health Insurance Portability and Accountability Act (HIPAA):* Medical facilities must put in place policies and procedures regarding the release of patient information
- *Do not resuscitate (DNR) order:* May be placed on file when the quality of life has seriously declined or the patient's condition is terminal; also called *no code*
- *Advance directive:* Patient provides directives regarding medical care before becoming incapacitated
- *Durable power of attorney:* Patient provides for another person (personal representative) to make decisions regarding medical care if the patient is unable to communicate

---

SCHEDULING OF RADIOGRAPHIC EXAMINATIONS

A. General considerations
   1. Schedule in an appropriate and timely sequence to ensure patient comfort and fiscal responsibility
   2. Sequence so that examinations do not interfere with one another
   3. Schedule barium studies last
   4. Schedule several examinations in a single day if the patient is able to tolerate them
   5. Seriously ill or weak patients may be able to tolerate only one examination per day or must have a rest between examinations
   6. If sedation is used, patient must be given time to recover from sedation before beginning fluoroscopic studies
   7. Thyroid assessment must precede any examinations involving iodinated contrast media
   8. Schedule radiographic examinations not requiring contrast agents first
   9. Total doses of iodinated contrast media should be calculated if they are to be used in a series of examinations
   10. Schedule patients who have been held NPO (nothing by mouth) first
   11. Schedule pediatric and elderly patients early
   12. Schedule diabetic patients early because of their need for insulin
B. Sequence of examinations
   1. Fiberoptic (endoscopy) studies are conducted first in a series
   2. Radiography of the urinary tract
   3. Radiography of the biliary system

4. CT studies should be scheduled before examinations involving the use of barium sulfate
5. Lower gastrointestinal (GI) series (check for residual contrast material from previous examinations before proceeding)
6. Upper GI series

KEY REVIEW POINTS
Scheduling of Radiographic Examinations

- Schedule so that examinations do not interfere with one another, with barium studies last
- Schedule radiographic examinations not requiring contrast agents first
- Schedule patients who have been held NPO (nothing by mouth) first; schedule pediatric and geriatric patients early; schedule diabetic patients early because of their need for insulin
- *Sequence of examinations:* Fiberoptic (endoscopy) studies; radiography of the urinary tract; radiography of the biliary system; CT studies before examinations involving the use of barium sulfate; lower GI series; upper GI series

PATIENT PREPARATION

A. GI system or urinary system
1. Low-residue diet
2. NPO for 8 to 12 hours before procedure
3. Cathartics and enemas are used to cleanse the GI system
4. If scheduled as an outpatient
   a. Patient must clearly understand the routine for proper preparation
   b. Patient should be asked to explain the procedure back to the radiographer to verify understanding
B. All procedures
1. Clothing is removed from area to be radiographed and replaced by patient gown when appropriate
2. All radiopaque objects are removed from area of interest

KEY REVIEW POINTS
Patient Preparation

- *GI system or urinary system:* Low-residue diet; NPO for 8 to 12 hours before the procedure; cathartics and enemas used to cleanse GI system; patient must clearly understand the routine for proper preparation
- *All procedures:* Clothing removed from area to be radiographed; all radiopaque objects removed from area of interest

PATIENT HISTORY

A. Provides information for the radiographer about the extent of the patient's injury and the range of motion the patient can tolerate

B. Assists the radiologist during interpretation of the radiographs
C. History should begin with the radiographer introducing himself or herself and verifying the patient's name
D. Types of questions asked to obtain a patient's history (depending on type and site of injury)
1. How did your injury occur?
2. When did your injury occur?
3. Where is your pain?
4. Do you have tingling or numbness?
5. Do you have any weakness?
6. Were you unconscious after your injury?
7. Why did your physician order this examination?
8. Have you experienced shortness of breath or been coughing?
9. Have you experienced a fever or heart problems?
10. Have you experienced any nausea, vomiting, or diarrhea?
11. Have you had previous surgery on this area?
12. Is there any family history of problems in this area?

KEY REVIEW POINTS
Patient History

- *Purpose:* Provides information for the radiographer; assists the radiologist during interpretation of the radiographs
- *Types of questions asked to obtain a patient's history:* How did your injury occur? When did your injury occur? Where is your pain? Do you have tingling or numbness? Do you have any weakness? Were you unconscious after your injury? Why did your physician order this examination? Have you experienced shortness of breath or been coughing? Have you experienced a fever or heart problems? Have you experienced any nausea, vomiting, or diarrhea?

PATIENT TRANSFER

A. Check identification bracelet to ensure that correct patient is being transferred
B. Ask patient to state his or her name to double-check identity; ask date of birth as a backup
C. Explain the transfer procedure to the patient to gain cooperation and alleviate fear
D. The radiographer must always use proper body mechanics for patient transfer
1. Keep knees slightly bent
2. Keep back straight
3. Use legs, not back, to perform all lifting

TRANSFER FROM WHEELCHAIR TO X-RAY TABLE

A. Wheelchair is parallel to table
B. Brakes are applied with step stool nearby
C. Using face-to-face method, assist the patient to a standing position

D. Have patient place one hand on step stool handle, place the other hand on your shoulder, and step up onto the stool

E. Patient pivots with back against the table into a sitting position on the edge of the table

F. Place one arm around patient's shoulder and the other arm under the knees

G. Assist patient to a supine position

TRANSFER FROM X-RAY TABLE TO WHEELCHAIR

A. Check to see that brakes of wheelchair have been applied

B. Assist patient to a sitting position

C. Allow patient to sit up for a short time to regain sense of balance

D. Ambulatory patient
1. Assist to a standing position and pivot
2. Have patient reach back with both hands and grab arms of wheelchair
3. Assist patient to sit in the wheelchair

E. Nonambulatory patients
1. Stand facing the patient
2. Reach around patient and place your hands on each scapula
3. Lift patient upward to a standing position with your knees bent
4. Pivot so that the back of the patient's leg is touching the edge of the wheelchair; ensure the wheels on the wheelchair are locked
5. Ease patient down to a sitting position with your knees bent
6. Position foot and leg rests into place
7. Cover patient's lap with a sheet

CART TRANSFER

A. Place cart near and parallel to the x-ray table, and lock wheels

B. Do not attempt patient transfer from cart to x-ray table without assistance

C. One person supports the neck and shoulders at the head of the cart; the second person lifts the pelvis and knees; if available, other individuals support patient at both sides

D. Transfer sheet or draw sheet should be used under patient; a slide board should be used when available

E. On signal, all persons involved in transfer move patient in one fluid motion to the x-ray table

PATIENT COMFORT

A. Taking into account the patient's physical condition, carefully position pillows or radiolucent sponges so that they do not interfere with the examination

B. Evaluate patient's condition
1. Ability to breathe
2. Presence of nausea
3. Allow patient to remain partially upright when possible
4. Special care must be given to older patients, who may have decubitus ulcers or particularly sensitive or thin skin

KEY REVIEW POINTS
Patient Transfer

- Check identification bracelet to ensure that correct patient is being transferred
- Explain transfer procedure to patient to gain cooperation and alleviate fear
- Always use proper body mechanics
- Ensure all appropriate brakes are applied
- Make creative use of sheets and helpers when moving patient

INFECTION CONTROL

ROUTES OF TRANSMISSION

A. Contact transmission
1. *Direct contact:* Infected person touches susceptible host, allowing the infectious organisms to come in contact with susceptible tissues
2. *Indirect contact:* Inanimate object containing pathogenic organisms is placed in contact with susceptible person

B. *Airborne transmission:* Droplets and dust

C. *Droplet transmission:* Transmitted primarily by coughs, sneezes, or other methods of spraying onto a nearby host

D. *Common vehicle transmission:* Transmitted primarily by contaminated items such as food, water, medications, devices, and equipment

E. *Vectorborne transmission:* Animal or insect contains and transmits infectious organism to humans

STANDARD PRECAUTIONS

A. First tier of transmission-based isolation precautions

B. System that uses barriers to prevent contact with blood, all body fluids, nonintact skin, and mucous membranes if there is a chance of transmission of infection

C. Assumes all body fluids are sources of infection

D. Assumes all patients are infected

E. Guidelines
1. Always wear gloves when any chance of being in contact with body substances exists
2. Protect clothing by wearing a protective gown or plastic apron if a chance of coming in contact with body substances exists

3. Masks or eye protection must be worn if a chance of body substances splashing exists
4. Handwashing is the most effective method to prevent the spread of infection
5. Uncapped needle syringe units and all sharps must be discarded in biohazard containers
6. If any contact is made with body substances, the entire area contacted must be washed completely with bleach
7. Contaminated articles must be disposed of properly
8. Needles should never be recapped but should be placed with the syringe in a sharps container
9. Protective masks or mouthpieces should be used when performing cardiopulmonary resuscitation (CPR) if providing breaths in addition to chest compression.

MEDICAL ASEPSIS

A. Microorganisms have been eliminated as much as possible
B. Water and chemicals are used for the disinfection

SURGICAL ASEPSIS

A. Complete removal of all organisms from equipment and the environment in which patient care is conducted
B. Includes complete sterilization of equipment and appropriate skin preparation
    1. *Chemical sterilization:* Soaking objects in germicidal solution
    2. *Boiling:* Sterilization with moist heat
    3. *Dry heat:* Placing objects in an oven at temperatures greater than 300° F
    4. *Gas sterilization:* Items are exposed to a mixture of gases, which do not harm the materials
    5. *Autoclaving:* Steam sterilization under pressure; most convenient way to sterilize materials

STERILE TECHNIQUE

A. Steps to follow in opening sterile packs
    1. Place pack on a clean surface
    2. Break the seal and open the pack
    3. Unfold first corner of the pack away from you
    4. Unfold both sides
    5. Pull front portion of the wrap toward you and drop it
    6. Never touch the inner surface
    7. If there is an inner wrap, open it using the same method
    8. Separately wrapped sterile items may be added to the sterile field by opening the pack and allowing the items to drop onto the sterile field
    9. Never allow the container to touch the sterile field

B. Pouring liquids into containers in a sterile field
    1. Carefully determine the contents of the container
    2. Pour a small amount into a waste receptacle to cleanse the lip of the bottle
    3. Pour the medium into the receptacle, being careful not to touch the sterile field in the process
C. Sterile objects or fields touched by unsterile objects or persons are immediately contaminated
D. Avoid reaching across sterile fields
E. If you suspect that an object is contaminated, assume that it is contaminated
F. Always assume that damp items are contaminated
G. Do not invade the space between a physician and the sterile field
H. Never abandon a sterile field; it must be under direct observation at all times
I. Never turn your back on a sterile field
J. *Remember:* Only from your waist up and in front is sterile

GLOVING

A. Wash hands thoroughly
B. Open outer package containing gloves
C. Open inner package, exposing gloves
D. Approach glove from open end, and touch only inner surface with opposite hand
E. Put on glove, touching only the folded cuff
F. Pick up other glove with gloved hand under the cuff
G. Place second glove on other hand, and unfold cuff
H. Carefully unfold cuff on both gloves
I. Always keep hands in front of the body without touching body covering or placing hands under arms

TYPES OF ISOLATION PRECAUTIONS

A. Transmission-based precautions
    1. Airborne precautions
        a. Respiratory protection required for individuals entering patient's room
        b. Gowns required to prevent contamination of clothing
        c. Use of standard precautions
    2. Droplet precautions
        a. Masks required for persons coming in close contact with patient
        b. Use of standard precautions
    3. Contact precautions
        a. Masks, gloves, and gowns are indicated for individuals coming in contact with patient
        b. Use of standard precautions
B. Empirical use
    1. Routine use of standard precautions
    2. Each patient condition is evaluated
    3. Appropriate isolation precaution guidelines are put in place

ISOLATION TECHNIQUE

Mobile Radiography

A. If protective cap is indicated, it should be put on and all hair should be tucked inside

B. Mask should be put on next, completely covering the nose and mouth

C. Gown should be put on and tied securely at the back and neck

D. Gloves should be put on and pulled over the end of the sleeve of the gown

E. Radiographic IR should be placed in a protective plastic cover

F. Enter patient's room and follow all isolation guidelines that have been posted

G. When possible, have a second "clean" radiographer handle the portable x-ray machine and controls while the first "dirty" radiographer touches only the patient

H. After the radiographic exposure is made
1. Remove IR from the vicinity of the patient
2. Open the end of the protective covering
3. "Clean" radiographer handling the equipment should remove cassette from the open end of the cover

I. When leaving the patient's isolation room, carefully remove attire and leave it in room
1. Untie waist belt of protective gown
2. Remove gloves
   a. Pull off one glove by grasping the cuff and inverting it as it is pulled off
   b. Remove second glove by inserting clean fingers inside the cuff and inverting it as it is removed
3. Untie neck and back strings from gown
4. Remove mask by using strings only
5. Remove gown by holding it away from the body as it is removed
6. Carefully wash hands
7. Use paper towels to touch faucet handles
8. After portable x-ray unit is moved safely outside the room, it should be cleaned thoroughly before it is returned to the radiology department

Patients in Radiology Departments

A. Identify isolation category and follow guidelines

B. Isolation patients should never spend time waiting in the hallway

C. Carefully cover x-ray table with a sheet

D. Work in pairs so that only one radiographer is in contact with the patient while the other radiographer manipulates the equipment

E. Carefully cover patient with protective sheets and blankets when returning patient to the wheelchair or cart

F. All contaminated materials must be placed in an appropriate discard bag

G. Carefully clean off x-ray table and any other equipment with which the patient came in contact

H. Remove gloves and carefully wash hands

📱 KEY REVIEW POINTS
Infection Control

- *Routes of transmission:* May be direct or indirect
- *Direct contact:* Infected person touches susceptible host, allowing infectious organisms to come in contact with susceptible tissues
- *Indirect contact:* Inanimate object containing pathogenic organisms is placed in contact with susceptible person
- *Airborne transmission:* Droplets and dust
- *Droplet transmission:* Transmitted primarily by coughs, sneezes, or other methods of spraying onto a nearby host
- *Common vehicle transmission:* Transmitted primarily by contaminated items such as food, water, medications, devices, and equipment
- *Vectorborne transmission:* Animal contains and transmits an infectious organism to humans
- *Standard precautions:* System that uses barriers to prevent contact with blood, all body fluids, nonintact skin, and mucous membranes of all individuals and susceptible persons; assumes all body fluids are sources of infection; assumes all patients are infected
- *Gloves:* Should always be worn
- *Protective gown:* Wear to protect clothing
- *Masks or eye protection:* Must be worn if there is a chance that body substances will be splashed
- *Protective masks or mouthpieces:* Wear when performing CPR
- *Handwashing:* Most effective method to prevent spread of infection
- *Uncapped needle syringe units and all sharps:* Must be discarded in biohazard containers
- *Medical asepsis:* Microorganisms have been eliminated as much as possible
- *Surgical asepsis:* Complete removal of all organisms
- *Chemical sterilization:* Soaking of objects in germicidal solution
- *Boiling:* Sterilization with moist heat
- *Dry heat:* Placing objects in an oven at temperatures greater than 300° F
- *Gas sterilization:* Items are exposed to a mixture of gases, which do not harm the materials
- *Autoclaving:* Steam sterilization under pressure; most convenient way to sterilize materials
- *Sterile technique:* Several steps required to maintain integrity of sterile field; review each step and be able to place them in order
- *Gloving:* Several steps required for proper gloving; review each step and be able to place them in order
- *Transmission-based precautions:* Airborne precautions; droplet precautions; contact precautions
- *Isolation technique during mobile radiography:* Specific steps are required; know each step and the order in which steps occur
- *Isolation technique in the imaging department:* Specific steps are required; know each step and the order in which steps occur

ASSESSMENT OF CHANGING PATIENT CONDITIONS

A. Visual observation of patient
B. Changes in skin color to cyanotic or waxen pallor
C. Patient verbalizations of discomfort or dizziness
D. Cyanosis of lips or nail beds
E. Patient is cool and diaphoretic to touch

VITAL SIGNS

A. *Temperature:* Normal oral temperature is 98° F to 99° F
B. Pulse
  1. Taken at radial or carotid artery
  2. *Tachycardia:* More than 100 beats per minute
  3. *Bradycardia:* Less than 60 beats per minute
C. *Respiration:* Normal respiratory rate is 12 to 16 breaths per minute
D. Blood pressure
  1. Measured with sphygmomanometer
  2. *Systolic pressure:* Measurement of pumping action of the heart
  3. *Diastolic pressure:* Measures the blood pressure of the heart at rest
  4. Diastolic pressure greater than 90 mm Hg indicates increasing level of hypertension
  5. Diastolic pressure less than 50 mm Hg gives some indication of shock
  6. Always expressed as systolic pressure over diastolic pressure (e.g., 120/80 mm Hg)

MEDICAL EMERGENCIES

A. Oxygen administration
  1. Generally administered via a mask or nasal cannula
  2. Usual oxygen flow rate is 3 to 5 L/minute
  3. Care must be taken while radiographing patients who are on portable oxygen support; avoid pinching or kinking oxygen tubing
  4. Radiographers must know how to operate oxygen tanks or wall oxygen outlets so that they can administer oxygen to a patient in the event of an emergency
B. Suction unit
  1. Used to maintain patient's airway
  2. Must be used anytime the airway becomes obstructed by fluids
  3. If the radiographer is working alone and the patient's airway needs suctioning, the radiographer should call for help before beginning procedure
C. Cardiac arrest
  1. Cessation of heart function
  2. Specific routine for announcing cardiac arrest must be followed
  3. Emergency medical assistance must be called immediately
  4. CPR must begin immediately
  5. Radiographer must be familiar with location and contents of crash cart
    a. Medications
    b. Airways
    c. Sphygmomanometers
    d. Stethoscopes
    e. Defibrillators
    f. Cardiac monitors
D. Respiratory arrest
  1. Cessation of breathing
  2. Possible causes of respiratory arrest
    a. Upper respiratory tract swelling
    b. Failure of the central nervous system
    c. Choking
  3. Tracheolaryngeal edema
    a. Tracheolaryngeal edema may follow injection of iodinated contrast material
    b. May necessitate an emergency tracheotomy
    c. Radiographer should know location of tracheotomy tray
  4. Respiratory arrest caused by central nervous system failure necessitates calling a respiratory arrest code
  5. Respiratory arrest secondary to choking necessitates use of suction or the Heimlich maneuver
E. Shock
  1. Failure of circulation in which blood pressure is inadequate to oxygenate tissues and remove by-products of metabolism
  2. *Hypovolemic shock:* Follows loss of large amount of blood or plasma
  3. *Septic shock:* Occurs when toxins produced during massive infection cause a dramatic decrease in blood pressure
  4. *Neurogenic shock:* Causes blood to pool in peripheral vessels
  5. *Cardiogenic shock:* Results from cardiac failure or other interference with heart function
  6. Allergic shock (anaphylaxis)
    a. Allergic reaction to foreign proteins after injections
    b. Marked by extremely low pressure, dyspnea, and possible death
    c. May follow injection of iodinated contrast media
  7. Symptoms of shock
    a. Restlessness, apprehension
    b. Accelerated pulse
    c. Pale skin
    d. Weakness

e. Alteration in ability to think

f. Cool, clammy skin

g. Systolic blood pressure less than 30 mm Hg

8. Radiographer's response to shock

a. Stop procedure

b. Place patient in recumbent (Trendelenburg) position

c. Immediately obtain help, calling a code if necessary

d. Determine blood pressure

e. Administer oxygen

f. Accurately document the time and occurrence of each symptom

F. Trauma

1. Serious, potentially life-threatening injuries

2. Be careful to do no additional harm to the patient

3. Be prepared to work with other health care professionals present in the radiography room

4. Be prepared to perform a lateral cross-table cervical spine examination as soon as possible

5. Regardless of which area of the body is to be radiographed, assume that a serious internal injury is present

6. Patient is at one of four levels of consciousness

a. Alert and conscious

b. Drowsy

c. Unconscious but reactive to stimuli

d. Comatose

7. Carefully observe the condition of the patient when first brought to the radiography room

8. Note any changes in patient's condition during the course of radiographic procedures

9. Trauma patients should not be left alone under any circumstances

10. Until otherwise informed by a physician, assume the presence of serious spinal injuries

11. Slight movement of a patient with spinal injuries may result in paralysis or death

12. Immobilization devices such as cervical collars or splints must never be removed unless permission is granted by a physician

13. Be prepared to alter routine positions and projections because of the inability to move the anatomical part

14. Adjust radiographic technique to compensate for the presence of splints, spine boards, and other immobilization devices

15. Work carefully with patients who have wounds, making certain to wear gloves

16. Observe condition of wounds when patient is brought for radiography, and immediately notify emergency department personnel of any changes in wounds, including fresh bleeding

17. Patients with severe burns require protective isolation

a. Patients with severe burns experience either no sensation at all or extreme pain

b. Care must be exercised when working with burn patients under either condition

PATIENT MONITORING AND SUPPORT EQUIPMENT

A. Ventilators

1. Mechanical respirators attached to tracheostomies

2. Patient with a ventilator has been intubated (a tube inserted into the trachea)

3. Care must be taken not to dislodge tubing connected to tracheostomy

B. Nasogastric (NG) tubes

1. Tube inserted through the nose and down the esophagus into the stomach

2. Used to feed the patient or to conduct gastric suction

3. Care must be taken by the radiographer not to pull on the NG tube while moving patient or performing the examination

C. Chest tube

1. In place to remove fluid or air from pleural space

2. May be connected to a suction device

3. Radiographer must be careful not to disturb the chest tube or suction devices or bottles to which tube may be attached

4. Bottle must never be raised above chest level

5. Tubing must not be pinched

D. Venous catheters

1. May be kept in place for patients requiring long-term chemotherapy or nutrition

2. Must not be disturbed or pulled in any way

E. Urinary catheters (Foley and suprapubic)

1. Care must be taken during transfer and radiography of patients with urinary catheters in place

2. Urinary catheter tubing must not be bent, pinched, or caught on other equipment and pulled out of the bladder

3. Bag attached to urinary catheters must always be kept below the level of the bladder

4. Allowing urine to flow retrograde into the urethra and bladder can cause urinary tract infections

a. Urinary tract infections are the number one cause of nosocomial infections (infections acquired in the hospital)

F. Oxygen

1. Oxygen should not be removed during radiographic examinations (but care should be taken to remove tubing away from anatomy being radiographed)

2. Oxygen may be removed only with a physician's order

3. Care should be taken to avoid pinching the tubing

KEY REVIEW POINTS
Assessment of Changing Patient Conditions

The radiographer should be able to observe changes in patient condition and understand the ramifications of each. Review those listed in the outline.

- *Temperature:* Normal oral temperature is 98° to 99° F
- *Pulse:* Normal is around 60 beats per minute; greater than 100 beats per minute indicates tachycardia; less than 60 beats per minute indicates bradycardia
- *Respiration:* Normal rate of respiration is 12 to 16 breaths per minute
- *Blood pressure:* Always expressed as systolic pressure over diastolic pressure (e.g., 120/80 mm Hg)
- *Systolic pressure:* Measurement of the pumping action of the heart
- *Diastolic pressure:* Measures the blood pressure of the heart at rest
- *Oxygen administration:* Generally administered using mask or nasal cannula; usual oxygen flow rate is 3 to 5 L/minute
- *Suction unit:* Used to maintain patient's airway
- *Cardiac arrest:* Cessation of heart function; CPR must begin immediately
- *Crash cart:* Medications, airways, sphygmomanometers, stethoscopes, defibrillators, cardiac monitors
- *Respiratory arrest:* Cessation of breathing; CPR must begin immediately
- *Respiratory arrest caused by choking:* Necessitates the use of suction or the Heimlich maneuver
- *Shock:* Failure of circulation in which blood pressure is inadequate to oxygenate tissues and remove by-products of metabolism
- *Hypovolemic shock:* Follows loss of large amount of blood or plasma
- *Septic shock:* Occurs when toxins produced during massive infection cause a dramatic decrease in blood pressure
- *Neurogenic shock:* Causes blood to pool in peripheral vessels
- *Cardiogenic shock:* Caused by cardiac failure or other interference with heart function
- *Allergic shock (anaphylaxis):* Allergic reaction to foreign proteins after injections
- *Symptoms of shock:* Restlessness, apprehension, accelerated pulse, pale skin, weakness, alteration in ability to think, cool clammy skin, systolic blood pressure less than 30 mm Hg
- *Radiographer's response to shock:* Stop procedure, place patient in a recumbent (Trendelenburg) position, immediately obtain help, call a code if necessary, determine blood pressure, administer oxygen
- *Trauma:* Serious, potentially life-threatening injuries; do no additional harm to the patient
- *Four levels of consciousness:* Alert and conscious, drowsy, unconscious but reactive to stimuli, comatose
- *Ventilators:* Mechanical respirators attached to tracheostomies
- *NG tube:* Tube inserted through the nose and down the esophagus into the stomach
- *Chest tube:* In place to remove fluid or air from the pleural space
- *Venous catheters:* May be kept in place for patients requiring long-term chemotherapy or nutrition
- *Urinary catheters (Foley and suprapubic):* Do not bend, pinch, or catch tubing; bag attached to urinary catheters must always be kept below the level of the bladder
- *Urinary tract infections:* Number one cause of health care–acquired infections

CONTRAST MEDIA

A. Negative contrast agent
 1. Most commonly used agent is air
 2. Requires fewer x-rays and produces a higher density on the radiograph
 3. Air may be used in combination with a positive contrast agent on double-contrast studies
 4. Most common examination performed using a negative contrast agent is a routine chest radiograph
B. Positive contrast agents
 1. Examples
  a. Iodine (atomic number 53)
  b. Barium (atomic number 56)
 2. Relatively high atomic numbers
  a. Result in greater attenuation of x-rays
  b. Provide lower density on radiograph
  c. Provide an increase in contrast between structure to be visualized and surrounding structures
C. Barium
 1. Administered to patient in the form of barium sulfate, an inert salt
 2. For upper GI series and esophagogram, barium is most palatable when mixed with very cold water
 3. For barium enema, barium powder is mixed with water at a temperature of approximately 100° F
 4. For some studies of esophagus, barium sulfate paste, which is much thicker and more difficult to swallow, may be administered
 5. Barium tends to absorb water
 6. Patients must be given careful instructions regarding fluid intake after barium studies so that the barium does not cause an impaction
 7. Barium sulfate escaping into the peritoneal cavity can cause peritonitis
D. Aqueous iodine compounds
 1. Used for contrast studies of GI tract
 2. Used when barium could be a surgical contaminant
  a. Perforated ulcers
  b. Ruptured appendix
 3. Aqueous iodine compounds may also be used in patients at high risk for impactions
 4. These compounds may cause significant dehydration
E. Iodinated contrast media
 1. Ionic contrast agents
  a. Salts of organic iodine compounds
  b. Composed of positively and negatively charged ions
 2. Nonionic contrast agents
  a. Similar to ionic contrast agents
  b. Do not ionize into separate positive and negative charges, which negates their primary advantage over ionic contrast agents
  c. Provide far lower incidence of contrast agent reactions

3. Contraindications to use of iodinated contrast media
   a. Previous sensitivity to contrast agents
   b. Known sensitivity to iodine
4. Both ionic and nonionic contrast agents are iodinated (i.e., both contain various concentrations of iodine—nonionic does not mean noniodinated)

PHARMACOLOGY

History and Patient Care Preceding Injection of Iodinated Contrast Media

A. Determine history of allergies or previous hypersensitivity to contrast media
B. Determine extent of patient's medical problems, including medications being taken
C. Review possible reactions to contrast medium being used; determine the presence of contraindications
D. Verify pertinent laboratory values (blood urea nitrogen, creatinine, and glomerular filtration rate) per department and contrast agent protocol
E. Verify appropriate dosage related to patient weight and age
F. Know the location of all emergency equipment
G. Obtain informed consent from patient per department protocol
H. Carefully observe and evaluate the patient, noting color of skin, tone and pitch of voice, and presence of apprehension or anxiety, so that changes from these baseline observations may be noted after injection

Patient Care After Injection of Iodinated Contrast Media

A. Continue conversation with patient
   1. Encourage patient to speak
   2. Laryngeal swelling as a contrast agent reaction first manifests as a change in the tone and pitch of the patient's voice
B. Continue to observe the patient for early signs of urticaria, profuse sweating, or extreme anxiety
C. If patient becomes overanxious, take patient's pulse to determine whether tachycardia is present
D. If patient becomes faint, immediately check respirations, pulse, and blood pressure, and observe for signs of cyanosis
E. Be aware of the location of a physician in the event of an emergency, such as a contrast agent reaction
F. Remain with the patient (except when at the control panel to make exposures)
   1. Patient should never be left alone after injection or at any time during the procedure
   2. Although most contrast media reactions are noticeable and may even be violent, others are more difficult to observe
      a. A patient who appears to be resting comfortably or sleeping may have experienced cardiac arrest

3. Summon help immediately on observing the onset of a contrast agent reaction
   a. Although a calm response is required to avoid alarming the patient, urgency is important because a mild contrast agent reaction may quickly accelerate into a more serious reaction

Contrast Media Complications and Reactions

A. *Overdose:* May occur in infants or adults with renal, cardiac, or hepatic failure
B. *Anaphylactic reactions:* Flushing, hives, nausea
C. *Cardiovascular reactions:* Hypotension, tachycardia, cardiac arrest
D. *Psychogenic factors:* May be caused by patient anxiety or suggested by the possible reactions described during the informed consent process
E. Other symptoms of contrast agent reactions
   1. Nausea and vomiting
   2. Sneezing
   3. Sensation of heat
   4. Itching
   5. Hoarseness (or change in pitch of voice during conversation)
   6. Coughing
   7. Urticaria
   8. Dyspnea
   9. Loss of consciousness
   10. Convulsions
   11. Cardiac arrest
   12. Paralysis
   13. Any change in level of orientation
F. Complications may occur at site of injection
   1. Local irritation may occur if contrast material extravasates
   2. Phlebitis may occur in the vein in which contrast material was injected

---

KEY REVIEW POINTS
Contrast Media

- *Negative contrast agent:* Air
- *Positive contrast agents:* Iodine and barium
- *Barium:* As barium sulfate; in cold water for upper GI, 100° F for lower GI
- *Aqueous iodine compounds:* Used for contrast studies of GI tract when barium could prove to be a surgical contaminant (perforated ulcers, ruptured appendix)
- *Iodinated ionic contrast media:* Contain positively and negatively charged ions
- *Iodinated nonionic contrast agents:* Do not ionize into separate positive and negative charges, which is their primary advantage over ionic contrast agents; far lower incidence of contrast agent reactions
- *Contrast agent reaction:* Anaphylactic (flushing, hives, nausea); cardiovascular reaction (hypotension, tachycardia, cardiac arrest); psychogenic factors (may be caused by patient anxiety)

- *Other symptoms of contrast agent reactions:* Nausea and vomiting, sneezing, sensation of heat, itching, hoarseness (or change in pitch of voice during conversation), coughing, urticaria, dyspnea, loss of consciousness, convulsions, cardiac arrest, paralysis, any change in level of orientation
- Determine patient history of allergies or previous hypersensitivity to contrast media and extent of medical problems
- Continue talking with and observing patient after injection; be prepared to recognize any signs of a reaction

VENIPUNCTURE

A. Use of hypodermic needle
1. May be used for small injections
2. Described by gauge
   a. Unit of measurement that indicates diameter
   b. The larger the gauge, the smaller the diameter of the needle opening
   c. Higher gauge needles are useful for intravenous (IV) injection of contrast agents because they make a smaller hole and limit bleeding at the site
   d. Higher gauge needles limit the rate at which contrast material may be injected and consequently limit the size of the bolus that may be injected
3. If a hypodermic needle is used, the contrast medium must fill the needle before venipuncture so that air is not injected
B. IV catheter
1. Combination unit with a needle inside a flexible plastic catheter
2. Combination unit is inserted into the vein, needle first
3. Once in place, catheter is pushed in over the needle
4. Afterward, needle is withdrawn
5. Catheter may be connected to syringe containing contrast medium
6. Entire system is more flexible than a hypodermic needle or butterfly
7. Also allows attachment to IV tubing leading to bag or bottle, which can be used in the event of a serious contrast agent reaction
C. Procedure for performing venipuncture
1. Wash hands
2. Always wear gloves
3. Secure tourniquet in place
4. Select vein
5. Thoroughly cleanse the skin using departmental protocol
6. Insert needle into vein
7. Observe blood return into catheter, plastic tubing, or syringe depending on equipment used; remove tourniquet
8. Begin injection immediately
9. If using hypodermic needle, remove needle at conclusion of injection

a. Place small piece of gauze or alcohol wipe on puncture site, and bend patient's arm
b. Dispose of needle and syringe correctly; never recap
10. If using catheter, continue until all contrast medium has been injected, then disconnect syringe, and observe site for swelling
11. Do not discard vial of injected agent until examination is completed and patient has left the area

---

📱 **KEY REVIEW POINTS**
Venipuncture

Specific steps and knowledge are required when performing venipuncture; know each step and the order in which it occurs. Review the equipment used and the procedure.

HAZARDOUS MATERIALS

HANDLING AND DISPOSAL OF BIOHAZARDOUS MATERIALS (Figure 6-1)

A. General chemicals
1. Chemicals may cause harm if taken into the body by any route
2. Possible routes of entry
   a. Inhalation
   b. Swallowing
   c. Absorption through the skin or mucous membranes
3. Material safety data sheets (MSDS) must be available, and radiographers should be familiar with their content and warnings
4. MSDS provide direction for the following
   a. Handling precautions
   b. Safe use of the product
   c. Cleanup and disposal
5. Guidelines for handling chemicals
   a. Use only if container is clearly labeled
   b. Read container label several times before using the contents to be certain of what is being handled
   c. Handle carefully to prevent contact with skin, eyes, and mucous membranes
   d. Wear personal protective equipment (PPE)
   e. Use chemicals only as directed
   f. Never mix chemicals unless compatibility can be verified
   g. Store chemicals only as directed on label
   h. Never pour toxic chemicals down the drain; this includes irritating or flammable materials
   i. Clean up spills immediately according to written procedures

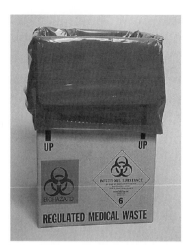

FIGURE 6-1 Biohazardous waste container and symbol.

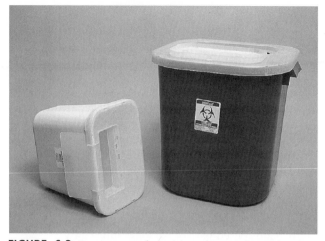

FIGURE 6-2 Puncture-proof container for needle and syringe disposal.

   j. After contact with the skin, rinse immediately with cool water for at least 5 minutes

   k. After contact with eyes, rinse for at least 15 minutes

   l. Always notify the supervisor on duty, and follow guidelines for medical follow-up and incident reports

B. Infectious waste

  1. Anything that has the potential to transmit disease

  2. Handle using U.S. Centers for Disease Control and Prevention (CDC) guidelines for standard precautions

  3. Place in containers or bags properly labeled with the type of waste therein

  4. Know the facility's procedures for handling, containment, and disposal of all infectious waste

  5. Exposure to infectious waste must be reported for medical follow-up and incident reports

  6. Gloves must always be worn in the following activities

    a. Handling used needles and syringes

    b. Handling bandages and dressing

    c. Assisting patients with urinals or bedpans

  7. Needles and syringes must be disposed of in special sharps containers (Figure 6-2)

  8. Needles should not be recapped

  9. Used bandages and dressings must be placed into waterproof bags and sealed

  10. Bedpans and urinals must be emptied immediately and rinsed

---

KEY REVIEW POINTS
Hazardous Materials

- *Route of entry:* May enter the body by any route—inhalation, swallowing, absorption through skin or mucous membranes
- *MSDS:* Radiographers should be familiar with their content and warnings
- *Handling chemicals:* Know all guidelines and be able to explain each step

---

- *Infectious waste:* Handle using CDC guidelines for standard precautions; place in containers or bags properly labeled with type of waste therein
- *Gloves:* Must always be worn when handling used needles and syringes; handling bandages and dressing; assisting patients with urinals or bedpans
- *Needles and syringes:* Must be disposed of in special sharps containers; must not be recapped
- *Used bandages and dressings:* Must be placed into waterproof bags and sealed
- *Bedpans and urinals:* Must be emptied immediately and rinsed

---

REVIEW QUESTIONS

1. Routes of entry of toxic chemicals may include:
  a. Swallowing
  b. Inhalation
  c. Absorption through skin or mucous membranes
  d. All of the above

2. Written instructions for handling of biohazardous materials, safe use of the product, and clean-up and disposal directions are called:
  a. Package inserts
  b. HIPAA
  c. MSDS
  d. Biohazardous warning systems

3. Older patients should be scheduled:
  a. Late in the day to give them time to build their strength
  b. For one examination at a time
  c. As early in the day as possible
  d. Only when no one else is in the department

4. Patients who have been NPO should be scheduled:
  a. Last
  b. First
  c. Just before lunch
  d. In any way that helps the work flow

5. Patients with diabetes should be scheduled:
   a. Late in the day to give them time to build their strength
   b. Only after they have had their insulin
   c. As early in the day as possible
   d. Immediately after a full breakfast

6. Endoscopic procedures should be scheduled:
   a. After ingestion of barium for increased contrast
   b. First in a series of procedures
   c. After a series of procedures so as to verify the diagnosis
   d. Only by the endoscopy department

7. What describes torts?
   a. Violations of civil law
   b. Considered part of personal injury law
   c. Provide for compensation for injury
   d. All of the above

8. Which of the following may be considered an example of battery?
   a. Touching the patient without consent
   b. Threatening the patient
   c. Radiographing the wrong patient
   d. All of the above

9. Assault means:
   a. Threatening the patient or causing the patient to be apprehensive
   b. Striking the patient
   c. Touching the patient without consent
   d. Performing radiography against the patient's will

10. Which of the following is *not* an example of invasion of privacy?
    a. Violation of confidentiality, such as discussing the patient's case in public
    b. Unjustified restraint of patient
    c. Improperly exposing the patient's body
    d. Improperly touching the patient's body

11. Unintentional misconduct is also called:
    a. Negligence
    b. An accident
    c. Libel
    d. Slander

12. The concept of the reasonably prudent person is interpreted as:
    a. How a reasonable jury member would perform the act
    b. How a professional with similar education, training, and experience would perform the act
    c. How a prudent attorney would interpret the act
    d. How a reasonable and prudent judge would rule on the act

13. *Respondeat superior* means:
    a. "The thing speaks for itself"
    b. A radiographer has no need to carry malpractice insurance
    c. The reasonable and prudent person should make the decision
    d. "Let the master answer"

14. Gross negligence is:
    a. A case that includes the injured person as a contributing party to the injury
    b. Loss of life or limb
    c. An act that shows reckless disregard for life or limb
    d. Found in criminal cases only

15. Which of the following conditions must be met to prove malpractice?
    a. The injury actually occurred and is a result of negligence
    b. The standard of care was violated
    c. The injury was caused by the person being sued
    d. All of the above

16. A case involving obvious negligence would be defined by the doctrine of:
    a. *Respondeat superior*
    b. Slander
    c. Libel
    d. *Res ipsa loquitur*

17. Which of the following statements are true concerning valid (informed) consent?
    1. Patient must be of legal age
    2. Patient must be given a brochure describing the risks of the procedure in lay terms
    3. Consent must be offered voluntarily
    4. Patient must be mentally competent
    5. Patient must completely understand all aspects of the procedure
       a. 1, 3, 4
       b. 1, 2, 3, 4, 5
       c. 1, 2, 3, 4
       d. 1, 2, 3, 5

18. Patient transfers from cart to x-ray table and back to cart should be performed:
    a. By the radiographer alone if the patient is ambulatory
    b. By two or more radiographers to ensure patient and radiographer safety
    c. By the radiographer alone if the department is short staffed
    d. By the radiographer alone so as not to frighten the patient

19. A patient history should be taken by the radiographer:
    a. To assist the radiologist with interpretation of the radiographs
    b. To verify patient name and condition
    c. To assist the radiographer in understanding the patient's injury and range of motion
    d. All of the above

20. Direct contact allows an infectious organism to move:
    a. From the susceptible host directly to the infected person
    b. From the infected person directly to the susceptible host
    c. In either direction

21. MSDS provide directions for:
    a. Housekeeping only
    b. Engineering only
    c. Radiology only
    d. All persons exposed to hazardous materials
22. If the radiographer touches hazardous chemicals, what must be done first?
    a. Rinse immediately with warm water
    b. Rinse immediately with cool water for at least 5 minutes
    c. Rinse immediately with cool water for at least 15 minutes
    d. Rinse with the warmest water that can be tolerated
23. Vectors may be:
    a. Animals such as rabid dogs and bats
    b. Persons
    c. Plants
24. Common vehicle transmission involves:
    a. The spread of infection in crowded forms of public transportation such as jet aircraft, subways, and trains
    b. Food, water, medications, equipment
    c. Animals
    d. Plants
25. Airborne transmission of infection may occur as a result of contact with:
    a. Bird droppings, acid rain, or air pollution
    b. Droplets and dust
    c. Animals
    d. Other humans
26. Indirect contact involves:
    a. Coughs or sneezes
    b. An inanimate object containing pathogenic organisms
    c. Plants and animals
    d. Other humans
27. A system that emphasizes the placement of barriers between the health care worker and the patient is called:
    a. Universal precautions
    b. Standard precautions
    c. Universal safety
    d. Infection barriers
28. The placement of barriers between the health care worker and the patient assumes that:
    a. There is always a contagion present
    b. No one wants to be touched
    c. Every patient should be in isolation
    d. Every health care worker is carrying something contagious
29. The most effective method used to prevent the spread of infection is:
    a. Wearing of gloves
    b. Wearing of gowns
    c. Distance
    d. Handwashing

30. Because barium enemas increase the possibility of contact between body substances and clothing, the radiographer should always wear:
    a. Disposable gowns or surgical scrubs
    b. Head covering
    c. Shoe covering
    d. A regular hospital uniform
31. A radiographer should wear eye protection:
    a. Anytime blood may be present
    b. Anytime an injection is being made
    c. Anytime there is a possibility of blood splashing
    d. With nearly all patients
32. Needles should be recapped after use:
    a. Never
    b. Always
    c. In a nonsterile field
    d. Only during procedures involving a sterile field
33. Any area that is touched by body fluids:
    a. Must be washed completely
    b. Must be covered and isolated for the remainder of the day
    c. Must be evaluated by infection control
    d. Must be reported to risk management
34. Hands should be washed:
    a. At least five times during each shift to help stop the spread of infections
    b. After contact with each patient and before touching equipment and other patients
    c. Every hour regardless of patient contact
    d. Both with and without gloves
35. The process of eliminating as many organisms as possible by the use of water and chemical disinfectants is called:
    a. Surgical asepsis
    b. Sterilization
    c. Medical asepsis
    d. Boiling
36. The process of eliminating all organisms from the environment by gas sterilization, use of germicides, or use of dry heat is called:
    a. Surgical asepsis
    b. Sterilization
    c. Medical asepsis
    d. Autoclaving
37. When putting on gloves for a procedure, which of the following should occur first?
    a. Carefully open glove package, and avoid touching outside of gloves
    b. Wash hands
    c. Place glove package in center of sterile field in preparation for the procedure
    d. Put on one glove immediately so that one hand is protected and the other is free
38. After a radiographer is gowned and gloved for a procedure, hands may not be placed:
    a. Anywhere on the body because the gown and gloves are sterile

b. Anywhere on the front or sides of the gown

c. Anywhere on the table containing the sterile field

d. Under the arms or on the sides or back of the gown

39. A radiographer who is assisting with a sterile procedure but is not gloved and gowned:
    a. Should never step between the physician and the sterile field
    b. Should carefully place all utensils needed in the center of the sterile field by dropping them from above out of their packages
    c. Should not come in contact with the sterile field under any circumstances
    d. All of the above

40. What route of transmission involves touching a susceptible person with a contaminated object (e.g., a radiographic cassette)?
    a. Droplet transmission
    b. Indirect contact
    c. Direct contact
    d. Airborne transmission

41. Which of the following transmission-based precautions also require the use of standard precautions?
    a. Airborne precautions
    b. Droplet precautions
    c. Contact precautions
    d. All of the above

42. Which of the following rules must always be followed regardless of the route of transmission of infection?
    a. Gloves must be worn
    b. Gowns must be worn
    c. Patient must not have any direct contact with the health care worker
    d. Handwashing must be performed

43. Which of the following does *not* require the use of gloves?
    a. Strict isolation
    b. Respiratory isolation
    c. Enteric isolation
    d. Body substance precautions

44. Which of the following requires that all equipment and personnel be carefully covered?
    a. Strict isolation
    b. Respiratory isolation
    c. Enteric isolation
    d. Reverse isolation

45. What is used for total protection of the health care worker from every method of transmission possible in the work setting?
    a. Strict isolation
    b. Respiratory isolation
    c. Enteric isolation
    d. Body substance precautions

46. Which of the following is used if there is any chance of coming in contact primarily with products of the GI system of an infected person?
    a. Strict isolation
    b. Respiratory isolation
    c. Enteric isolation
    d. Body substance precautions

47. When are gowns and gloves *not* required?
    a. Strict isolation
    b. Respiratory isolation
    c. Enteric isolation
    d. Reverse isolation

48. When are masks not required, but needle-stick injuries must be avoided?
    a. Strict isolation
    b. Respiratory isolation
    c. Enteric isolation
    d. Body substance precautions

49. Which of the following is used to protect the health care worker from airborne droplets?
    a. Strict isolation
    b. Respiratory isolation
    c. Enteric isolation
    d. Body substance precautions

50. Which of the following is used with patients who are not infectious?
    a. Strict isolation
    b. Respiratory isolation
    c. Enteric isolation
    d. Body substance precautions

51. Assessment of changing patient conditions includes observing for:
    a. Skin that becomes cool and diaphoretic
    b. Patient expressions of discomfort or dizziness
    c. Lips or nail beds that become cyanotic
    d. All of the above indicate changing patient conditions

52. The normal adult body temperature taken orally is:
    a. 98.6° C
    b. 98° to 99° C
    c. 99.6° F
    d. 98° to 99° F

53. Which of the following may be ingested by a patient who has been placed on a clear liquid diet?
    1. Bouillon
    2. Gelatin
    3. Tea
       a. 1 and 2 only
       b. 1 and 3 only
       c. 2 and 3 only
       d. 1, 2, and 3

54. Barium sulfate is classified as a(n):
    a. Dissolvable organic salt
    b. Inert inorganic salt
    c. Nonionic contrast agent
    d. Iodinated contrast agent

55. A sphygmomanometer is used to:
    a. Hear the heartbeat
    b. Hear the blood pressure
    c. Measure blood pressure
    d. Measure body temperature
56. A blood pressure of 120/80 mm Hg reveals that:
    a. The pressure is 120 mm Hg when the heart is at rest
    b. The diastolic pressure is 120 mm Hg
    c. The systolic pressure is 80 mm Hg
    d. The pressure is 80 mm Hg when the heart is at rest
57. When oxygen is administered, the usual rate is:
    a. 3 to 5 lb/minute
    b. 3 to 5 L/hour
    c. 3 to 5 L/minute
    d. 5 to 7 L/minute
58. A mechanical method used to clear the patient's airway is called:
    a. The Heimlich maneuver
    b. CPR
    c. Suctioning
    d. NG tube insertion
59. Which of the following contains all the instruments and medications necessary for dealing with cardiac arrest?
    a. Crash cart
    b. Tackle box
    c. IVP cabinet
    d. Code blue cabinet
60. What condition is caused by loss of a large amount of blood or plasma?
    a. Anaphylaxis
    b. Cardiogenic shock
    c. Hypovolemic shock
    d. Septic shock
61. What causes blood to pool in peripheral vessels?
    a. Anaphylaxis
    b. Cardiogenic shock
    c. Hypovolemic shock
    d. Neurogenic shock
62. What follows an allergic reaction to foreign proteins?
    a. Anaphylaxis
    b. Cardiogenic shock
    c. Hypovolemic shock
    d. Septic shock
63. What is caused by infection that results in extremely low blood pressure?
    a. Anaphylaxis
    b. Cardiogenic shock
    c. Hypovolemic shock
    d. Septic shock
64. What condition occurs secondary to heart failure or interference with heart function?
    a. Anaphylaxis
    b. Cardiogenic shock
    c. Hypovolemic shock
    d. Septic shock
65. What condition may occur after injection of an iodinated contrast agent?
    a. Anaphylaxis
    b. Cardiogenic shock
    c. Hypovolemic shock
    d. Septic shock
66. Which of the following is a symptom of shock?
    a. Accelerated pulse
    b. Cool, clammy, pale skin
    c. Systolic pressure less than 30 mm Hg
    d. All of the above
67. What should the radiographer do first when it is suspected a patient is going into shock?
    a. Call for assistance
    b. Place patient in Trendelenburg position
    c. Take patient's blood pressure to confirm shock status
    d. Administer oxygen
68. Which of the following statements apply when radiography is performed on trauma patients?
    1. Work quickly and efficiently
    2. Patient may be left alone if unconscious
    3. Spinal injury may be ruled out if patient is not on a spine board or wearing a cervical collar
    4. Observe for changes in wound dressing while performing radiography
    5. Document in writing changes in patient condition
    a. 1, 3, 4
    b. 1, 2, 3
    c. 1, 4, 5
    d. 1, 2, 3, 4, 5
69. Which of the following is used to feed a patient or conduct gastric suction?
    a. Urinary catheter
    b. Chest tube
    c. Ventilator
    d. NG tube
70. Which of the following is used to administer nutrition or long-term chemotherapy?
    a. Urinary catheter
    b. Chest tube
    c. Ventilator
    d. Venous catheter
71. What is the site of most nosocomial infections?
    a. Urinary catheter
    b. Chest tube
    c. NG tube
    d. Venous catheter
72. What is another name for a mechanical respirator?
    a. Urinary catheter
    b. Chest tube
    c. Ventilator
    d. Venous catheter

73. The most frequently performed examination using a contrast medium is a(n):
   a. Small bowel study
   b. IVP
   c. Barium enema
   d. Chest x-ray study

74. Which of the following statements are true concerning positive contrast media?
   1. Air is the most commonly used
   2. Aqueous iodine compounds may be used if perforations are suspected
   3. Barium should be mixed with cold water for retrograde administration
   4. Nonionic contrast media are ideal for injection because they do not contain iodine, reducing the risk of reactions
   5. Barium is an inert substance
   6. Aqueous iodine compounds may cause serious dehydration
   7. Barium is a surgical contaminant
   a. 2, 5, 6, 7
   b. 1, 2, 3, 4, 5, 6, 7
   c. 1, 2, 3, 4, 7
   d. 1, 2, 4, 5, 6, 7

75. Which of the following is a legitimate contraindication to the use of iodinated contrast media?
   a. Allergy to seafood
   b. Known sensitivity to proteins
   c. Previous sensitivity to contrast agents
   d. Allergy to any medications

76. A reaction at the site of injection of iodinated contrast media may be caused by:
   a. Extravasation of contrast agent
   b. Allergy to seafood
   c. Anaphylaxis
   d. Allergy to certain medications

77. Which of the following is a symptom (are symptoms) of a contrast agent reaction?
   a. Hoarseness
   b. Sneezing
   c. Urticaria
   d. All are symptoms

78. After injection of iodinated contrast media, the radiographer should:
   a. Leave the patient to rest
   b. Remain with the patient and have a conversation with the patient, listening for signs of laryngeal swelling
   c. Tell the patient a funny story as a means of allaying anxiety about the procedure
   d. Alert a radiologist

79. At the first indication of a contrast agent reaction, the radiographer should:
   a. Immediately shout for help
   b. Stop the examination and obtain help so as not to alarm the patient

   c. Continue with the examination because most reactions turn out to be minor
   d. Call a code blue

80. Hypodermic needles are described by their gauge, which is a:
   a. List of the uses of the needle
   b. Measure of the length of the needle
   c. Measure of the diameter of the needle
   d. Measure of the diameter of the needle opening— the larger the gauge, the smaller the diameter

81. Air must not be injected when performing venipuncture because:
   a. An air embolus would form that may be fatal to the patient
   b. Most examinations requiring injection are not air contrast studies
   c. It would interfere with the iodine
   d. It would prevent visualization of the iodine

82. A smaller, easier-to-handle injection set that includes plastic projections on both sides of the needle and may be used for venipuncture is called a:
   a. Venous catheter
   b. Butterfly
   c. Hypodermic needle
   d. Single-injection needle

83. A venous catheter:
   a. Consists of a long plastic tube that is inserted into the artery during angiography
   b. Is more flexible and easier to use than a needle or butterfly
   c. Is a combination unit with a needle inside a flexible plastic catheter; both the needle and the catheter are inserted into the vein, after which the needle is withdrawn
   d. b and c

84. Place the following steps for performing venipuncture in the proper order.
   1. Secure tourniquet in place
   2. Thoroughly cleanse the skin
   3. Wash hands
   4. Select vein
   5. Put on gloves
   6. Perform puncture
   7. Cover wound and compress site
   8. Inject contrast agent
   9. Check wound for swelling
   10. Observe blood return
   a. 5, 4, 1, 6, 8, 7
   b. 3, 1, 4, 5, 2, 6, 10, 8, 7, 9
   c. 3, 5, 1, 4, 2, 6, 10, 8, 7, 9
   d. 4, 1, 3, 5, 2, 6, 8, 9, 10, 7

85. Venipuncture:
   a. May be performed by a radiographer only where allowed by state law
   b. May be performed by a nurse only

c. Must be performed by a radiology supervisor

d. May be performed by a radiographer under any circumstances

86. A contrast medium overdose:
    a. Cannot occur because a contrast medium is not a drug
    b. May occur in infants
    c. May occur if contrast material was injected during the week before the examination
    d. May occur in infants or adults with renal, cardiac, or hepatic failure

87. If medication needs to be ordered for a patient in the radiology department, a physician *always*:
    1. Chooses the drug and the dosage
    2. Selects the route of administration
    3. Administers the drug
       a. 1 and 2 only
       b. 1 and 3 only
       c. 2 and 3 only
       d. 1, 2, and 3

88. A patient who has sustained a head injury in a motor vehicle accident arrived in the radiology department alert and well oriented. While radiographing the patient, the radiographer observed that the patient was becoming drowsy, irritable, and less coherent. Which of the following would be the correct action for the radiographer to take?
    a. Continue the radiographic examination
    b. Ignore the changes in the patient's condition, and place the patient back on the stretcher after completing the examination
    c. Notify the department supervisor or the attending physician of the change in the patient's condition
    d. Sound an emergency code alert

89. A reaction that causes the patient's skin to turn cyanotic means:
    a. The skin is turning yellow
    b. The skin is turning pale
    c. The skin is turning blue
    d. The skin is turning red

90. What degree of reaction is vomiting?
    a. Mild to moderate reaction to contrast agent
    b. Severe reaction to contrast agent
    c. Not considered a reaction to contrast agent

91. In patient care, the radiographer must be constantly aware of the myriad of variations among people of all backgrounds and experiences. This involves the study and understanding of:
    a. Nonverbal communication
    b. Diversity
    c. Verbal communication only
    d. Patient preferences

92. What degree of reaction is dyspnea?
    a. Mild to moderate reaction to contrast agent
    b. Severe reaction to contrast agent
    c. Not considered a reaction to contrast agent

93. Which of the following is always a part of the radiographer's scope of practice?
    a. Patient education
    b. Administration of medications
    c. Serve as a resource person for referring physicians
    d. Serving on the hospital's radiation safety committee

94. What degree of reaction is cardiac arrest?
    a. Mild to moderate reaction to contrast agent
    b. Severe reaction to contrast agent
    c. Not considered a reaction to contrast agent

95. A document that provides instructions regarding medical care that a patient may prepare prior to incapacitation is called a(n):
    a. Pre-planning order
    b. Advance directive
    c. Physician notice
    d. Informed consent

96. The formal term for 'no code' is:
    a. Advance directive
    b. Right to die
    c. Do not resuscitate order (DNR)
    d. Euthanasia

97. Which of the following contains points that are enforceable?
    a. ARRT Mission Statement
    b. ARRT Code of Ethics
    c. ARRT Exam Content Specifications
    d. ARRT Rules of Ethics

98. Which of the following serves as a guide to professional conduct?
    a. ARRT Mission Statement
    b. ARRT Code of Ethics
    c. ARRT Exam Content Specifications
    d. ARRT Rules of Ethics

99. The patient may be left alone following injection of a contrast agent:
    a. Never
    b. After several minutes have passed and there is no sign of a reaction
    c. Immediately since contrast agent reactions are rare
    d. If they are of legal age

100. The study of contrast agents, their administration, and possible reactions fall under the category of:
    a. Nursing
    b. Pharmacology
    c. Emergency care
    d. Respiratory care

7

Challenge Tests

The review tests in this chapter are constructed using the same proportion of questions contained on the radiography certification exam. The computer-based certification exam asks you questions at random; however, these printed tests are sorted by category.

After you complete your review work and take these challenge tests, you are ready to move on to the online questions. There you will find hundreds of additional multiple choice questions presented randomly in 200-question blocks, sectioned to simulate the actual American Registry of Radiologic Technologists (ARRT) examination. The online questions are your best practice and preparation. You will be answering questions on a computer at random, just as you will when you take the ARRT exam. There are enough questions to give you many different exams with countless combinations of questions, always according to ARRT test specifications. By drilling yourself using this test bank, you will be as prepared as possible for test day.

CHALLENGE TEST NUMBER 1

Radiation Protection (Questions 1-45)

1. Attenuation:
   a. Is radiation that emerges from the patient
   b. Describes changes in the x-ray beam as it travels through the patient
   c. Produces only scatter radiation
   d. Occurs only at doses used in radiation therapy
2. Which photon-tissue interaction makes radiography possible because of its creation of contrast?
   a. Compton
   b. Coherent
   c. Photoelectric
   d. Pair production
3. Which photon-tissue interaction produces radiation that may expose others in the room during fluoroscopy?
   a. Compton
   b. Coherent
   c. Photoelectric
   d. Pair production
4. The traditional unit of absorbed dose is:
   a. Coulombs/kilogram
   b. Gray

c. Curie
d. Rad
5. The traditional unit of activity is:
   a. Becquerel
   b. Gray
   c. Quality factor
   d. Curie
6. Measurement of positive and negative particles created when radiation ionizes atoms in the air helps define the:
   a. Becquerel
   b. Gray
   c. Roentgen
   d. Curie
7. Linear energy transfer:
   a. Is the same for all types of radiation
   b. Is the same for wave and particulate radiations used in diagnosis and treatment
   c. Occurs only during x-ray procedures
   d. Varies for different types of radiation
8. The unit of the curie would be used in what imaging modality?
   a. Radiography
   b. CT
   c. MRI
   d. Nuclear medicine
9. Graphs that show the relationship between radiation received and the organism's response are called:
   a. Response curves
   b. H & D curves
   c. Dose-response curves
   d. Radiation-threshold curves
10. Medical x-rays are an example of:
    a. Natural background radiation
    b. Artificially produced radiation
    c. Nonionizing radiation
    d. Ionizing, natural background radiation
11. Cataractogenesis does not occur at low levels of radiation exposure; it is best expressed by which of the following dose-response relationships?
    a. Threshold
    b. Nonthreshold
    c. Low dose
    d. Occupational dose

12. *Increased dose equals increased probability of effects* best describes which of the following?
    a. Stochastic effects
    b. Deterministic effects
    c. Direct effect
    d. Indirect effect
13. The cumulative occupational exposure for a 22-year-old radiographer is:
    a. 22 mrem
    b. 55 rem
    c. 11 mrem
    d. 22 rem
14. The annual effective dose limit for the general public, assuming frequent exposure, is:
    a. 0.5 mrem
    b. 500 mrem
    c. 0.05 rem
    d. 0.1 rem
15. The secondary protective barrier used in room shielding must be at least how thick?
    a. $1/32$ inch Al equivalent
    b. $1/16$ inch Al equivalent
    c. $1/16$ inch Pb equivalent
    d. $1/32$ inch Pb equivalent
16. The intensity of the scattered beam is $1/1000$ the intensity of the primary beam at a _____ angle 1 m from the patient.
    a. 45-degree
    b. 25-degree
    c. 90-degree
    d. 10-degree
17. If the radiation dose 6 feet from the x-ray table is 5 R, what is the dose at a distance of 3 feet?
    a. 20 R
    b. 10 R
    c. 1.25 R
    d. 2.5 R
18. The minimum source-to-skin distance for fixed fluoroscopes is:
    a. 15 inches
    b. 12 inches
    c. 10 inches
    d. 18 inches
19. The use of gonadal shielding on female patients may reduce gonad dose by:
    a. 50%
    b. 75%
    c. 85%
    d. 95%
20. Cells that are oxygenated are more susceptible to radiation damage; this describes:
    a. Target theory
    b. Direct effect
    c. Doubling dose
    d. Oxygen enhancement ratio
21. The blood count is depressed after a whole-body dose equivalent of at least how many rads?

a. 10
b. 25
c. 5
d. 1

22. Highly reactive ions that have unpaired electrons in the outer shell are called:
    a. Electrified
    b. Radiolytic
    c. Hydrogen peroxide
    d. Free radicals
23. The master molecule that directs cell activities is:
    a. RNA
    b. Hydrogen peroxide
    c. A free radical
    d. DNA
24. The process of somatic cell division is called:
    a. Mitosis
    b. Spermatogenesis
    c. Organogenesis
    d. Cytogenesis
25. The most common effect from exposure to ionizing radiation is:
    a. Mutations
    b. Ionization of atoms in the cells
    c. Cell death
    d. Nothing
26. Most radiation-induced damage to cells occurs:
    a. At diagnostic levels of radiation
    b. During fluoroscopy
    c. At doses of radiation much higher than doses used in radiography
    d. From background radiation
27. Radiation doses up to _____ are considered relatively low risk to the embryo and fetus.
    a. 5 rads
    b. 5 to 10 rads
    c. 1 rad
    d. 15 to 20 rads
28. A concept of radiologic practice that encourages radiation users to adopt measures that keep the dose to the patient and themselves at minimum levels is called:
    a. LET
    b. RBE
    c. MPD
    d. ALARA
29. Which of the following is(are) relatively insensitive to radiation?
    a. Nerve tissue
    b. Reproductive cells
    c. Epithelial tissue
    d. Immature sperm cells
30. Somatic effects of radiation:
    a. Are common
    b. Are caused when a large dose of high-LET radiation is received by a large area of the body
    c. Are caused after exposure of DNA
    d. Include genetic mutations

31. The best way to keep radiation dose to the patient low is:
    a. Distance
    b. Shielding
    c. Time
    d. Avoidance of repeat exposures

32. X-rays may remove electrons from atoms in the body by a process called:
    a. Electrification
    b. Exposure
    c. Ionization
    d. Radicalizing

33. Ionization may cause:
    a. Stable atoms
    b. Production of high-energy x-rays
    c. Formation of new molecules beneficial to the cell
    d. Unstable atoms

34. Cell damage may be exhibited as:
    a. Loss of function or abnormal function
    b. Nothing
    c. Enhanced function

35. Damage to the cell being irradiated is called:
    a. Genetic
    b. Exposed cell
    c. Somatic
    d. Molecular

36. Radiation effects that show up in the next generation are called:
    a. Genetic
    b. Exposed cell
    c. Somatic
    d. Molecular

37. Radiation that is contained in the environment is called:
    a. Man-made
    b. Artificial
    c. Natural background
    d. Artificial background

38. Background radiation is the source of what percent of human exposure?
    a. 95%
    b. 82%
    c. 50%
    d. 35%

39. The annual effective dose per person from natural background radiation is approximately:
    a. 100 mrem
    b. 295 mrem
    c. 50 mrem
    d. 900 mrem

40. The greatest source of natural background radiation to humans is:
    a. X-rays
    b. Delta rays
    c. Radon
    d. Radium

41. According to NCRP Report #160, the increase in total exposure is primarily attributed to increased use of:
    a. MRI
    b. Diagnostic medical ultrasound
    c. Fluoroscopy and interventional procedures
    d. CT

42. According to NCRP Report #160, interventional fluoroscopy contributes approximately what amount to the annual dose to the population?
    a. 1.5 mSv
    b. 0.7 mSv
    c. 0.43 mSv
    d. 2.0 mSv

43. CT accounts for approximately what percent dose to the population (NCRP Report #160)?
    a. 24%
    b. 50%
    c. 15%
    d. 80%

44. Using data from NCRP Report #160, the typical dose for an upper GI is:
    a. 1.5 mSv
    b. 6.0 mSv
    c. 3.5 mSv
    d. 10.3 mSv

45. NCRP Report #160 indicates the dose for an examination of the extremities is:
    a. Negligible—0.005 to 0.008 mSv
    b. 1.0 to 3.0 mSv
    c. Negligible—0.10 to 0.15 mSv
    d. Too low to be accurately measured

Equipment Operation and Quality Control (Questions 46-67)

46. The smallest particle of an element that retains the characteristics of the element is a(n):
    a. Element
    b. Atom
    c. Molecule
    d. Neutron

47. Atomic mass refers to:
    a. The number of protons plus the number of neutrons
    b. The number of electrons
    c. The number of electron shells
    d. The number of protons

48. X-rays travel as bundles of energy called:
    a. Protons
    b. Phasers
    c. Particles
    d. Photons

49. The height of a sine wave is called:
    a. Wavelength
    b. Altitude
    c. Amplitude
    d. Frequency

50. The number of x-ray waves passing a given point per unit time is called:
    a. Wavelength
    b. Altitude
    c. Amplitude
    d. Frequency

51. The transformer that operates on the principle of self-induction is the:
    a. Step-up transformer
    b. Step-down transformer
    c. Induction transformer
    d. Autotransformer

52. Electronic timers used in x-ray equipment allow for exposure times of:
    a. $\frac{1}{100}$ second
    b. $\frac{1}{1000}$ second
    c. 1 µs
    d. There is no limit to how short the exposure can be

53. To ensure consistency of radiographic quality from one exposure to the next, what device may be used?
    a. Electronic timer
    b. Automatic collimation
    c. Automatic exposure control
    d. Falling load generator

54. What happens when a predetermined level of ionization is reached in the ionization chamber?
    a. The unit shuts off because of a malfunction
    b. The maximum allowable time has been reached
    c. The highest allowable dose to the patient has been reached
    d. The exposure is terminated

55. An x-ray machine that uses a continually decreasing mA for the shortest times possible uses a(n):
    a. Ionization chamber
    b. Phototimer
    c. AEC
    d. Falling load generator

56. An x-ray machine that makes maximum use of heat loading potential uses a(n):
    a. Ionization chamber
    b. Phototimer
    c. AEC
    d. Falling load generator

57. Devices in the x-ray circuit that operate on the principle of mutual induction are called:
    a. Rectifiers
    b. Generators
    c. Timers
    d. Transformers

58. The high-voltage section of the x-ray circuit makes use of what type of transformer?
    a. Step-up
    b. Autotransformer
    c. Step-down
    d. Falling load

59. The device in the x-ray circuit that changes AC to DC is the:
    a. Autotransformer
    b. Step-up transformer
    c. Rectifier
    d. Falling load generator

60. What type of current is required for proper operation of the x-ray tube?
    a. Direct
    b. Falling load
    c. Alternating
    d. Fluctuating

61. Modern rectifiers are made of:
    a. Silicone-based semiconductors
    b. Transistors
    c. Cathode ray tubes
    d. Silicon-based semiconductors

62. The result of thermionic emission is a(n):
    a. Recoil electron
    b. Electron cloud
    c. Scattered photon
    d. Characteristic photon

63. The focusing cup is located at the:
    a. Cathode
    b. Anode
    c. X-ray tube window
    d. Control panel

64. An interaction that produces x-rays at the anode as a result of outer shell electrons filling holes in the K-shell is called:
    a. Characteristic
    b. Photoelectric
    c. Compton
    d. Brems

65. When a quality control test is performed to ensure that adjacent mA stations are accurate, the results must be within this amount of one another:
    a. 2% of SID
    b. 4%
    c. 10%
    d. 5%

66. When a quality control test is performed to ensure that the same exposure factors produce consistent x-ray output, successive exposures must be within this amount of one another:
    a. 2% of SID
    b. 4%
    c. 10%
    d. 5%

67. When a quality control test is performed to ensure that the collimator is providing appropriate radiation protection, the result must be within this amount:
    a. 2% of SID
    b. 4%
    c. 10%
    d. 5%

**Image Acquisition and Evaluation
(Questions 68-112)**

68. In digital fluoroscopy, the image should be viewed on what device to take advantage of the digital capabilities?
    a. Digital viewbox
    b. High-resolution monitor
    c. High-definition TV
    d. Plasma TV

69. A primary advantage of digital fluoroscopy is:
    a. Postprocessing manipulation of the image
    b. No radiation dose to the patient
    c. No fluoroscopist required
    d. Lower cost

70. The active portion of a CR imaging plate is:
    a. Intensifying screen phosphor
    b. Photostimulable phosphor
    c. Silver halide crystals
    d. Rare earth phosphor

71. Energy in a CR imaging plate is released after exposure to:
    a. Developer solution
    b. White light
    c. Ultrasound
    d. Laser beam

72. In digital fluoroscopy and computed radiography, the energy must be changed to digital form by a(n):
    a. Digital-to-analog converter
    b. Flux capacitor
    c. Analog-to-digital converter
    d. DVD-ROM

73. An algorithm is:
    a. A mathematical hypothesis used in imaging
    b. A mathematical formula used to reconstruct the image in digital imaging
    c. An advanced imaging procedure
    d. The mathematical basis for film-screen imaging

74. In computed radiography, each pixel corresponds to a shade of gray representing an area in the patient known as a(n):
    a. Pathology
    b. Density
    c. Voxel
    d. Artifact

75. A digital image is composed of rows and columns known as a:
    a. Photonic image
    b. Matrix
    c. Digital
    d. Cyborg assimilator

76. Image brightness in computed radiography may be adjusted by:
    a. Doubling the kVp
    b. Changing the window level
    c. Repeating the exposure
    d. Using digital fluoroscopy

77. The window level in computed radiography is the:
    a. Area of the patient being irradiated
    b. Amount of radiation needed to obtain the image
    c. Midpoint of densities
    d. Toe of the H & D curve

78. Radiographic contrast in computed radiography may be adjusted by changing the:
    a. Window level
    b. Window width
    c. Area of the patient being irradiated
    d. Imaging plate

79. The amount of darkness on a radiograph is controlled primarily by:
    a. kVp
    b. Focal spot size
    c. AEC
    d. mAs

80. The visible image may also be called the:
    a. Manifest image
    b. Image-in-waiting
    c. Preprocessed image
    d. Latent image

81. The quantity of x-rays produced is directly controlled by:
    a. kVp
    b. OID
    c. SID
    d. mAs

82. The rule or law that governs changing technique using kVp is the:
    a. Inverse square law
    b. Density maintenance law
    c. Reciprocity law
    d. 15% rule

83. Given an original technique of 10 mAs and 70 kVp, which of the following would produce a radiograph with double the density?
    a. 20 mAs, 80 kVp
    b. 30 mAs, 92 kVp
    c. 20 mAs, 70 kVp
    d. 15 mAs, 82 kVp

84. If SID is halved, what may be said about radiographic density?
    a. Density doubles
    b. Density is reduced by half
    c. Density is reduced by one-half of the mAs
    d. Density is quadrupled

85. The letters *TFT* stand for:
    a. To formulate text translation
    b. Thin film transistor
    c. Test scheduled for tomorrow
    d. Thin film text

86. Distortion that affects the size of the object as represented on the radiographic image is called:
    a. Minification
    b. Foreshortening
    c. Elongation
    d. Magnification

87. Shape distortion may take the form of:
    a. Magnification and minification
    b. Size and shape distortion
    c. Elongation and foreshortening
    d. Magnification and elongation
88. A longer than usual OID may cause:
    a. Elongation
    b. Foreshortening
    c. Minification
    d. Magnification
89. CR cassettes *should* be erased:
    a. Every 24 hours
    b. Every 48 hours
    c. Every 3 months
    d. Weekly
90. The equation *H/D* describes:
    a. Grid radius
    b. Contrast
    c. Grid ratio
    d. Reciprocity law
91. If the exposure field is not accurately recognized, the histogram:
    a. Narrows
    b. Widens
    c. Remains the same
92. Noise increases with an increase in:
    a. mAs
    b. Speed class
    c. SID
    d. OID
93. Edge enhancement provides:
    a. Artificial increase in display contrast at an edge of the image
    b. Artificial increase in display density at an edge of the image
    c. Artificial increase in recorded detail at an edge of the image
    d. Artificial increase in spatial resolution at an edge of the image
94. Which of the following grid errors would result in an image that shows normal density in the middle but decreased density on the sides and may follow removal and replacement of the grid?
    a. Upside down
    b. Off-level
    c. Lateral decentering
    d. Grid-focus decentering
95. Grid frequency is described as the:
    a. Height of the lead strips divided by the distance between the lead strips
    b. Distance between the lead strips divided by the height of the lead strips
    c. Number of lead strips per inch or centimeter
    d. SID at which the grid may be used
96. When working with CR and DR, one must be aware that their response to scatter radiation is:
    a. Very sensitive

b. Minimally sensitive
    c. Irrelevant
97. The images on radiologists' monitors appear:
    a. The same as on radiographers' monitors
    b. In greater detail than on radiographers' monitors
    c. In less detail than on radiographers' monitors
98. A histogram analysis error may be caused by:
    a. Excessive mAs
    b. Pixel unresponsiveness
    c. Inappropriate collimation
    d. Excessive kVp
99. Smoothing provides:
    a. Higher spatial resolution
    b. Equalization
    c. Evenness in brightness
    d. Higher contrast resolution
100. Consistency of image appearance is achieved through the use of:
    a. Higher speed class
    b. Uniform processing codes
    c. More effective postprocessing
    d. Lower exposure index numbers
101. As kVp is decreased:
    a. Density increases
    b. Contrast decreases
    c. Recorded detail decreases
    d. Contrast increases
102. As kVp is increased:
    a. Density decreases
    b. Contrast increases
    c. Recorded detail increases
    d. Scale of contrast lengthens
103. Which of the following sets of exposure factors would produce a radiograph with the poorest recorded detail?
    a. 60 mAs, 80 kVp, 40-inch SID, 4-inch OID
    b. 30 mAs, 92 kVp, 40-inch SID, 4-inch OID
    c. 120 mAs, 92 kVp, 20-inch SID, 4-inch OID
    d. 15 mAs, 100 kVp, 40-inch SID, 4-inch OID
104. Which of the following sets of exposure factors would produce a radiograph with the lowest contrast?
    a. 60 mAs, 80 kVp, 40-inch SID, 4-inch OID
    b. 30 mAs, 92 kVp, 40-inch SID, 4-inch OID
    c. 120 mAs, 92 kVp, 20-inch SID, 4-inch OID
    d. 15 mAs, 100 kVp, 40-inch SID, 4-inch OID
105. Beam restriction has the following effect on contrast:
    a. Decreases contrast
    b. Longer scale of contrast
    c. Shorter scale of contrast
    d. No effect on contrast
106. As kVp increases, there is an increased production of:
    a. Long wavelengths
    b. Low-energy waves
    c. Short wavelengths
    d. Electrons

107. The relationship between kVp and density is:
   a. Indirect
   b. Directly proportional
   c. Direct, although not proportional
   d. Inverse

108. Grids that have strips angled to coincide with divergence of the x-ray beam are called:
   a. Parallel
   b. Crosshatch
   c. Focused
   d. Rhombic

109. In digital imaging, the radiographer must be aware that:
   a. mAs is the primary controlling factor
   b. The image is determined by the total exposure
   c. Speed class is the primary controlling factor
   d. kVp is the primary controlling factor

110. When a grid is used, what technical factor must be increased to compensate for the loss of image-forming rays?
   a. kVp
   b. Time
   c. mAs
   d. Distance

111. Filters that even out density of irregular anatomy are called:
   a. Inherent
   b. Compensating
   c. Eveners
   d. Thoraeus

112. Any misrepresentation of an anatomical structure on an image receptor that alters its size or shape defines:
   a. Elongation
   b. Magnification
   c. Definition
   d. Distortion

Imaging Procedures (Questions 113-170)

Using Figure 7-1, identify the radiographic anatomy of the urinary system.

113. Structure *A* is the:
   a. Renal pelvis
   b. Ureter
   c. Minor calyces
   d. Major calyces

114. Structure *B* is the:
   a. Renal pelvis
   b. Urethra
   c. Minor calyces
   d. Major calyces

115. Structure *C* is the:
   a. Renal pelvis
   b. Ureter
   c. Urethra
   d. Renal pyramids

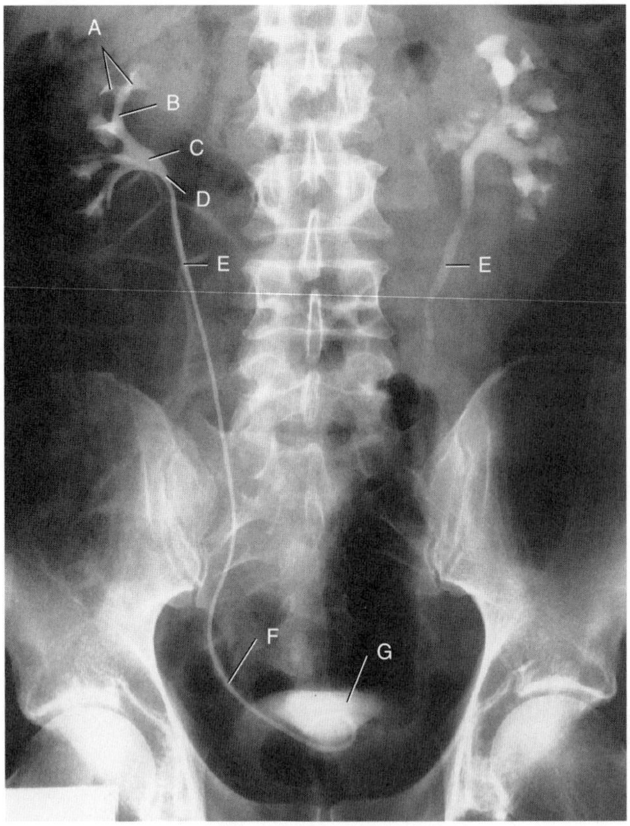

FIGURE 7-1 Retrograde pyelogram.

Using Figure 7-2, identify the radiographic anatomy of the colon.

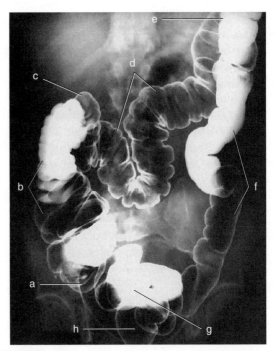

FIGURE 7-2 AP projection, barium enema (double-contrast enema).

116. Structure *B* is the:
a. Transverse colon
b. Ascending colon
c. Hepatic flexure
d. Descending colon

117. Structure *C* is the:
a. Transverse colon
b. Ascending colon
c. Hepatic flexure
d. Splenic flexure

118. Structure *D* is the:
a. Transverse colon
b. Splenic flexure
c. Hepatic flexure
d. Descending colon

119. Structure *F* is the:
a. Jejunum
b. Ascending colon
c. Hepatic flexure
d. Descending colon

Using Figure 7-3, identify the radiographic anatomy visualized during an upper GI series.

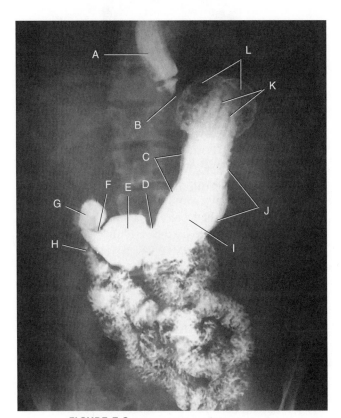

FIGURE 7-3 PA projection of the stomach.

120. Structure *D* is the:
a. Rugae
b. Haustra
c. Pylorus
d. Incisura angularis

121. Structure *E* is the:
a. Rugae
b. Fundus
c. Pylorus
d. Cardiac sphincter

122. Structure *K* is the:
a. Rugae
b. Haustra
c. Pylorus
d. Incisura angularis

123. Structure *L* is the:
a. Rugae
b. Fundus
c. Pylorus
d. Incisura angularis

Using Figure 7-4, identify the anatomy of a lumbar vertebra:

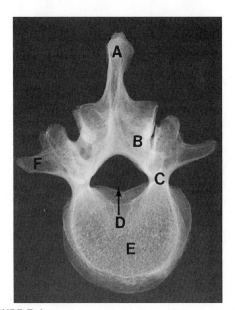

FIGURE 7-4 Lumbar vertebra (superoinferior projection).

124. Structure *A* is the:
a. Pedicle
b. Spinous process
c. Transverse process
d. Lamina

125. Structure *B* is the:
a. Pedicle
b. Spinous process
c. Coracoid process
d. Lamina

126. Structure *C* is the:
a. Pedicle
b. Coronoid process
c. Transverse process
d. Lamina

127. Structure *F* is the:
a. Pedicle
b. Spinous process
c. Transverse process
d. Lumbar angle

Using Figure 7-5, identify the radiographic anatomy of the cervical spine.

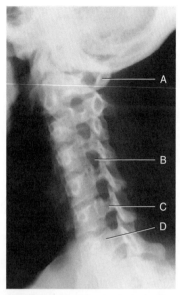

FIGURE 7-5 Oblique cervical spine.

128. Structure *B* is the:
a. Intervertebral foramen
b. Spinous process
c. Pedicle
d. Lamina
129. Structure *C* is the:
a. Intervertebral foramen
b. Spinous process
c. Pedicle
d. Lamina

Using Figure 7-6, identify the radiographic anatomy of the hip.

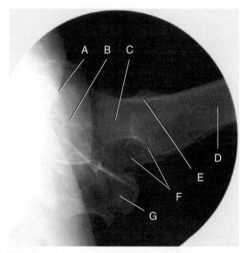
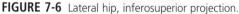

FIGURE 7-6 Lateral hip, inferosuperior projection.

130. Structure *E* is the:
a. Acetabulum
b. Ischial tuberosity
c. Greater trochanter
d. Lesser trochanter
131. Structure *F* is the:
a. Obturator foramen
b. Ischial tuberosity
c. Greater trochanter
d. Lesser trochanter
132. Structure *G* is the:
a. Acetabulum
b. Ischial tuberosity
c. Superior trochanter
d. Lesser trochanter

Using Figure 7-7, identify the radiographic anatomy of the knee.

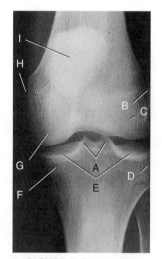

FIGURE 7-7 AP knee.

133. Structure *B* is the:
a. Medial condyle
b. Lateral epicondyle
c. Lateral condyle
d. Lateral plateau
134. Structure *D* is the:
a. Medial condyle
b. Lateral epicondyle
c. Lateral condyle
d. Tibial plateau
135. Structure *E* is the:
a. Tibial condyle
b. Lateral epicondyle
c. Lateral condyle
d. Tibial plateau
136. Structure *G* is the:
a. Medial condyle
b. Lateral epicondyle
c. Lateral condyle
d. Tibial plateau

Using Figure 7-8, identify the radiographic anatomy of the hand.

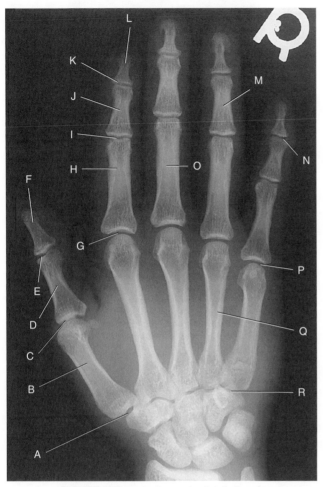

FIGURE 7-8 PA radiograph of right hand.

137. Structure *A* is the:
   a. First proximal interphalangeal joint
   b. First carpometacarpal joint
   c. Second distal interphalangeal joint
   d. Second metacarpophalangeal joint
138. Structure *G* is the:
   a. Second proximal interphalangeal joint
   b. First carpometacarpal joint
   c. Second distal interphalangeal joint
   d. Second metacarpophalangeal joint
139. Structure *I* is the:
   a. Second proximal interphalangeal joint
   b. First carpometacarpal joint
   c. Second distal interphalangeal joint
   d. Second metacarpophalangeal joint
140. Structure *K* is the:
   a. Second proximal interphalangeal joint
   b. First carpometacarpal joint
   c. Second distal interphalangeal joint
   d. Second metacarpophalangeal joint

Using Figure 7-9, identify the radiographic anatomy of the wrist.

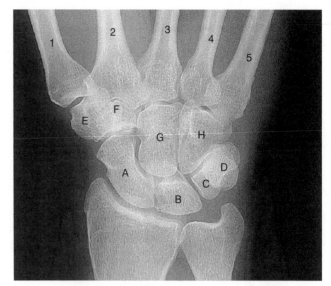

FIGURE 7-9 PA wrist.

141. Structure *A* is the:
   a. Pisiform
   b. Hamate
   c. Triquetral
   d. Scaphoid
142. Structure *B* is the:
   a. Hamate
   b. Lunate
   c. Triquetral
   d. Scaphoid
143. Structure *C* is the:
   a. Pisiform
   b. Lunate
   c. Triquetral
   d. Trapezium
144. Structure *D* is the:
   a. Pisiform
   b. Lunate
   c. Triquetral
   d. Hamate
145. Structure *E* is the:
   a. Hamate
   b. Trapezium
   c. Trapezoid
   d. Capitate
146. Structure *F* is the:
   a. Hamate
   b. Trapezium
   c. Trapezoid
   d. Capitate
147. Structure *G* is the:
   a. Hamate
   b. Trapezium
   c. Trapezoid
   d. Capitate

148. Structure *H* is the:
   a. Hamate
   b. Trapezium
   c. Trapezoid
   d. Capitate

Using Figure 7-10, identify the radiographic anatomy of the shoulder.

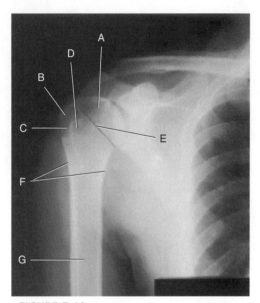

FIGURE 7-10 AP shoulder in external rotation.

149. Structure *B* is the:
   a. Surgical neck
   b. Glenoid fossa
   c. Anatomical neck
   d. Greater tubercle
150. Structure *D* is the:
   a. Surgical neck
   b. Lesser tubercle
   c. Scapula
   d. Greater tubercle
151. Structure *E* is the:
   a. Surgical neck
   b. Lesser tubercle
   c. Anatomical neck
   d. Greater tubercle
152. Structure *F* is the:
   a. Surgical neck
   b. Semilunar notch
   c. Anatomical neck
   d. Greater tubercle

Using Figure 7-11, identify the radiographic anatomy of the foot.

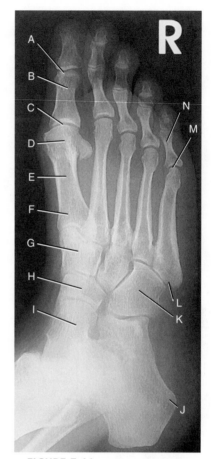

FIGURE 7-11 Oblique right foot.

153. Structure *G* is the:
   a. Talus
   b. Navicular
   c. Cuboid
   d. Second or intermediate cuneiform
154. Structure *H* is the:
   a. Talus
   b. Navicular
   c. First or intermediate cuneiform
   d. Second or intermediate cuneiform
155. Structure *I* is the:
   a. Talus
   b. Navicular
   c. Tuberosity
   d. Second or intermediate cuneiform
156. Structure *J* is the:
   a. Talus
   b. Tuberosity of the calcaneus
   c. Cuboid
   d. Second or intermediate cuneiform

157. Structure *K* is the:
  a. Fifth metatarsophalangeal joint
  b. Navicular
  c. Cuboid
  d. Second or intermediate cuneiform
158. Structure *M* is the:
  a. Talus
  b. Navicular
  c. Cuboid
  d. Fifth metatarsophalangeal joint

Using Figure 7-12, identify the radiographic anatomy of the elbow.

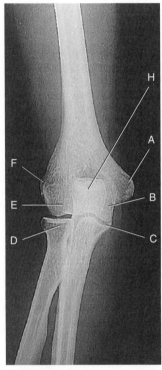

FIGURE 7-12 AP elbow.

159. Structure *A* is the:
  a. Lateral epicondyle
  b. Olecranon process
  c. Radial head
  d. Medial epicondyle
160. Structure *D* is the:
  a. Capitulum
  b. Olecranon process
  c. Radial head
  d. Ulnar head
161. Structure *E* is the:
  a. Capitulum
  b. Olecranon process
  c. Radial head
  d. Medial epicondyle

162. Structure *H* is the:
  a. Ulnar head
  b. Olecranon process
  c. Radial head
  d. Medial epicondyle

Using Figure 7-13, identify the radiographic anatomy of the skull.

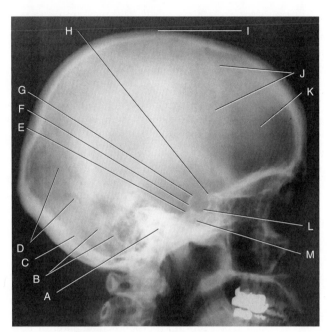

FIGURE 7-13 Lateral projection of skull.

163. Structure *C* is the:
  a. Body of sphenoid
  b. Occipital bone
  c. Dorsum sellae
  d. Anterior clinoid process
164. Structure *F* is the:
  a. Body of sphenoid
  b. Occipital bone
  c. Dorsum sellae
  d. Sella turcica
165. Structure *H* is the:
  a. Sella turcica
  b. Occipital bone
  c. Dorsum sellae
  d. Anterior clinoid process
166. Structure *M* is the:
  a. Body of sphenoid (sphenoid sinus)
  b. Occipital bone
  c. Dorsum sellae
  d. Anterior clinoid process

Using Figure 7-14, identify the radiographic anatomy of the facial bones.

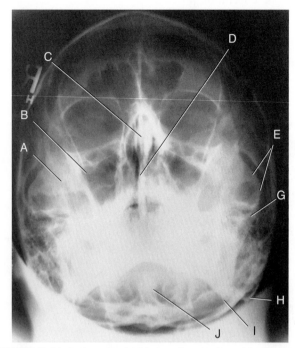

FIGURE 7-14 Parietoacanthial (Waters) projection of facial bones.

167. Structure *B* is the:
    a. Zygomatic arch
    b. Foramen magnum
    c. Bony nasal septum (perpendicular plate of ethmoid and vomer)
    d. Body of maxilla (contains the maxillary sinuses)
168. Structure *C* is the:
    a. Zygomatic arch
    b. Foramen magnum
    c. Bony nasal septum (perpendicular plate of ethmoid and vomer)
    d. Body of maxilla (contains the maxillary sinuses)
169. Structure *D* is the:
    a. Zygomatic arch
    b. Anterior nasal spine
    c. Bony nasal septum (perpendicular plate of ethmoid and vomer)
    d. Angle of mandible
170. Structure *E* is the:
    a. Zygomatic arch
    b. Foramen magnum
    c. Bony nasal septum (perpendicular plate of ethmoid and vomer)
    d. Body of maxilla (contains the maxillary sinuses)

Patient Care and Education (Questions 171-200)

171. The prefix that means "false" is:
    a. retro-
    b. endo-
    c. pseudo-
    d. epi-

172. The prefix that means "above" is:
    a. hypo-
    b. ex-
    c. ect-
    d. hyper-
173. Infectious waste is placed in containers:
    a. Made of lead
    b. Properly labeled with the type of waste therein
    c. That are incinerated
    d. Made of plastic only
174. Needles and syringes must be disposed of:
    a. Capped
    b. Weekly
    c. Uncapped
    d. Monthly
175. Causing a patient to become apprehensive of being injured is called:
    a. Assault
    b. Battery
    c. False imprisonment
    d. Invasion of privacy
176. Violation of confidentiality defines:
    a. Assault
    b. Battery
    c. False imprisonment
    d. Invasion of privacy
177. Neglect or omission of reasonable care defines:
    a. *Respondeat superior*
    b. *Res ipsa loquitur*
    c. Gross negligence
    d. Unintentional misconduct
178. Bradycardia indicates a pulse of:
    a. More than 100 beats per minute
    b. Fewer than 60 beats per minute
    c. Greater than 90
    d. Less than 50
179. Which of the following contains all equipment and drugs needed during respiratory arrest?
    a. Crash cart
    b. Suction unit
    c. Defibrillator
    d. Sphygmomanometer
180. Which of the following is used to measure blood pressure?
    a. Crash cart
    b. Suction unit
    c. Defibrillator
    d. Sphygmomanometer
181. A positive contrast agent that may be administered to a patient when barium sulfate is contraindicated is called:
    a. Barium thiosulfate
    b. Iodine
    c. Air
    d. Aqueous iodine compound

182. Flushing, urticaria, and nausea are symptoms of what type of contrast agent reaction?
  a. Local irritation
  b. Cardiovascular shock
  c. Anaphylactic shock
  d. Psychogenic shock

183. What is the type of infection control in which microorganisms have been eliminated as much as possible by the use of water and chemical disinfectants?
  a. Medical asepsis
  b. Surgical asepsis
  c. Standard precautions
  d. Gas sterilization

184. The abbreviation that means "history" is:
  a. hx
  b. bx
  c. hs
  d. MI

185. The abbreviation that means "heart attack" is:
  a. hx
  b. HA
  c. CVA
  d. MI

186. When scheduling radiographic examinations:
  a. Schedule barium studies first to get them over with
  b. Schedule special studies for the afternoon
  c. Schedule barium studies last
  d. Always schedule a scout CT scan first

187. Infectious waste must be handled according to which of the following?
  a. Radiation protection guidelines
  b. Radiology department rules
  c. CDC guidelines
  d. The condition of the patient

188. Normal adult respiration is measured by:
  a. Counting breaths
  b. Thermometer
  c. Sphygmomanometer
  d. Digital BP cuff

189. What item is used to administer oxygen through the nose?
  a. Crash cart
  b. Suction unit
  c. Defibrillator
  d. Nasal cannula

190. What type of infection transmission is defined as being spread primarily on contaminated items, food, or water?
  a. Contact transmission
  b. Airborne transmission
  c. Droplet transmission
  d. Common vehicle transmission

191. Which of the following is used to restore normal heartbeat?
  a. Crash cart
  b. Suction unit
  c. Defibrillator
  d. Sphygmomanometer

192. Shock is indicated when the diastolic pressure is:
  a. Greater than 100 beats per minute
  b. Less than 60 beats per minute
  c. Greater than 90
  d. Less than 50

193. The law governing patient confidentiality is abbreviated:
  a. CDC
  b. HHS
  c. ALARA
  d. HIPAA

194. The type of shock that occurs secondary to heart failure is called:
  a. Hypovolemic shock
  b. Septic shock
  c. Neurogenic shock
  d. Cardiogenic shock

195. Needles and syringes must be disposed of in:
  a. Lead containers
  b. Sharps containers
  c. Plastic bags
  d. Metal pans

196. Used bandages and dressings must be placed into:
  a. Lead containers
  b. Waterproof bags and sealed
  c. Plastic bags
  d. Metal pans

197. Infectious waste must be discarded:
  a. Immediately
  b. Monthly
  c. And burned
  d. With other hospital waste

198. Toxic chemicals may:
  a. Be poured down the drain if it does not enter the public water supply
  b. Never be poured down the drain
  c. Be poured down the same drain as the processing water
  d. Be poured down the drain in the restroom only

199. The suffix that means "pain" is:
  a. -itis
  b. -algia
  c. -ectomy
  d. -megaly

200. The suffix that means "puncture" is:
  a. -centesis
  b. -otomy
  c. -genic
  d. -osis

Scoring

Traditionally you have probably focused on how many questions you miss on an exam. As you prepare for the certification exam, I encourage you to focus on how many you answer correctly. Use Table 7-1 to calculate the percentage of questions you answered correctly in each category and on the test as a whole. Remember, a score of less

TABLE 7-1	**Calculating Your Score for Challenge Test Number 1**	
Topic	**Percentage Calculation**	**Your Score**
Radiation protection	Number correct _____ × 100, ÷ 45 =	
Equipment operation and quality control	Number correct _____ × 100, ÷ 22 =	
Image acquisition and evaluation	Number correct _____ × 100, ÷ 45 =	
Imaging procedures	Number correct _____ × 100, ÷ 58 =	
Patient care and education	Number correct _____ × 100, ÷ 30 =	
Total	Number correct _____ × 100, ÷ 200 =	

than 75% on any topic or on an entire test is an indication that more review is needed on that topic. Now go back and concentrate on the items that were missed and figure out the reason why. Then go on to Challenge Test Number 2.

CHALLENGE TEST NUMBER 2

Radiation Protection (Questions 1-45)

1. The amount of radiation deposited per unit length of tissue traversed by incoming photons is called:
   a. Tissue exposure
   b. Linear deposition of energy
   c. Linear energy transfer
   d. Effective dose limit
2. Cataractogenesis, life span shortening, embryological effects, and carcinogenesis are examples of:
   a. Short-term somatic effects
   b. Genetic effects
   c. Acute radiation syndrome
   d. Long-term somatic effects
3. Compton interaction:
   a. Increases contrast in the radiographic image
   b. Results in scattering of the incident electrons
   c. Decreases recorded detail in the radiographic image
   d. Decreases contrast in the radiographic image
4. Rem multiplied by a radiation weighting factor equals:
   a. Rads
   b. Roentgens
   c. Grays
   d. No such equation is used
5. Effective dose limit:
   a. Is the level of radiation that an organism can receive and probably sustain no appreciable damage
   b. Is a safe level of radiation that can be received with no effects
   c. Should be absorbed annually to maintain proper immunity to radiation
   d. Is 5000 mrem per year for the general public
6. Radiation with a high LET:
   a. Has low ionization
   b. Is highly ionizing
   c. Carries a low quality factor
   d. Equates with a low RBE

7. Radiation protection is based on which dose-response relationship?
   a. Linear-threshold
   b. Nonlinear-nonthreshold
   c. Linear-nonthreshold
   d. Nonlinear-threshold
8. Which of the following states that the radiosensitivity of cells is directly proportional to their reproductive activity and inversely proportional to their degree of differentiation?
   a. Inverse square law
   b. Law of Bergonié and Tribondeau
   c. Reciprocity law
   d. Ohm's law
9. Which of the following causes about 95% of the cellular response to radiation?
   a. Direct effect
   b. Law of Bergonié and Tribondeau
   c. Target theory
   d. Indirect effect
10. When radiation strikes DNA, which of the following occurs?
    a. Direct effect
    b. Law of Bergonié and Tribondeau
    c. Target theory
    d. Indirect effect
11. The amount of radiation that causes the number of genetic mutations in a population to double is called the:
    a. Threshold dose
    b. Doubling dose
    c. Mutagenic dose
    d. Genetic dose
12. The units of equivalent dose, activity, in-air exposure, and absorbed dose are:
    a. Roentgen, rad, rem, curie
    b. Rad, coulomb per kilogram, curie, becquerel
    c. Rem, curie, roentgen, rad
    d. Sievert, becquerel, gray, coulomb per kilogram
13. Medical x-rays are an example of:
    a. Natural background radiation
    b. Artificially produced radiation
    c. Nonionizing radiation
    d. Ionizing, natural background radiation

14. The equivalent dose limit for an embryo or fetus is:
    a. 500 mrem during gestation
    b. 5 rem per year
    c. 0.5 rem per month
    d. 50 mrem per year
15. The photoelectric effect:
    a. Results in absorption of the incident photon
    b. Results in absorption of the incident electron
    c. Produces contrast fog on the radiographic image
    d. Is the same as brems radiation
16. The effective dose limit for radiographers is:
    a. 3 rem per quarter
    b. 500 mrem per year
    c. 5000 mrem per year
    d. 100 mrem per month
17. The average dose to active bone marrow as an indicator of somatic effects on a population is called:
    a. Doubling dose
    b. Bone dose
    c. GSD
    d. Mean marrow dose
18. A radiation dose that if received by the entire population would cause the same genetic injury as the total of doses received by the members actually being exposed is called:
    a. Genetically significant dose
    b. Doubling dose
    c. Mean marrow dose
    d. Genetic dose
19. A lead apron of at least what thickness *should* be worn while being exposed to scatter radiation?
    a. 0.25-mm Pb equivalent
    b. 0.50-mm Pb equivalent
    c. 0.50-mm Al equivalent
    d. 0.10-mm Al equivalent
20. Use of a thyroid shield of at least what thickness should be used for fluoroscopy?
    a. 0.10-mm Pb equivalent
    b. 0.50-mm Pb equivalent
    c. 0.50-mm Al equivalent
    d. 0.10-mm Al equivalent
21. How thick are primary protective barriers?
    a. $\frac{1}{32}$-inch lead equivalent
    b. $\frac{1}{16}$-inch aluminum equivalent
    c. $\frac{1}{32}$-inch concrete
    d. $\frac{1}{16}$-inch lead equivalent
22. Primary protective barriers, if in the wall, must extend to a height of at least:
    a. 5 feet
    b. 6 feet
    c. 7 feet
    d. 10 feet
23. Secondary protective barriers must extend to a height of:
    a. 5 feet
    b. 6 feet
    c. The ceiling
    d. 10 feet
24. The protective curtain hanging from the fluoroscopy tower must be at least:
    a. 0.50-mm Pb equivalent
    b. 0.25-mm Al equivalent
    c. 0.10-mm Pb equivalent
    d. 0.25-mm Pb equivalent
25. The Bucky slot cover must be at least:
    a. 0.50-mm Pb equivalent
    b. 0.25-mm Al equivalent
    c. 0.10-mm Pb equivalent
    d. 0.25-mm Pb equivalent
26. Filters made of aluminum and copper are placed in the film badge to measure x-ray:
    a. Quantity
    b. Source
    c. Energy
    d. Type
27. Film badges are changed:
    a. Quarterly
    b. Weekly
    c. Yearly
    d. Monthly
28. Thermoluminescent dosimeters use what type of crystals to record dose?
    a. Dilithium crystals
    b. Lithium fluoride
    c. Flux
    d. Silver bromide
29. TLDs are heated and release what type of energy to indicate dose?
    a. Laser
    b. Visible light
    c. X-rays
    d. Gamma rays
30. Optically stimulated luminescence (OSL) dosimeters are sensitive to exposures as low as:
    a. 1 mrem
    b. 5 mrem
    c. 10 mrem
    d. 20 mrem
31. The recording material in an OSL dosimeter is:
    a. Film
    b. Lithium fluoride
    c. Aluminum oxide
    d. Silver halide
32. The energy stored in an OSL dosimeter is released when the dosimeter is exposed to:
    a. Heat
    b. White light
    c. Laser
    d. Ultrasound
33. OSL dosimeters may be worn for:
    a. 1 month
    b. 1 week
    c. 3 months
    d. 1 year

34. OSL dosimeters may be scanned and reanalyzed:
    a. Only once
    b. Monthly
    c. Five times
    d. An unlimited number of times
35. The most commonly used gonadal shield is the:
    a. Shadow shield
    b. Collimator
    c. Contact shield
    d. None of the above
36. For optimal radiation protection, what type of exposure technique should be used?
    a. Low kVp, high mAs
    b. Small focal spot
    c. All manual technique
    d. High kVp, low mAs
37. For optimal radiation protection, what speed of IR should be used?
    a. Slow
    b. Speed has no impact on dose
    c. Analog
    d. Fast
38. The minimum source-to-skin distance for portable radiography is:
    a. At least 12 inches
    b. At least 15 inches
    c. At least 72 inches
    d. At least 40 inches
39. How often is filtration adjusted by the radiographer?
    a. After several exposures
    b. Daily
    c. As part of weekly quality control
    d. Never
40. The personal dosimeter report reads in what unit of measurement?
    a. Rads
    b. Roentgens
    c. Curies
    d. Rem or mrem
41. According to NCRP Report #160, the effective dose for a typical CT examination is:
    a. 1.47 mSv
    b. 3.58 mSv
    c. 0.77 mSv
    d. 1.0 mSv
42. According to NCRP Report #160, the typical dose for a lumbar spine examination is:
    a. 1.0 mSv
    b. 3.75 mSv
    c. 1.5 mSv
    d. 0.78 mSv
43. Of the total radiation exposure, 36% involves:
    a. CT and nuclear medicine
    b. Fluoroscopy
    c. Mobile radiography and fluoroscopy
    d. CT

44. A typical chest x-ray involves a dose of:
    a. 0.77 mSv
    b. 0.1 mSv
    c. 1.67 mSv
    d. Negligible dose
45. According to NCRP Report #160, a typical dose for a pelvis and hip examination is:
    a. 0.7 mSv
    b. 1.67 mSv
    c. 3.0 mSv
    d. 0.1 mSv

Equipment Operation and Quality Control (Questions 46-67)

46. An ionization chamber circuit places:
    a. A photomultiplier tube between the IR and the patient
    b. An ionization chamber beneath or behind the IR
    c. An ionization chamber between the patient and the x-ray tube
    d. An ionization chamber between the IR and the patient
47. Full-wave rectification uses:
    a. A single semiconductor
    b. Four silicone-based semiconductors
    c. The x-ray tube as a semiconductor
    d. Four silicon-based semiconductors
48. A full-wave rectified, three-phase, 12-pulse x-ray machine produces approximately ____% more average photon energy than a full-wave rectified, single-phase x-ray machine.
    a. 35
    b. 50
    c. 41
    d. 100
49. According to the anode heel effect, the intensity of radiation is greater at the _____ side of the x-ray tube.
    a. Anode
    b. Central x-ray
    c. Neither side; the beam is of uniform intensity
    d. Cathode
50. The amount of time needed for an AEC to terminate the exposure is called:
    a. Exposure latitude
    b. Minimum reaction time
    c. Chamber response time
    d. Electronic time
51. A tube rating chart is used to determine:
    a. The safety of a single exposure
    b. The safety of a series of exposures such as performed in tomography
    c. Patient dose per mAs
    d. The number of exposures made on the anode

Using Figure 7-15, answer questions 52 through 55.

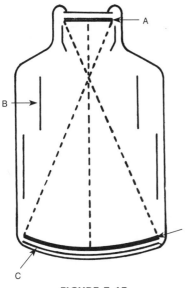

FIGURE 7-15

52. Where is the electron beam focused?
    a. *A*
    b. *B*
    c. *C*
    d. *D*
53. Where is the electronic image produced?
    a. *A*
    b. *B*
    c. *C*
    d. *D*
54. From where is the visible image distributed to viewing or recording media?
    a. *A*
    b. *B*
    c. *C*
    d. *D*
55. Where is x-ray energy converted to visible light?
    a. *A*
    b. *B*
    c. *C*
    d. *D*
56. A particular x-ray room is "shooting dark." The problem arises when a change is made from 200 to 300 mA using fixed kVp techniques at 0.16 second. Which of the following would lead to an accurate diagnosis of the problem?
    a. Wire mesh test
    b. Pinhole camera test
    c. Use of a digital dosimeter to determine HVL
    d. Use of a digital dosimeter to determine exposure linearity

57. An outpatient radiographic room is used primarily for tabletop radiography of the extremities. On a particularly busy afternoon, the radiographers find that similar exposure techniques on successive patients result in substantially different radiographs. Which of the following would lead to an accurate diagnosis of the problem?
    a. Wire mesh test
    b. Pinhole camera test
    c. Use of a digital dosimeter to determine HVL
    d. Use of a digital dosimeter to determine exposure reproducibility
58. Localized lack of sharpness on a radiograph may be diagnosed with which of the following tests?
    a. Wire mesh test
    b. Pinhole camera test
    c. Use of a digital dosimeter to determine HVL
    d. Use of a digital dosimeter to determine exposure linearity
59. X-ray beam quality is expressed in terms of:
    a. Half-value layer
    b. Exposure linearity
    c. Exposure reproducibility
    d. mAs
60. The accuracy of collimation at a 40-inch SID must be:
    a. ± 4 inches
    b. ± 8/10 inch
    c. ± 1 inch
    d. ± 1/10 inch
61. The accuracy of kVp at 80 kVp must be:
    a. No lower than 75 kVp and no higher than 85 kVp
    b. No lower than 79 kVp and no higher than 81 kVp
    c. No lower than 76 kVp and no higher than 84 kVp
    d. No lower than 78 kVp and no higher than 82 kVp
62. The apparent size of the focal spot as viewed by the image receptor is called the:
    a. Actual focal spot
    b. Target angle spot
    c. Anode heel effect
    d. Effective focal spot
63. As the angle of the anode decreases, the:
    a. Actual focal spot decreases
    b. Effective focal spot increases
    c. Actual focal spot increases
    d. Effective focal spot decreases
64. Which of the following interactions is the primary source of diagnostic x-rays?
    a. Photoelectric effect
    b. Bremsstrahlung
    c. Compton
    d. Pair production
65. Which set of exposure factors would produce the greatest density?
    a. 100 mAs, 70 kVp, 0.5-mm focal spot, 60-inch SID
    b. 200 mAs, 60 kVp, 1.2-mm focal spot, 60-inch SID
    c. 100 mAs, 70 kVp, 1.2-mm focal spot, 60-inch SID
    d. 300 mAs, 90 kVp, 0.5-mm focal spot, 60-inch SID

66. Which set of exposure factors would produce the greatest density?
    a. 80 mAs, 85 kVp, 40-inch SID, 1.2-mm focal spot
    b. 40 mAs, 80 kVp, 40-inch SID, 0.5-mm focal spot
    c. 160 mAs, 70 kVp, 40-inch SID, 1.2-mm focal spot
    d. 160 mAs, 90 kVp, 40-inch SID, 0.5-mm focal spot

67. The components of a grid are:
    a. Pb strips and Pb interspacers
    b. Al strips and Pb interspacers
    c. Pb strips and Al interspacers
    d. Pb strips and cardboard interspacers

Image Acquisition and Evaluation (Questions 68-112)

68. What is the purpose of a grid?
    a. To remove scatter radiation from the primary beam
    b. To decrease radiographic contrast
    c. To decrease dose to the patient
    d. To remove scatter radiation from the remnant beam

69. Which of the following lists of substances that make up the human body best places them in increasing order of density?
    a. Air, fat, water, muscle, bone
    b. Bone, muscle, water, fat, air
    c. Air, fat, muscle, water, bone
    d. Air, fat, water, muscle, bone, tooth enamel

70. Bit depth describes:
    a. The available gray scale of an imaging system
    b. Window level
    c. Spatial resolution
    d. Optimum exposure needed for an imaging system

71. If it is necessary to reduce radiographic density by half, and it is impossible to do so by changing mAs, the radiographer may:
    a. Reduce SID by half
    b. Double SID
    c. Decrease kVp by 15%
    d. Decrease kVp by 50%

72. Compared with film, the dynamic range for digital imaging is:
    a. Wider
    b. Narrower
    c. The same

73. Grid cutoff may be described as:
    a. Grid efficiency
    b. Absorption of scatter radiation
    c. H/D
    d. Absorption of primary rays

74. Dynamic range is defined as:
    a. The range of exposures over which a detector can acquire image data
    b. Exposure latitude
    c. Window width
    d. Window level

75. Modulation transfer function (MTF) is:
    a. The controlling factor of contrast resolution
    b. A measure of the ability of the imaging system to preserve signal contrast as a function of the spatial resolution.
    c. A function of exposure
    d. A function of pixel density

76. $2n$ (where n equals the number of bits) defines:
    a. Pixel density
    b. Shades of gray
    c. Bit depth
    d. Detector element size

77. A scintillator:
    a. Absorbs x-ray energy and emits part of that energy as visible light
    b. Absorbs x-ray energy and emits that energy as electrons
    c. Converts visible light to electrons
    d. Converts electrons into visible light

78. The magnitude of the signal differences in the remnant beam refers to:
    a. Subject contrast
    b. IP contrast
    c. Window level
    d. Spatial resolution

79. A term used to describe the mathematical formula used by the computer to reconstruct the image is:
    a. Bit depth
    b. Algorithm
    c. Mathematical function
    d. Exposure equation

80. When speed is essential in completing an imaging examination, the preferred IR is:
    a. CR
    b. Film-screen
    c. DDR
    d. Wireless DDR plate

81. Pixel is an acronym meaning:
    a. Detector element
    b. Picture element
    c. Volume element
    d. Bit element

82. Improper use of grids with a digital imaging system may cause an artifact known as:
    a. Moiré pattern
    b. Grid cutoff
    c. Motion artifact
    d. Quantum mottle

83. An integrated system of images and information is called:
    a. DICOM
    b. DDR
    c. CR/DDR
    d. PACS

84. Image noise may be described as:
    a. Undesirable fluctuations in brightness
    b. Undesirable fluctuations in contrast
    c. Inadequate spatial resolution
    d. A function of mAs

85. The measurement of the luminance of a monitor is called:
    a. Density
    b. Contrast
    c. Brightness
    d. Detail visibility
86. Grid radius is:
    a. The total amount of lead in a grid
    b. The range of SIDs that may be used with a focused grid
    c. The objective plane
    d. H/D
87. Visibility of an object's edge may be limited by:
    a. Speed class
    b. Modulation transfer function
    c. Contrast resolution
    d. Quantum noise
88. Detective quantum efficiency indicates:
    a. Patient dose
    b. Potential speed class
    c. Spatial resolution
    d. Contrast resolution
89. Digital receptors have what kind of response to exposure?
    a. Nonlinear
    b. Linear
    c. Curvilinear
    d. Hyperlinear
90. If the angle on the anode is decreased, what effect is there on recorded detail?
    a. Increase
    b. Decrease
    c. No appreciable effect
91. If mAs is increased by four times, what is the effect on radiographic contrast?
    a. Increase
    b. Decrease
    c. No appreciable effect
92. If SID is increased, what is the effect on density?
    a. Increase
    b. Decrease
    c. No appreciable effect
93. If OID is decreased, what is the effect on recorded detail?
    a. Increase
    b. Decrease
    c. No appreciable effect
94. A photodiode converts:
    a. AC to DC
    b. Light into a charge
    c. Electrons into light
    d. MRI signal into PACS data
95. If kVp is increased, what happens to radiographic contrast?
    a. Increase
    b. Decrease
    c. No appreciable effect

96. Amorphous silicon is used in:
    a. AECs
    b. OSL badges
    c. Flat panel detectors
    d. Rectifier diodes
97. In a conversion from nongrid to a 12:1 grid, what happens to radiographic contrast?
    a. Increase
    b. Decrease
    c. No appreciable effect
98. If SID is decreased from 60 inches to 30 inches, what happens to magnification?
    a. Increase
    b. Decrease
    c. No appreciable effect
99. If kVp is decreased, what happens to recorded detail?
    a. Increase
    b. Decrease
    c. No appreciable effect
100. If the IR is moved from tabletop to Bucky, what happens to recorded detail?
    a. Increase
    b. Decrease
    c. No appreciable effect
101. If there is a decrease in source-to-object distance, what happens to recorded detail?
    a. Increase
    b. Decrease
    c. No appreciable effect
102. The amount of lead in a grid is referred to as:
    a. Grid frequency
    b. Grid ratio
    c. Grid radius
    d. Grid cleanup ability
103. If there is an increase in added filtration, what happens to contrast?
    a. Increase
    b. Decrease
    c. No appreciable effect
104. If collimation is severely tightened, what happens to radiographic density?
    a. Increase
    b. Decrease
    c. No appreciable effect
105. If a cylinder cone is added, what effect is there on radiographic contrast?
    a. Increase
    b. Decrease
    c. No appreciable effect

106. If the focal spot is changed from large to small, what happens to radiographic density?
   a. Increase
   b. Decrease
   c. No appreciable effect

107. If kVp is changed when using an AEC, what happens to radiographic density?
   a. Increase
   b. Decrease
   c. No appreciable effect

108. What occurs when an incident electron interacts with the force field of an atomic nucleus?
   a. Characteristic radiation
   b. Photoelectric effect
   c. Pair production
   d. Bremsstrahlung

109. What occurs when an incident photon interacts with an outer shell electron, producing a scatter photon and a recoil electron?
   a. Characteristic radiation
   b. Photoelectric effect
   c. Pair production
   d. Compton interaction

110. What occurs when an incident electron dislodges a *K*-shell electron?
   a. Characteristic radiation
   b. Photoelectric effect
   c. Pair production
   d. Bremsstrahlung

111. A low signal to noise ratio (SNR) provides an image with:
   a. Poor spatial resolution
   b. Higher spatial resolution
   c. Poor contrast
   d. Higher distortion

112. Degraded visibility of anatomy on a digital image may be caused by:
   a. Narrow bit depth
   b. Excessive window level
   c. Extremely narrow window width
   d. Excessive processing of the image

Imaging Procedures (Questions 113-170)

113. For the parietoacanthial projection (Waters) for the sinuses, the OML forms an angle of how many degrees with the cassette?
   a. 53
   b. 45
   c. 25
   d. 37

114. For the PA axial projection for the colon, the central ray is angled caudad how many degrees?
   a. 10 to 20
   b. 20 to 30
   c. 30 to 40
   d. 25 to 45

115. The carpal bones are arranged in two rows as follows:
   a. Proximal row (scaphoid, lunate, triquetral, pisiform) and distal row (trapezium, trapezoid, capitate, hamate)
   b. Distal row (scaphoid, lunate, triquetral, pisiform) and proximal row (trapezium, trapezoid, capitate, hamate)
   c. Proximal row (scaphoid, triquetral, capitate, pisiform) and distal row (trapezium, trapezoid, lunate, hamate)
   d. The carpals are not arranged in rows

116. The prominent point of the elbow is called the:
   a. Olecranon, part of the radius
   b. Semilunar notch
   c. Trochlea
   d. Olecranon, part of the ulna

117. Imaging of what pathological condition would require radiography of the cervical spine?
   a. Talipes
   b. Colles' fracture
   c. Ankylosing spondylitis
   d. Jefferson's fracture

118. Imaging of what pathological condition would require radiography of the hand?
   a. Talipes
   b. Colles' fracture
   c. Boxer's fracture
   d. Ankylosing spondylitis

119. Imaging of what pathological condition would require radiography of the distal forearm?
   a. Talipes
   b. Colles' fracture
   c. Boxer's fracture
   d. Ankylosing spondylitis

120. Imaging of what pathological condition would require radiography of the feet?
   a. Talipes
   b. Colles' fracture
   c. Boxer's fracture
   d. Ankylosing spondylitis

121. Imaging of what pathological condition would require radiography of the entire spine?
   a. Talipes
   b. Colles' fracture
   c. Boxer's fracture
   d. Ankylosing spondylitis

Using Figure 7-16, answer questions 122 through 127.

127. The structure designated as *VI* is the:
   a. Lunate
   b. Triquetrum
   c. Capitate
   d. Scaphoid

Using Figure 7-17, answer questions 128 through 132.

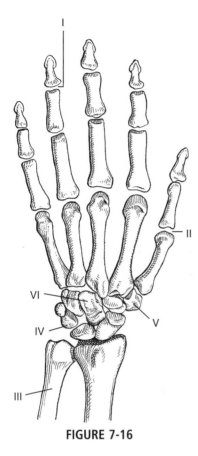

FIGURE 7-16

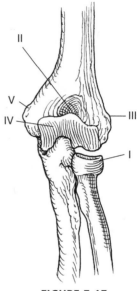

FIGURE 7-17

122. The structure designated as *I* is the:
   a. Carpometacarpal joint
   b. Interphalangeal joint
   c. Proximal phalanx
   d. Distal interphalangeal joint
123. The structure designated as *II* is the:
   a. Carpometacarpal joint
   b. Interphalangeal joint
   c. Proximal phalanx
   d. Metacarpophalangeal joint
124. The structure designated as *III* is the:
   a. Ulna
   b. Metacarpal
   c. Radius
   d. Humerus
125. The structure designated as *IV* is the:
   a. Lunate
   b. Triquetral
   c. Capitate
   d. Pisiform
126. The structure designated as *V* is the:
   a. Lunate
   b. Scaphoid
   c. Trapezium
   d. Trapezoid

128. The structure designated as *I* is the:
   a. Head of ulna
   b. Radial head
   c. Medial epicondyle
   d. Lateral epicondyle
129. The structure designated as *II* is the:
   a. Coronoid fossa
   b. Olecranon
   c. Semilunar notch
   d. Radial head
130. The structure designated as *III* is the:
   a. Head of the ulna
   b. Radial head
   c. Medial epicondyle
   d. Lateral epicondyle
131. The structure designated as *IV* is the:
   a. Medial epicondyle
   b. Trochlea
   c. Lateral epicondyle
   d. Ulnar head
132. The structure designated as *V* is the:
   a. Medial epicondyle
   b. Trochlea
   c. Lateral epicondyle
   d. Ulnar head

Using Figure 7-18, answer questions 133 through 137.

Using Figure 7-19, answer questions 138 through 141.

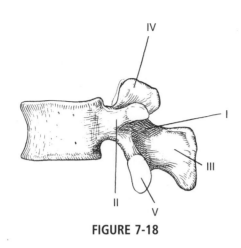

FIGURE 7-18

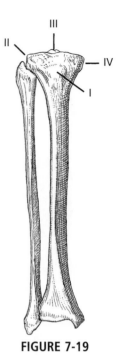

FIGURE 7-19

133. The structure designated as *I* is the:
a. Pedicle
b. Superior vertebral notch
c. Interior vertebral notch
d. Lamina

134. The structure designated as *II* is the:
a. Pedicle
b. Superior vertebral notch
c. Interior vertebral notch
d. Spinous process

135. The structure designated as *III* is the:
a. Lamina
b. Spinous process
c. Superior articular process
d. Pedicle

136. The structure designated as *IV* is the:
a. Superior vertebral notch
b. Superior articular process
c. Transverse process
d. Spinous process

137. The structure designated as *V* is the:
a. Lamina
b. Spinous process
c. Inferior vertebral notch
d. Inferior articular process

138. The structure designated as *I* is the:
a. Head of the fibula
b. Head of the tibia
c. Tuberosity
d. Styloid process

139. The structure designated as *II* is the:
a. Medial condyle
b. Lateral condyle
c. Intercondylar eminence
d. Head of the fibula

140. The structure designated as *III* is the:
a. Tubercle
b. Lateral condyle
c. Medial condyle
d. Intercondylar eminence

141. The structure designated as *IV* is the:
a. Tubercle
b. Lateral condyle
c. Medial condyle
d. Intercondylar eminence

Using Figure 7-20, answer questions 142 through 147.

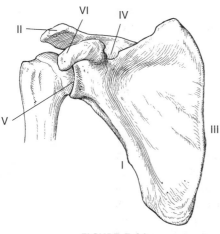

FIGURE 7-20

142. The structure designated as *I* is the:
a. Vertebral border
b. Scapular notch
c. Body
d. Axillary border

143. The structure designated as *II* is the:
a. Humeral head
b. Acromion
c. Coracoid process
d. Coronoid process

144. The structure designated as *III* is the:
a. Vertebral border
b. Scapular notch
c. Body
d. Subscapular fossa

145. The structure designated as *IV* is the:
a. Coracoid process
b. Coronoid process
c. Scapular notch
d. Glenoid fossa

146. The structure designated as *V* is the:
a. Glenoid fossa
b. Acromion
c. Coronoid process
d. Coracoid process

147. The structure designated as *VI* is the:
a. Glenoid fossa
b. Acromion
c. Coronoid process
d. Coracoid process

148. Critique Figure 7-21.
a. Radiograph is unacceptable; radius and ulna should be superimposed
b. Radiograph is unacceptable; tibia and fibula should be superimposed
c. Radiograph is acceptable, but only one joint is needed
d. Radiograph is acceptable

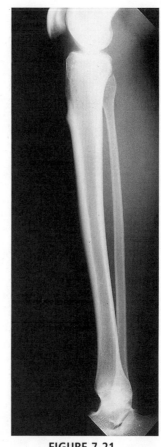

FIGURE 7-21

149. The radiograph in Figure 7-22 illustrates what region?
- a. Genitourinary
- b. Cardiovascular
- c. Hepatobiliary
- d. Gastrointestinal

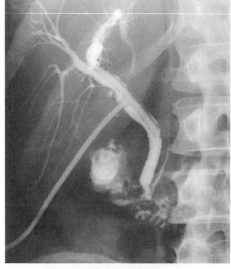

FIGURE 7-22

150. Critique Figure 7-23.
- a. Radiograph unacceptable; arm rotated
- b. Radiograph acceptable for medial oblique
- c. Radiograph acceptable for lateral oblique
- d. Radiograph unacceptable; humerus and forearm must be in same plane

151. Critique Figure 7-24.
- a. Radiograph was taken with interpupillary line parallel to IR
- b. Radiograph was taken with MSP perpendicular to IR
- c. Radiograph was taken with interpupillary line perpendicular to IR
- d. Radiograph was taken with MSP parallel to central ray

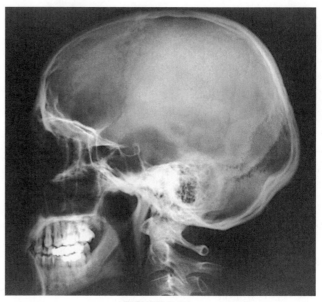

FIGURE 7-24

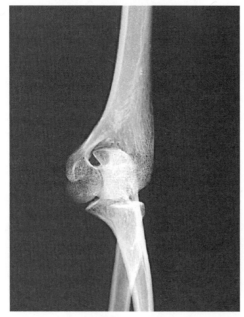

FIGURE 7-23

152. Critique Figure 7-25.
   a. Radiograph was taken with central ray angled 15 degrees caudad
   b. Radiograph was taken with central ray angled 0 degrees
   c. Radiograph was taken with central ray angled 15 degrees cephalad
   d. Radiograph was taken with MSP perpendicular to central ray

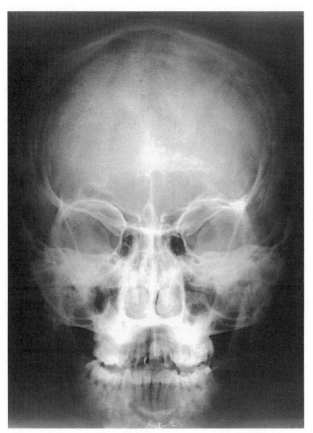

FIGURE 7-25

Using Figure 7-26, answer questions 153 through 157.

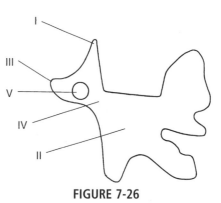

FIGURE 7-26

153. The structure designated as *I* is the:
   a. Pars interarticularis
   b. Superior articular process
   c. Pedicle
   d. Lamina
154. The structure designated as *II* is the:
   a. Pars interarticularis
   b. Superior articular process
   c. Pedicle
   d. Lamina
155. The structure designated as *III* is the:
   a. Spinous process
   b. Transverse process
   c. Pedicle
   d. Inferior articular process
156. The structure designated as *IV* is the:
   a. Spinous process
   b. Transverse process
   c. Pedicle
   d. Pars interarticularis
157. The structure designated as *V* is the:
   a. Spinous process
   b. Transverse process
   c. Pedicle
   d. Inferior articular process
158. The lateral transthoracic humerus, oblique sternum, and lateral thoracic spine may be imaged best by using a technique called:
   a. Tomography
   b. Zonography
   c. Autotomography
   d. CT

159. A patient unable to supinate the hand for an anteroposterior (AP) projection of the forearm:
    a. Should be made to do so to provide a diagnostic radiograph
    b. Probably has a fracture of the radial head and must be handled carefully
    c. Probably has a low pain tolerance and must be handled carefully
    d. May require radiographs with and without weights

160. When a posteroanterior (PA) axial projection of the clavicle is performed, the central ray should be angled:
    a. 15 degrees cephalad
    b. 15 degrees caudad
    c. 25 to 30 degrees cephalad
    d. 25 to 30 degrees caudad

161. When a lateral projection of the knee is performed, the knee should be:
    a. Extended 20 to 30 degrees
    b. Flexed to a 90-degree angle
    c. Flexed 20 to 30 degrees
    d. Fully extended

162. When a tangential projection of the patella is performed with the patient prone, the central ray should be angled:
    a. 15 degrees cephalad
    b. 15 degrees caudad
    c. 25 degrees cephalad
    d. 45 degrees cephalad

163. Use of which of the following would provide an improved image of the femur?
    a. Trough filter
    b. Anode heel effect
    c. Short SID
    d. Long OID

164. When an AP projection of the hip is performed, the central ray is directed:
    a. Perpendicular to a point 2 inches medial to the anterior superior iliac spine (ASIS) at the level of the superior margin of the greater trochanter
    b. Parallel to a point 2 inches medial to the ASIS at the level of the superior margin of the greater trochanter
    c. At a 15-degree cephalad angle
    d. To the level of the ASIS

165. When an AP oblique projection is performed for the cervical vertebrae, the central ray is directed:
    a. 25 to 30 degrees cephalad
    b. 15 to 20 degrees caudad
    c. 5 to 10 degrees cephalad
    d. 15 to 20 degrees cephalad

166. When the AP oblique projection is performed for the lumbar vertebrae, the side of interest is:
    a. Farthest from the film
    b. Closest to the film
    c. Rotated 30 degrees
    d. Rotated 20 degrees

167. When the PA oblique projection for the sacroiliac joints is performed, the side of interest is:
    a. Farthest from the film
    b. Closest to the film
    c. Rotated 10 degrees
    d. Rotated 45 degrees

168. Routine chest radiography is performed:
    a. At the end of full inspiration
    b. At the end of full expiration
    c. At the end of the second full inspiration
    d. With the patient supine or upright

169. The primary purpose of performing oblique projections of the ribs is:
    a. To image the axillary portion of the ribs
    b. To image the ribs above the diaphragm
    c. To image the ribs below the diaphragm
    d. To determine the extent of the patient's pain tolerance

170. When the PA projection of the skull is performed to image the frontal bone:
    1. The central ray is directed perpendicular to the cassette
    2. The OML is perpendicular to the cassette
    3. The central ray exits at the glabella
    4. MSP is parallel to cassette
    a. All are true
    b. 1, 2
    c. 1, 3, 4
    d. 1, 3

Patient Care and Education (Questions 171-200)

171. The suffix that means "condition" is:
    a. -pathy
    b. -itis
    c. -osis
    d. -tomy

172. The suffix that means "disease" is:
    a. -osis
    b. -pathy
    c. -rhaphy
    d. -scopy

173. Bradycardia indicates a pulse of:
    a. Greater than 100 beats per minute
    b. Greater than 60 beats per minute
    c. Greater than 90
    d. Less than 60 beats per minute

174. Normal adult respiration is:
    a. Greater than 100 beats per minute
    b. Less than 60 beats per minute
    c. 12 to 16 breaths per minute
    d. 12 to 16 beats per minute

175. The radiographer must be proficient in the use of which of the following medical instruments?
    a. Angiography catheter
    b. Sphygmomanometer
    c. Thermometer
    d. Oxygen administration equipment

176. A tube used to feed a patient or to perform gastric suction is called a:
a. Tracheostomy tube
b. Tracheotomy tube
c. Nasogastric tube
d. Ventilator tube

177. Nosocomial infections are acquired:
a. In radiology
b. Through the nose
c. During cold and flu season
d. In the health care setting

178. During movement and transfer of patients, urinary catheter bags should be:
a. Safely placed on the patient's abdomen
b. Kept below the level of the urinary bladder
c. Kept below the level of the x-ray table
d. Kept on the cart or wheelchair

179. The first task that must be performed when beginning a radiographic examination of a patient is to:
a. Verify patient identity
b. Determine accuracy of physician's orders
c. Verify the examination to be performed
d. Remove radiopaque objects from the area of interest

180. Which of the following is *not* required for valid consent?
a. Patient must be of legal age
b. Patient must be adequately informed and sign a consent form
c. Patient must be mentally competent
d. Consent must be offered voluntarily

181. The prefix that means "around" is:
a. poly-
b. peri-
c. retro-
d. trans-

182. Prefix that means "many" is:
a. peri-
b. poly-
c. hemi-
d. epi-

183. A system that uses barriers between individuals and assumes all patients are infectious is called:
a. Standard precautions
b. Whole-body isolation
c. Sterile technique
d. Surgical asepsis

184. When you are performing patient care in radiology:
a. Hands should be washed after each procedure
b. Gowns and gloves should always be worn
c. Hands should be washed only after you care for obviously infectious patients
d. Gloves should be worn only when you perform gastrointestinal procedures or venipuncture

185. Patient transfer from cart to x-ray table should be performed:
a. Alone when working evenings or nights
b. By radiographers working in pairs at all times
c. Alone when the department is busy or has a staff shortage
d. In pairs only when other radiographers are available to assist

186. Your best source for the latest information regarding standard precautions is the:
a. Radiology administrator
b. Radiology purchasing manager
c. Infection control department
d. Radiologist

187. After all radiographic or fluoroscopic procedures, the radiographer should use _____ to clean surfaces with which the patient was in contact.
a. Alcohol
b. Surgical asepsis
c. Soap and water
d. Medical asepsis

188. When sterile fields are prepared, damp packages:
a. Are always considered contaminated
b. Are always considered sterile because the dampness confirms they were cleaned
c. Should be unwrapped first and placed in the center of the sterile field
d. Are always considered sterile; the dampness is a remnant of the gassing process

189. When mobile radiography is performed, the mobile unit:
a. Does not have to be cleaned because it is never in contact with sterile fields
b. Must be cleaned before and after each use
c. Must be cleaned before it is brought into surgical areas or reverse isolation units
d. Must be cleaned before it is brought into surgical areas or reverse isolation units and after its removal from most isolation units

190. When radiography is performed on patients in isolation, the IR:
a. Should be placed in a protective covering only if the patient is in reverse isolation
b. Must always be placed in a protective covering
c. Should be placed in a protective covering to keep it free of microbes
d. Should be placed in a protective covering so that no microbes leave the room

191. Which of the following procedures should a radiographer be prepared to assist with at any time?
a. Cardiac massage
b. Defibrillation
c. Feeding tube insertion
d. CPR

192. In addition to performing radiography on a trauma victim, the radiographer should be:
1. Assessing the patient's condition continually
2. Interpreting the radiographs for the emergency department physician
3. Taking additional projections as indicated by the patient's condition or preliminary radiographs
4. Keeping all other health care workers out of the room because of radiation protection standards
5. Providing comfort and communicating quietly with the patient, whether the patient is conscious or unconscious
   a. 1, 3
   b. All are true
   c. 1, 3, 5
   d. 1, 3, 4, 5

193. For a barium enema, the contrast agent should be mixed with:
a. Cold water
b. Water at or below body temperature
c. Water at approximately 120° F
d. Water at approximately 100° F

194. All iodinated contrast media used today contain:
a. Iodine and free ions
b. Free ions
c. Only iodine
d. Salts of organic iodine compounds

195. The highest incidence of contrast agent reactions occurs with the use of:
a. Negative contrast media
b. Ionic iodinated contrast media
c. Nonionic iodinated contrast media
d. Barium sulfate

196. It is important for the radiographer to obtain the recent history of radiographic examinations performed on a patient so that:
a. An overdose of iodinated contrast media does not occur from examinations recently performed
b. An overdose of radiation is not administered
c. Unnecessary examinations may be avoided
d. Costs may be contained

197. For a patient with a history of intravenous urography and no contrast agent reactions:
a. The radiographer may assume there would be no reaction on subsequent intravenous urograms
b. The radiographer must assume there is a chance of a reaction on other contrast examinations
c. The radiographer must assume there is a chance of a reaction on subsequent intravenous urograms
d. There is no chance of reactions on subsequent intravenous urograms

198. A negative contrast agent used in chest radiography and some arthrography is:
a. Barium sulfate
b. Iodine
c. Perforated ulcers or ruptured appendix
d. Air

199. A positive contrast agent administered to the patient who is going to surgery is:
a. Barium sulfate
b. Iodine
c. Perforated ulcers or ruptured appendix
d. Aqueous iodine compound

200. In an attempt to maintain the quality of patient care at the highest level possible over time, proof of continuing education is mandatory for renewal of certification with:
a. State licensing board in all 50 states
b. American Society of Radiologic Technologists
c. The Joint Commission
d. ARRT

Scoring

Use Table 7-2 to calculate the percentage of questions you answered correctly in each category and on the test as a whole. Remember, a score of less than 75% on any topic or the entire test is an indication that more review is needed on that topic. Now go back and concentrate on which items were missed and the reason why. When you are done reviewing, go on to Challenge Test Number 3.

TABLE 7-2	Calculating Your Score for Challenge Test Number 2	
Topic	**Percentage Calculation**	**Your Score**
Radiation protection	Number correct _____ × 100, ÷ 45 =	
Equipment operation and quality control	Number correct _____ × 100, ÷ 22 =	
Image acquisition and evaluation	Number correct _____ × 100, ÷ 45 =	
Imaging procedures	Number correct _____ × 100, ÷ 58 =	
Patient care and education	Number correct _____ × 100, ÷ 30 =	
Total	Number correct _____ × 100, ÷ 200 =	

CHALLENGE TEST NUMBER 3

Read each question and the answer choices carefully. Choose the best, most complete answer for each item. Use the results of this test to assess your strengths and weaknesses. Do not look up any of the answers until you have completed the entire test. Correct the test using the answer key in the back of the book. Then compute your scores using Table 7-3 to see where you are strong and where you need additional review. Refer to the appropriate chapter in this book for review of the questions you miss.

Radiation Protection (Questions 1-45)

For the following questions, choose the single best answer.

1. Radiation that exits the x-ray tube from the anode is called:
   a. Remnant radiation
   b. Gamma radiation
   c. Nonionizing radiation
   d. Primary radiation

2. The photon-tissue interaction in diagnostic radiography that results in the total absorption of an x-ray photon and the production of contrast in the radiographic image is:
   a. Compton
   b. Coherent
   c. Photoelectric
   d. Pair production

3. Which photon-tissue interaction produces a recoil electron and a scattered photon in diagnostic radiography?
   a. Compton
   b. Coherent
   c. Photoelectric
   d. Pair production

4. The traditional unit of in-air exposure is the:
   a. Coulombs/kilogram
   b. Rem
   c. Becquerel
   d. Roentgen

5. The SI unit of absorbed dose is the:
   a. Coulombs/kilogram
   b. Gray
   c. Curie
   d. LET

6. The traditional unit of dose equivalency is the:
   a. Rem
   b. Gray
   c. Quality factor
   d. LET

7. The SI unit of equivalent dose and effective dose is the:
   a. Rem
   b. Gray
   c. Quality factor
   d. Sievert

8. The traditional unit of activity is the:
   a. Becquerel
   b. Gray
   c. Quality factor
   d. Curie

9. _____ refers to 100 ergs of energy deposited per 1 g of tissue.
   a. Becquerel
   b. Gray
   c. Quality factor
   d. Rad

10. The amount of radiation deposited per unit length of tissue traversed by incoming photons is called:
    a. REM
    b. RADS
    c. LET
    d. RPU

11. Rads multiplied by a radiation weighting factor equals:
    a. Rem
    b. Roentgens
    c. Grays
    d. No such equation is used

12. Compton interaction:
    a. Produces poorer recorded detail in the radiographic image
    b. Results in absorption of the incident photon
    c. May produce higher contrast on the radiograph
    d. May produce a gray fog on the image, lowering contrast

13. The radiation weighting factor for x-rays is:
    a. 10
    b. 1
    c. 20
    d. 5

14. Mutations are examples of:
    a. Short-term somatic effects
    b. Genetic effects
    c. Acute radiation syndrome
    d. Long-term somatic effects

15. Effective dose limit:
    a. Is the level of radiation that an organism can receive before formation of cancer
    b. Is age × 1 REM
    c. Is 50 mrem per month
    d. Is 5000 mrem per year for occupationally exposed individuals

16. What agency publishes radiation protection recommendations?
    a. ICRP
    b. NCRP
    c. NRC
    d. ASRT

17. Radiation safety standards assume what relationship between dose and response?
    a. Linear-threshold
    b. Nonlinear-nonthreshold
    c. Linear-nonthreshold
    d. Nonlinear-threshold

18. Which of the following would be applicable to radiation therapy?
    a. Inverse square law
    b. Law of Bergonié and Tribondeau
    c. Reciprocity law
    d. Ohm's law

19. Which of the following causes about 5% of the cellular response to radiation?
    a. Direct effect
    b. Law of Bergonié and Tribondeau
    c. Target theory
    d. Indirect effect

20. When radiation strikes the cytoplasm, which of the following occurs?
    a. Direct effect
    b. Law of Bergonié and Tribondeau
    c. Target theory
    d. Indirect effect

21. The equivalent dose limit for the embryo-fetus is:
    a. 500 mrem per year
    b. 5 rem per year
    c. 0.05 rem per month
    d. 500 mrem during gestation

22. The effective dose limit for radiographers is:
    a. 3 rem per quarter
    b. 500 mrem per year
    c. 5 rem per year
    d. 100 mrem per month

23. The cumulative occupational exposure for a 29-year-old radiographer is:
    a. 29 mrem
    b. 55 rem
    c. 11 mrem
    d. 29 rem

24. The annual effective dose limit for the general public, assuming infrequent exposure, is:
    a. 0.5 mrem
    b. 500 rem
    c. 0.5 rem
    d. 50 mrem

25. The upper boundary dose that can be absorbed that carries a negligible risk of somatic or genetic damage to the individual defines:
    a. Maximum permissible dose
    b. ALARA
    c. Law of Bergonié and Tribondeau
    d. Effective dose limit

26. Film badges are generally accurate down to the level of:
    a. 10 rem
    b. 5 rem
    c. 0.1 mrem
    d. 10 mrem

27. The exposure switch on a portable x-ray machine must be attached to a cord that is at least how many feet long?
    a. 3
    b. 6
    c. 12
    d. 2

28. Under what conditions can the radiographer be exposed to the primary beam?
    a. When performing mobile radiography, as long as the exposure is low
    b. Never, under any conditions
    c. When performing cross-table projections, if needed to hold the cassette in place
    d. When assisting with fluoroscopy

29. For purposes of radiation protection, the x-ray beam is filtered. X-ray tubes operating above 70 kVp must have total filtration of:
    a. At least 0.25-mm aluminum equivalent
    b. At least 0.25-mm lead equivalent
    c. No more than 2.5-mm aluminum equivalent
    d. At least 2.5-mm aluminum equivalent

30. Gonadal shielding should be used:
    a. On every examination performed
    b. Whenever it does not obstruct the area of clinical interest
    c. Only on children and women of childbearing age
    d. Only during pregnancy

31. The secondary protective barrier must overlap the primary protective barrier by at least:
    a. $\frac{1}{10}$ inch
    b. 1 inch
    c. 1 foot
    d. ½ inch

32. The x-ray control booth is considered a:
    a. Secondary protective barrier
    b. Primary protective barrier
    c. Mobile barrier
    d. Nonbarrier

33. The exposure switch must keep the radiographer behind the:
    a. Primary protective barrier
    b. Secondary protective barrier
    c. X-ray tube
    d. Door

34. Areas for the general public such as waiting rooms and stairways are considered:
    a. Controlled areas
    b. Uncontrolled areas
    c. Off-limits areas
    d. Radiation areas

35. An uncontrolled area must be kept under what dose annually?
    a. 0.10 rem
    b. 0.50 rem
    c. 500 rem
    d. 5000 mrem

36. Areas occupied by persons trained in radiation safety and wearing personnel monitoring devices are called:
a. Controlled areas
b. Uncontrolled areas
c. Off-limits areas
d. Radiation areas

37. Which of the following takes into account the volume and types of examinations performed in the room?
a. Use factor
b. Shielding factor
c. Volume factor
d. Workload

38. How is workload factor measured?
a. Half-value layer
b. Amount of time the beam is on
c. mA minutes per week
d. Average kVp per week

39. The amount of time the beam is on and directed at a particular barrier is called:
a. Use factor
b. Shielding factor
c. Occupancy
d. Workload

40. Leakage radiation from a diagnostic x-ray tube may not exceed:
a. 100 mrad per hour, measured at 1 m from the housing
b. 10 R per hour
c. 100 mR per hour, measured at 1 m from the housing
d. 100 R per hour, measured at 1 m from the housing

41. According to NCRP Report #160, nuclear medicine procedures add approximately what dose?
a. 1.0 mSv
b. 0.77 mSv
c. 0.2 mSv
d. 3.5 mSv

42. The typical dose for a KUB is:
a. 0.7 mSv
b. Negligible
c. 1.0 mSv
d. 0.2 mSv

43. NCRP Report #160 indicates that a typical dose for a cervical spine examination is:
a. 0.77 mSv
b. 2.56 mSv
c. 1.0 mSv
d. 0.2 mSv

44. The typical dose for a thoracic spine examination is:
a. 0.75 mSv
b. 2.0 mSv
c. 1.0 mSv
d. 0.2 mSv

45. According to NCRP Report #160, conventional radiography and fluoroscopy contribute what dose overall?
a. 0.33 mSv
b. 3.5 mSv
c. 1.0 mSv
d. 0.77 mSv

Equipment Operation and Quality Control (Questions 46-67)

46. Devices in the x-ray circuit that increase or decrease voltage are called:
a. Rectifiers
b. Generators
c. Timers
d. Transformers

47. The filament circuit makes use of what type of transformer?
a. Step-up
b. Autotransformer
c. Step-down
d. Falling load

48. Because the x-ray tube requires DC to operate properly, what device is required in the x-ray circuit?
a. Autotransformer
b. Step-up transformer
c. Rectifier
d. Falling load generator

49. Where is the rectifier located in the x-ray circuit?
a. Between the timer and the step-up transformer
b. Between the step-up transformer and the step-down transformer
c. Between the primary and secondary coils of the step-up transformer
d. Between the step-up transformer and the x-ray tube

50. Thermionic emission occurs at the:
a. Anode
b. Control panel
c. Rectifier
d. Cathode

51. At the time of exposure, the charge on the focusing cup is:
a. Irrelevant
b. Positive
c. Negative
d. Alternating

52. An interaction that produces heat at the anode and also produces x-rays is called:
a. Characteristic
b. Photoelectric
c. Compton
d. Bremsstrahlung

53. Examples of video tubes that may be used in fluoroscopy are:
a. Brems and characteristic
b. Vidicon and Plumbicon
c. Digital and analog
d. Anode and cathode

54. When a quality control test for exposure linearity is performed, adjacent mA stations must be within _____ of one another.
    a. 2% of SID
    b. 4%
    c. 10%
    d. 5%

55. When a quality control test for exposure reproducibility is performed, successive exposures must be within _____ of one another.
    a. 2% of SID
    b. 4%
    c. 10%
    d. 5%

56. When a quality control test for collimator accuracy is performed, the result must be within _____.
    a. 2% of SID
    b. 4%
    c. 10%
    d. 5%

57. When a quality control test for accuracy of kVp is performed, the result must be within _____ of the control panel setting.
    a. 2% of SID
    b. 4%
    c. 10%
    d. 4

58. When a spinning top test is performed on single-phase equipment, a radiograph exhibiting six dots would indicate:
    a. An accurate timer, if set on $\frac{1}{20}$ second
    b. A malfunctioning timer, if set on $\frac{1}{20}$ second
    c. A malfunctioning autotransformer, if set on $\frac{1}{20}$ second
    d. An accurate timer, if set on $\frac{1}{6}$ second

59. When a spinning top test is performed on three-phase equipment, a timer setting of 0.5 second should indicate the following on the resultant radiograph:
    a. 180 dots
    b. 90 dots
    c. A 180-degree arc
    d. A 90-degree arc

60. The accuracy of collimation at a 72-inch SID must be:
    a. ± 1.44 inches
    b. ± 7.2 inches
    c. ± 3.6 inches
    d. ± 0.02 inch

61. The accuracy of kVp at 90 kVp must be:
    a. No lower than 85 kVp and no higher than 95 kVp
    b. No lower than 89 kVp and no higher than 91 kVp
    c. No lower than 86 kVp and no higher than 94 kVp
    d. No lower than 88 kVp and no higher than 92 kVp

62. The feature of the image intensifier that ensures the radiation dose striking the input phosphor is constant is the:
    a. Photocathode
    b. Electron focusing lens
    c. Automatic brightness control
    d. Vidicon tube

63. Instead of Vidicon or Plumbicon tubes, what device may be used in the television system?
    a. Charge-coupled device (CCD)
    b. C-arm
    c. Automatic brightness control
    d. Output phosphor

64. The electronic device that may be used for many quality control tests on x-ray equipment is the:
    a. Automatic exposure control
    b. Digital dosimeter
    c. Penetrometer
    d. Densitometer

For the following questions, choose the single best answer.

65. The amount of darkness on a radiograph is best described as:
    a. Contrast
    b. Detail
    c. Brightness
    d. mAs

66. The smallest particle of a compound that retains the characteristics of the compound is a(n):
    a. Element
    b. Atom
    c. Molecule
    d. Neutron

67. The equation mAs = mAs describes which of the following?
    a. Inverse square law
    b. mAs-density law
    c. Reciprocity law
    d. 15% law

Image Acquisition and Evaluation (Questions 68-112)

68. Given an original technique of 20 mAs and 80 kVp, which of the following would produce a radiograph with double the density?
    a. 40 mAs, 90 kVp
    b. 30 mAs, 92 kVp
    c. 40 mAs, 80 kVp
    d. 15 mAs, 92 kVp

69. Distance and density are governed by what law or rule?
    a. Reciprocity law
    b. 15% rule
    c. Inverse square law
    d. Density maintenance rule

70. Unwanted markings on a radiograph are called:
    a. Processing irregularities
    b. Processing artifacts
    c. Artifacts
    d. Plus-density markings
71. Manual manipulation of the digital image after acquisition is referred to as:
    a. Digital coding
    b. Postprocessing
    c. Leveling
    d. Archiving
72. As speed class decreases, patient dose:
    a. Increases
    b. Decreases
    c. Remains the same
73. Because the digital system software ultimately controls contrast, kVp may be:
    a. Increased
    b. Decreases
    c. Kept the same
74. Image acquisition, image display, and image storage are the primary components of what system?
    a. DICOM
    b. CR/DR
    c. PACS
    d. HIS
75. What "language" is used by PACS?
    a. DICOM
    b. Base 10
    c. HIS
    d. RIS
76. Which exposure factor causes excessive image noise if set too high?
    a. kVp
    b. mAs
    c. AEC
    d. Time
77. Which of the following can be documented as an indication of patient dose?
    a. AEC
    b. Exposure indicator
    c. System speed class
    d. Histogram
78. Choosing the anatomical region on a touch screen display to set technique is called:
    a. Phototiming
    b. Anatomically programmed radiography
    c. AEC imaging
    d. Automatic radiography
79. What is used to reduce both patient dose and the production of scatter radiation?
    a. Grids
    b. High speed class
    c. Collimation
    d. Filtration
80. Image artifacts are usually classified as:
    a. Scatter
    b. Plus density and minus density
    c. Compton and photoelectric
    d. Patient motion and equipment motion
81. Grid ratio is expressed as:
    a. Length of the lead strips to the space between them
    b. Height of the aluminum strips to the space between them
    c. Height of the interspacers to the lead strips
    d. Height of the lead strips to the space between them
82. The primary type of grid used in diagnostic imaging is:
    a. Crosshatch
    b. Parallel
    c. Rhombic
    d. Focused
83. Which of the following does *not* belong in the definition of matter?
    a. Travels at the speed of light
    b. Has shape
    c. Has form
    d. Occupies space
84. The accuracy of collimation at a 60-inch SID must be:
    a. ± 6 inches
    b. ± 3 inches
    c. ± 2 inches
    d. ± 1.2 inches
85. Which of the following is true regarding frequency and wavelength of electromagnetic radiation?
    a. Frequency and wavelength are directly proportional
    b. Frequency and wavelength are unrelated
    c. Wavelength and frequency are inversely proportional to the square of the distance between wave crests
    d. Wavelength and frequency are inversely proportional
86. Beam restrictors reduce the amount of scatter produced by reducing which of the following?
    a. Characteristic rays
    b. Photoelectric effect
    c. Compton's interactions
    d. Pair production
87. What effect does increasing filtration have on contrast?
    a. Increase contrast
    b. Decrease contrast
    c. No effect
    d. Varying effect
88. Decreased SID causes image:
    a. Minification
    b. Foreshortening
    c. Elongation
    d. Magnification

89. Grid ratio is expressed as:
    a. Length of the lead strips to the space between them
    b. Height of the aluminum strips to the space between them
    c. Height of the interspacers to the lead strips
    d. Height of the lead strips to the space between them

90. The primary type of grid used in diagnostic imaging is:
    a. Crosshatch
    b. Parallel
    c. Rhombic
    d. Focused

91. The measure of a grid's ability to enhance contrast is called:
    a. Grid ratio
    b. Grid selectivity
    c. Speed
    d. Contrast improvement factor

92. Which of the following grid errors would result in an image that shows normal density in the middle but decreased density on the sides, assuming the correct side of the grid faces the x-ray tube?
    a. Upside down
    b. Off-level
    c. Lateral decentering
    d. Grid-focus decentering

93. Which of the following grid errors would result in an image that shows decreased density more to one side than the other?
    a. Upside down
    b. Off-level
    c. Lateral decentering
    d. Grid-focus decentering

94. Grid ratio is described by which of the following?
    a. H & D
    b. H/D
    c. mAs = mAs
    d. 15% rule

95. Grid radius is described as:
    a. The height of the lead strips divided by the distance between the lead strips
    b. The distance between the lead strips divided by the height of the lead strips
    c. The number of lead strips per inch or centimeter
    d. The SID at which the grid may be used

96. Structures seen outside of the collimated area on a radiograph, produced by "off-focus" (extrafocal) radiation, are the result of:
    a. Electron interaction within the x-ray tube at a point other than the focal spot
    b. Scatter radiation emanating from the patient or tabletop
    c. The use of an SID not recommended with the grid in use
    d. The x-ray tube positioned off-center to the grid

97. Geometric unsharpness within the radiographic image can be minimized by using the:
    1. Smallest focal spot
    2. Shortest object film distance
    3. Longest target film distance
    a. 1 and 2 only
    b. 1 and 3 only
    c. 2 and 3 only
    d. 1, 2, and 3

98. An *undistorted* radiographic image results when the object plane and the image plane are:
    a. Angled in relation to each other
    b. At right angles
    c. Parallel
    d. Perpendicular

99. A radiographic grid should be used when:
    1. The body area to be radiographed measures more than 10 cm
    2. A field size larger than 10 to 12 inches is used
    3. More than 60 kVp is required to penetrate a body part
    a. 1 and 2 only
    b. 1 and 3 only
    c. 2 and 3 only
    d. 1, 2, and 3

100. Twice as many electrons strike the target in the x-ray tube when:
    a. kVp is doubled
    b. mAs is doubled
    c. SID is reduced by one-half
    d. OFD is reduced by one-half

101. How does beam restriction affect contrast?
    a. Decreases contrast
    b. Longer scale of contrast
    c. Shorter scale of contrast
    d. No effect on contrast

102. Given an original technique of 10 mAs and 70 kVp, which of the following would produce a radiograph with double the density?
    a. 20 mAs, 80 kVp
    b. 30 mAs, 92 kVp
    c. 20 mAs, 70 kVp
    d. 15 mAs, 82 kVp

103. Grid conversion factor (Bucky factor) is described as the:
    a. Height of the lead strips divided by the distance between the lead strips
    b. Distance between the lead strips divided by the height of the lead strips
    c. Number of lead strips per inch or centimeter
    d. Amount of exposure increase necessary to compensate for the absorption of image-forming rays and scatter in the cleanup process

104. As the wavelength of the x-rays increases, penetrating ability:
    a. Decreases
    b. Increases
    c. Remains the same
    d. Fluctuates
105. If SID is doubled, density is:
    a. Doubled
    b. Halved
    c. Cut to one-fourth
    d. Quadrupled
106. As kVp is increased:
    a. Density decreases
    b. Contrast increases
    c. Recorded detail increases
    d. Contrast decreases
107. As kVp is decreased:
    a. Density increases
    b. Contrast decreases
    c. Recorded detail decreases
    d. Scale of contrast shortens
108. Which of the following sets of exposure factors would produce the radiograph with the best recorded detail?
    a. 60 mAs, 80 kVp, 40-inch SID, 4-inch OID
    b. 30 mAs, 92 kVp, 40-inch SID, 4-inch OID
    c. 120 mAs, 92 kVp, 40-inch SID, 4-inch OID
    d. All would produce equal recorded detail
109. Which of the following sets of exposure factors would produce the radiograph with the highest contrast?
    a. 60 mAs, 80 kVp, 40-inch SID, 4-inch OID
    b. 30 mAs, 92 kVp, 40-inch SID, 4-inch OID
    c. 120 mAs, 92 kVp, 40-inch SID, 4-inch OID
    d. 15 mAs, 100 kVp, 40-inch SID, 4-inch OID
110. Which of the following sets of exposure factors would produce the radiograph with the most magnification?
    a. 60 mAs, 80 kVp, 40-inch SID, 4-inch OID
    b. 30 mAs, 92 kVp, 40-inch SID, 4-inch OID
    c. 120 mAs, 92 kVp, 20-inch SID, 4-inch OID
    d. 15 mAs, 100 kVp, 40-inch SID, 4-inch OID
111. Which of the following is true?
    a. High kVp = low contrast = long-scale contrast = many gray tones
    b. Low kVp = low contrast = long-scale contrast = many gray tones
    c. When kVp is increased, there is an increase in the number of photoelectric interactions that occur
    d. When kVp is decreased, there is an increase in the number of Compton interactions that occur

112. Which of the following is true?
    a. High kVp = high contrast = short-scale contrast = few gray tones
    b. Low kVp = low contrast = long-scale contrast = many gray tones
    c. When kVp is increased, there is an increase in the number of photoelectric interactions that occur
    d. When kVp is decreased, there is an increase in the number of photoelectric interactions that occur

Imaging Procedures (Questions 113-170)

113. Differential absorption of the x-ray beam produces:
    a. Density
    b. Subject contrast
    c. Recorded detail
    d. Characteristic radiation
114. Beam restriction has the following effect on contrast:
    a. Decreases contrast
    b. Increases contrast
    c. Longer scale of contrast
    d. No effect on contrast
For the following questions, choose the single best answer.
115. An enlargement at the end of a bone is called a:
    a. Prominence
    b. Sharp prominence
    c. Tubercle
    d. Head
116. A rounded projection of moderate size is called a:
    a. Prominence
    b. Sharp prominence
    c. Tubercle
    d. Tuberosity
117. A spine describes a:
    a. Prominence
    b. Sharp prominence
    c. Tubercle
    d. Tuberosity
118. A pit is described as a:
    a. Fossa
    b. Groove
    c. Sulcus
    d. Sinus
119. A furrow is described as a:
    a. Fossa
    b. Groove
    c. Sulcus
    d. Sinus
120. A "typical" skull would be described as:
    a. Synarthroses
    b. Amphiarthroses
    c. Diarthroses
    d. Mesocephalic

121. Synovial joints are called:
     a. Synarthroses
     b. Amphiarthroses
     c. Diarthroses
     d. Mesocephalic
122. Fibrous joints are called:
     a. Synarthroses
     b. Amphiarthroses
     c. Diarthroses
     d. Mesocephalic
123. The radiocarpal joint has what type of movement?
     a. Hinge
     b. Pivot
     c. Saddle
     d. Condyloid
124. The proximal radioulnar articulation has what type of movement?
     a. Hinge
     b. Pivot
     c. Saddle
     d. Gliding
125. Which of the following bones has a temporal process?
     a. Sphenoid bone
     b. Ethmoid bone
     c. Mandible
     d. Zygomatic bone
126. Which of the following bones has an alveolar process?
     a. Sphenoid bone
     b. Ethmoid bone
     c. Mandible
     d. Maxilla
127. Which of the following bones has wings?
     a. Sphenoid bone
     b. Ethmoid bone
     c. Mandible
     d. Maxilla
128. Which of the following bones has a coronal suture?
     a. Frontal bone
     b. Temporal bone
     c. Occipital bone
     d. Parietal bone
129. Which of the following bones has an external protuberance?
     a. Frontal bone
     b. Temporal bone
     c. Occipital bone
     d. Mandible
130. Which of the following bones consists of five fused segments?
     a. Sacrum
     b. Axis
     c. Thoracic vertebra
     d. Lumbar vertebra

131. Which of the following bones has a dens?
     a. Atlas
     b. Axis
     c. Thoracic vertebra
     d. Lumbar vertebra
132. Which of the following individual vertebrae are larger and heavier than other individual vertebrae?
     a. Atlas
     b. Axis
     c. Thoracic vertebra
     d. Lumbar vertebra
133. The eleventh and twelfth pairs of ribs are called:
     a. Manubrium
     b. Floating
     c. Xiphoid
     d. Jugular notch
134. The blunt cartilaginous tip of the sternum is the:
     a. Manubrium
     b. Floating
     c. Xiphoid
     d. Jugular notch
135. Located between the greater and lesser tubercles of the humerus is(are) the:
     a. Greater and lesser tubercles
     b. Bicipital groove
     c. Capitulum
     d. Trochlea
136. Located below the tubercles of the humerus is(are) the:
     a. Greater and lesser tubercles
     b. Bicipital groove
     c. Capitulum
     d. Surgical neck
137. Which of the following parts of the humerus articulate(s) with the ulna?
     a. Greater and lesser tubercles
     b. Bicipital groove
     c. Capitulum
     d. Trochlea
138. Which bone is located in the wrist, between the trapezoid and the hamate?
     a. Scaphoid
     b. Hamate
     c. Pisiform
     d. Capitate
139. Which bone is located in the wrist, between the lunate and the pisiform?
     a. Scaphoid
     b. Hamate
     c. Pisiform
     d. Triquetrum
140. Which bone distributes body weight from the tibia to the other tarsal bones?
     a. Navicular
     b. Calcaneus
     c. Talus
     d. Cuboid

141. Which bone lies along the lateral border of the navicular bone?
    a. Navicular
    b. Calcaneus
    c. Talus
    d. Cuboid

142. Which of the following articulate(s) with the first, second, and third metatarsal bones?
    a. Navicular
    b. Calcaneus
    c. Talus
    d. Cuneiforms

143. This structure has superior, middle, and inferior lobes:
    a. Trachea
    b. Left lung
    c. Right lung
    d. Hilus

144. This structure is approximately 12 cm long and is located in front of the esophagus:
    a. Trachea
    b. Left lung
    c. Right lung
    d. Hilus

145. The narrow distal end of the stomach that connects with the small intestine is called the:
    a. Rugae
    b. Pylorus
    c. Fundus
    d. Greater curvature

146. The section of the stomach where the esophagus enters is called the:
    a. Rugae
    b. Pylorus
    c. Fundus
    d. Cardiac portion

147. The lateral surface of the stomach is called the:
    a. Rugae
    b. Pylorus
    c. Fundus
    d. Greater curvature

148. The portion of the colon located between the splenic flexure and the sigmoid portion is called the:
    a. Duodenum
    b. Descending
    c. Ileum
    d. Ascending

149. The portion of the small bowel that connects with the cecum is called the:
    a. Duodenum
    b. Jejunum
    c. Ileum
    d. Ascending

150. The portion of the small bowel that connects with the stomach is called the:
    a. Duodenum
    b. Jejunum
    c. Ileum
    d. Ascending

151. The outer part of the kidney is called the:
    a. Cortex
    b. Medulla
    c. Nephron
    d. Glomeruli

152. The part of the kidney through which blood is first filtered is called the:
    a. Cortex
    b. Medulla
    c. Nephron
    d. Glomeruli

153. For radiography of the fingers, the central ray enters:
    a. Perpendicular to the distal interphalangeal joint
    b. Parallel to the distal interphalangeal joint
    c. Parallel to the proximal interphalangeal joint
    d. Perpendicular to the proximal interphalangeal joint

154. For a PA projection of the hand, the central ray is centered:
    a. Perpendicular to the first metacarpophalangeal joint
    b. Perpendicular to the third metatarsophalangeal joint
    c. Parallel to the third metacarpophalangeal joint
    d. Perpendicular to the third metacarpophalangeal joint

155. For a lateral projection of the wrist, the elbow must be flexed:
    a. 45 degrees
    b. 90 degrees
    c. Only slightly
    d. Approximately 25 degrees

156. For PA axial projection of the clavicle, the central ray is angled:
    a. 25 to 30 degrees caudad
    b. 25 to 30 degrees cephalad
    c. 20 degrees caudad
    d. 20 degrees cephalad

157. For AP projection of the toes, the central ray enters at the:
    a. Third metatarsophalangeal joint
    b. Second metacarpophalangeal joint
    c. First metatarsophalangeal joint
    d. Second metatarsophalangeal joint

158. For AP projection of the foot, the central ray enters at the:
    a. Head of the third metatarsal
    b. Head of the second metatarsal
    c. Base of the first metatarsal
    d. Base of the third metatarsal

159. For axial projection of the calcaneus, the central ray is angled how many degrees to the long axis of the foot?
    a. 25
    b. 15
    c. 10
    d. 40

160. For AP projection of the ankle, the central ray is directed perpendicular to the:
    a. Lateral malleolus
    b. Ankle joint midway between malleoli
    c. Medial malleolus
    d. Tibia

161. For AP projection of the knee, the central ray is angled:
    a. 5 to 7 degrees cephalad
    b. 5 to 7 degrees caudad
    c. 10 degrees cephalad
    d. 10 degrees caudad

162. For AP projection of the cervical spine, the central ray is directed:
    a. 10 degrees cephalad
    b. Parallel to C4
    c. 15 to 20 degrees caudad
    d. 15 to 20 degrees cephalad

163. For lateral projection of the cervical spine, the central ray is directed:
    a. Perpendicular to C4
    b. Parallel to C4
    c. 15 to 20 degrees caudad
    d. 20 to 25 degrees cephalad

164. For AP projection of the thoracic spine, the central ray is directed:
    a. 5 degrees cephalad
    b. Parallel to T7
    c. 3 to 4 degrees caudad
    d. Perpendicular to T7

165. For AP projection of the lumbar spine, the central ray is directed:
    a. Parallel to midline, entering at the level of the iliac crests
    b. Perpendicular to L2
    c. Perpendicular to midline, entering at the level of the iliac crests
    d. Perpendicular to L4

166. For AP oblique projections of the sacroiliac joints, the central ray is directed:
    a. 1 inch lateral to elevated ASIS
    b. 1 inch medial to elevated ASIS
    c. 1 inch lateral to dependent ASIS
    d. 1 inch medial to dependent ASIS

167. For PA projection of the chest, the central ray is directed:
    a. Perpendicular to T10
    b. Parallel to the thoracic spine
    c. Perpendicular to T7
    d. Perpendicular to the posterior ribs

168. For AP projection of the lower ribs, the central ray is directed:
    a. Perpendicular to T10
    b. Perpendicular to T5
    c. Perpendicular to T7
    d. Perpendicular to T12

169. For AP axial (Towne) projection for the skull, the central ray is directed:
    a. 30 degrees to IOML
    b. 37 degrees to OML
    c. 25 degrees to IOML
    d. 30 degrees to OML

170. For lateral projection for the facial bones, the central ray enters at the:
    a. Glabella
    b. Medial surface of the zygomatic bone
    c. Medial surface of the nasal bone
    d. Lateral surface of the zygomatic bone

Patient Care and Education (Questions 171-200)

171. What must precede any examinations involving iodinated contrast media?
    a. Chest x-ray study
    b. Thyroid assessment
    c. Patient held NPO
    d. Pregnancy test

172. Diabetic patients should be scheduled:
    a. Later because of their need for insulin
    b. Early because of their need for insulin
    c. Just before mealtime
    d. Just after mealtime

173. The pelvocalyceal system reaches greatest visualization approximately how many minutes after injection?
    a. 1 to 2
    b. 2 to 5
    c. 2 to 8
    d. 15 to 20

174. For right posterior oblique and left posterior oblique projections for the kidneys, how many degrees is the patient's body rotated?
    a. 15
    b. 25
    c. 30
    d. 45

175. Violations of civil law are known as:
    a. Assault
    b. Battery
    c. False imprisonment
    d. Torts

176. Unjustified restraint of a patient defines:
    a. Assault
    b. Battery
    c. False imprisonment
    d. Invasion of privacy

177. The suffix that means "like" is:
    a. -oma
    b. -oid
    c. -osis
    d. -pathy
178. The suffix that means "tumor" is:
    a. -oid
    b. -pathy
    c. -oma
    d. -algia
179. A legal doctrine that states that the cause of the negligence is obvious is known as:
    a. *Respondeat superior*
    b. *Res ipsa loquitur*
    c. Gross negligence
    d. Slander
180. Tachycardia indicates a pulse of:
    a. Greater than 100 beats per minute
    b. Less than 60 beats per minute
    c. Greater than 90 beats per minute
    d. Less than 50 beats per minute
181. Some level of hypertension is indicated when diastolic pressure is:
    a. Greater than 100
    b. Less than 60
    c. Greater than 90
    d. Less than 50
182. When oxygen is administered to the patient, the usual flow rate is:
    a. 3 to 5 L/second
    b. 5 L/hour
    c. 1 to 3 L/minute
    d. 3 to 5 L/minute
183. This item is used to clear an obstructed airway:
    a. Crash cart
    b. Suction unit
    c. Defibrillator
    d. Sphygmomanometer
184. This item is used to restore the heart to normal rhythm:
    a. Crash cart
    b. Suction unit
    c. Defibrillator
    d. Sphygmomanometer
185. A type of shock that is caused by a severe allergic reaction is called:
    a. Hypovolemic shock
    b. Septic shock
    c. Neurogenic shock
    d. Anaphylactic shock
186. An item that is used to feed the patient or to suction gastric contents is a:
    a. Ventilator
    b. Nasogastric tube
    c. Chest tube
    d. Venous catheter
187. An item that must never be placed above the level of the bladder is a:
    a. Ventilator
    b. Nasogastric tube
    c. Chest tube
    d. Urinary catheter
188. A mechanical respirator is called a:
    a. Ventilator
    b. Nasogastric tube
    c. Chest tube
    d. Venous catheter
189. Barium sulfate should be mixed with water at what temperature for a barium enema?
    a. 100° C
    b. 75° F
    c. 85° C
    d. 100° F
190. A positive contrast agent administered to a patient in the form of an inert salt is:
    a. Barium sulfate
    b. Iodine
    c. Perforated ulcers or ruptured appendix
    d. Air
191. The most effective method to prevent the spread of infection is:
    a. Use of gloves
    b. Use of gowns
    c. Time, distance, and shielding
    d. Handwashing
192. If you suspect an object is contaminated, assume:
    a. That it is contaminated
    b. That it should be used immediately
    c. That it is not contaminated, so as not to waste supplies
    d. That your hands must be sterilized
193. Factors that may cause the patient to react to a contrast agent simply as a result of anxiety are termed:
    a. Local irritation
    b. Cardiovascular
    c. Anaphylactic
    d. Psychogenic
194. A reaction that may occur in the vein in which an injection occurred is:
    a. Local irritation
    b. Cardiovascular
    c. Anaphylactic
    d. Phlebitis
195. This type of infection transmission occurs when an animal contains and transmits an infectious organism to humans:
    a. Contact transmission
    b. Airborne transmission
    c. Droplet transmission
    d. Vectorborne transmission

196. This type of infection transmission occurs as a result of coughing or sneezing:
   a. Contact transmission
   b. Airborne transmission
   c. Droplet transmission
   d. Common vehicle transmission

197. This type of infection transmission occurs when an infected person or contaminated object touches a host:
   a. Contact transmission
   b. Airborne transmission
   c. Droplet transmission
   d. Common vehicle transmission

198. The complete removal of all organisms from equipment and the environment in which patient care is conducted is called:
   a. Medical asepsis
   b. Surgical asepsis
   c. Standard precautions
   d. Gas sterilization

199. The word part that means "organ" is:
   a. viscer
   b. megal
   c. trans
   d. emia

200. The word part that means "kidney" is:
   a. viscer
   b. megal
   c. trans
   d. nephr

Scoring

Traditionally you have probably focused on how many questions you miss on an exam. As you prepare for the certification exam, I encourage you to focus on how many you answer correctly. Use Table 7-3 to calculate the percentage of questions you answered correctly in each category and on the test as a whole. Remember, a score of less than 75% on any topic or the entire test is an indication that more review is needed on that topic. Now go back and concentrate on which items were missed and the reason why. When you are done reviewing, go on to the tutorials and tests found on the companion CD-ROM included with this book.

TABLE 7-3	Calculating Your Score for Challenge Test Number 3	
Topic	**Percentage Calculation**	**Your Score**
Radiation protection	Number correct _____ × 100, ÷ 45 =	
Equipment operation and quality control	Number correct _____ × 100, ÷ 22 =	
Image acquisition and evaluation	Number correct _____ × 100, ÷ 45 =	
Imaging procedures	Number correct _____ × 100, ÷ 58 =	
Patient care and education	Number correct _____ × 100, ÷ 30 =	
Total	Number correct _____ × 100, ÷ 200 =	

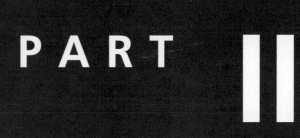

PART II

Career Planning

Career Paths

Do it now. You become successful the moment you start moving toward a worthwhile goal.

CAREER PLANNING INVENTORY

Individuals pursue chosen careers for a variety of reasons. Their sources of motivation for enrolling in an educational program and satisfying all of the graduation requirements may include the need for a stable income, the desire to become established in a career, or an interest in expanding their horizons. Incentives for undertaking such a process are unique to each individual and may clearly distinguish a 45-year-old from an 18-year-old. Also, incentives can change as you move toward a goal, so the circumstances that led you to select this educational program may differ considerably from circumstances that influence you to establish a career in this field.

Whether you are reading this chapter as a new radiography student, during your final year, or in your final semester, it is a good idea to examine your motivation for seeking employment and establishing a career in radiologic technology. You should reexamine your motivation and adjust your goals regularly—perhaps annually. The following questions can help with that process and assist you in establishing career goals.

1. Based on my studies and clinical education so far, what aspects of this profession am I really excited about?
2. Which aspects of patient care have I found the most satisfying?

Rationale: Questions 1 and 2 attempt to help you focus on what has brought you true satisfaction so far in the educational program. Being excited about what you do is critical to your longevity in the field. It is a daily reinforcement to your motivation. It helps you bring a positive attitude to class and to the clinical environment. Many individuals find certain aspects of patient care are particularly satisfying. Identifying yours can help you set goals for job placement or for continuing your education. For example, if you find great satisfaction working with children, pediatric radiography may be an excellent choice for a career. You could consider job possibilities at children's hospitals. Perhaps trauma radiography is particularly challenging and satisfying for you. Pursuing employment at an institution with a trauma center and a shift with a high level of trauma cases would

be a wise choice. Maybe teaching and working with students appeals to you. If so, your goals may include completing advanced academic degrees and finding a clinical job in a teaching institution.

Take time now to answer questions 1 and 2 in the space provided. Remember, you are examining situations you find motivating and exciting. You will have an opportunity to set your goals later in this chapter.

I am really excited about:

_____

_____

_____

_____

The aspects of patient care that have been most satisfying are:

_____

_____

_____

_____

3. Of the people with whom I have worked in clinical education, who has been most helpful?
4. Which characteristics do I want to emulate most?

Rationale: As a radiography student, you may be profoundly influenced by the personnel in the clinical department. It is important to identify people who have been particularly helpful to you as you have acquired your clinical skills. It is often tempting to think about, talk about, and remember only the people who have been hindrances to your education or who simply did not enjoy working with students. Concentrate instead on the positive people, and prepare a list of their names. Describe the personal and professional characteristics they possess. Explain why you enjoy working with them. Everyone benefits from role models. Describe why you wish to emulate, or pattern your professional attitudes and demeanor after, certain people with whom you have worked.

The most helpful individuals in clinical education have been:

_____

_____

_____

They have been great to work with because:

_____

_____

_____

I will emulate the following positive behaviors (also explain why):

_____

_____

_____

5. When during the educational process have I been most satisfied?
6. When during the educational process have I been least satisfied?

Rationale: An awareness of events, people, or situations that have caused you to feel happy or unhappy can be helpful in setting goals for employment. It is impossible to be satisfied or happy on the job all of the time or to avoid all unpleasant situations; however, being aware of such times can help you decide where you may or may not wish to work. In addition, addressing these issues now can help you understand how you respond to positive and negative situations and how to alter your responses if necessary. You may also wish to consider ways to maintain a positive outlook when dealing with unpleasant situations or individuals by recalling successful self-motivating strategies from the past. The mark of a true professional is the ability to summon the highest level of performance from yourself and the people around you even during difficult times.

I have been most satisfied during my education when:

_____

_____

_____

I have been most dissatisfied during my education when:

_____

_____

_____

7. What employment needs will I have after graduation?

8. What financial needs will I have after graduation?
9. What housing needs and living conditions will I seek after graduation?
10. Do I want or need to stay in this geographic area, or do I want or need to relocate?

Rationale: Individuals often do little or no planning for their employment, financial needs, or living conditions.

Consider what your needs will be for employment when you graduate. Decide whether you will need to begin work immediately and have to accept the first job offer you receive or whether you can wait a short time to scout the job market more thoroughly. It is crucial to have some idea of what your financial needs will be. Be aware of the cost of setting up your own living arrangements, paying back school loans, or providing for your family. If you are not currently responsible for your own housing, decide how it will be arranged. With a fluctuating job market, you must consider whether you will remain rooted where you are or relocate to find the type of position you desire. Perhaps relocating is something you have wanted to do all along or maybe relocating is simply not possible at this point in your life.

Answer each question in the space that follows. Describe what your needs and wants will be after graduation.

Employment:

_____

_____

_____

Financial:

_____

_____

_____

Housing:

_____

_____

_____

Location:

_____

_____

_____

Use the financial planning worksheet shown in Figure 8-1 to determine your actual salary needs. Be sure to base your compensation needs on your individual obligations, regardless of any domestic relationship that may include a combination of incomes.

Annual Living Expenses

These are for the *entire year;* be sure to calculate *annual* figures.

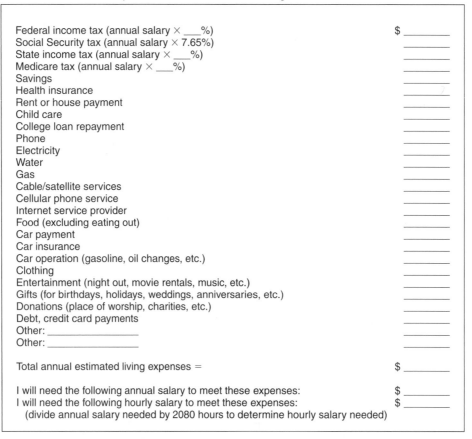

Federal income tax (annual salary × ___%)	$ _____
Social Security tax (annual salary × 7.65%)	_____
State income tax (annual salary × ___%)	_____
Medicare tax (annual salary × ___%)	_____
Savings	_____
Health insurance	_____
Rent or house payment	_____
Child care	_____
College loan repayment	_____
Phone	_____
Electricity	_____
Water	_____
Gas	_____
Cable/satellite services	_____
Cellular phone service	_____
Internet service provider	_____
Food (excluding eating out)	_____
Car payment	_____
Car insurance	_____
Car operation (gasoline, oil changes, etc.)	_____
Clothing	_____
Entertainment (night out, movie rentals, music, etc.)	_____
Gifts (for birthdays, holidays, weddings, anniversaries, etc.)	_____
Donations (place of worship, charities, etc.)	_____
Debt, credit card payments	_____
Other: _____	_____
Other: _____	_____
Total annual estimated living expenses =	$ _____
I will need the following annual salary to meet these expenses:	$ _____
I will need the following hourly salary to meet these expenses:	$ _____
(divide annual salary needed by 2080 hours to determine hourly salary needed)	

This form is not meant to be a substitute for guidance provided by a financial counselor or tax advisor. Scholarships or sign-on bonuses are not included in salary because they are one-time payments, not hourly salary. Taxes could be reduced with personal exemptions, deductions, credits, etc. Consider these factors when calculating actual tax liability.

FIGURE 8-1 Annual living expenses.

11. Am I more excited about working with the *high-touch* (people-oriented) aspects of this profession or the *high-tech* (equipment) aspects of the field?

Rationale: Some individuals work in this field because they truly love working with people and assisting with the diagnosis of their conditions. Others prefer working with complex electronic and computerized equipment and would rather not be involved in direct patient care. There is room for both types of people in this profession and for people who truly enjoy blending high touch with high tech. Identifying the aspects of the field that excite you can help with your career planning.

Perhaps you wish to continue providing direct patient care. Maybe you would rather work in areas involving significant use of equipment, such as in quality control, medical physics, or the sale and service of equipment. You may also serve patients indirectly in a position such as PACS administrator. Nothing will cause you to become more dissatisfied with your career choice than working in an area of radiologic technology to which you are not suited. Develop awareness now of what you most enjoy

doing. There is no right or wrong answer, and your choice does not make you "good" or "bad." Most important, be honest with yourself. You will have much to contribute to this field if you work where you are happiest and most productive.

Take some time and write in the space that follows your honest preferences based on your experiences so far. Remember, you are not setting a goal at this point, and your answer may change over time.

High tech versus high touch—my preference and why:

_____

_____

_____

12. Do I enjoy learning all I can about this field, or do I want to learn only what I need to graduate?

Rationale: Your answer to this question is very important. The field you have chosen changes rapidly. You must be honest with yourself about your desire to study and learn. The equipment currently used in clinical education did not even exist a few years ago. You will use equipment a few years after you graduate that does not exist today. If you are content to learn only what you need to graduate, you will soon possess outdated skills. You should also consider whether you truly enjoy learning or tend to regard it as a burden. Your education in this field will have barely begun by the time you graduate. Be aware you will need to set a course for lifelong learning. Understanding this reality now can assist you in developing your professional attitude and planning for continuing education. Realizing the importance of a commitment to learning may also serve to motivate you through the remainder of your educational program.

Take time to assess your motivation for learning. In the space that follows, describe your honest feelings and attitudes about the enjoyment of learning for its own sake as opposed to learning just enough to perform your job.

I want to learn all I can or just enough to get by. Here are my reasons and motivations:

_____

_____

_____

_____

13. Which aspect(s) of the specialty of radiography do I enjoy the most (e.g., general, fluoroscopy, mobile, surgical, trauma, pediatric)?
14. Have I particularly enjoyed any other radiologic specialties (e.g., angiography, mammography, CT, MRI, sonography, nuclear medicine, fusion imaging, radiation therapy, quality control)?

Rationale: You may not yet realize radiography is a specialty within which are areas of further specialization (e.g., general, fluoroscopy, mobile, digital/PACS). You are probably already familiar with the other specialties listed in question 14. By being aware of what you enjoy, you will have little difficulty later setting goals for employment or education. If you have not yet had the opportunity to spend clinical time in some of the areas mentioned, you may need to postpone answering this question. However, when such an opportunity arises, prepare yourself for the clinical experience by reading about the specialty area in your textbook and taking careful notes about your experiences. This field has countless opportunities for you in the practice of radiography or any of the other special imaging or therapy modalities.

Use the space provided to list the areas in which you are particularly interested, and describe why you have enjoyed them. Also list the areas you look forward to exploring, and explain why they are important to you.

I particularly enjoy working in the following area(s):

_____

_____

_____

I want to explore the following areas further:

_____

_____

_____

15. Are there any special projects I have done that brought me satisfaction (e.g., research papers, exhibits, in-class presentations, participation in radiography scholar bowls)?
16. Am I interested in pursuing positions of leadership or membership in local, state, or national radiologic technology organizations?

Rationale: This profession needs you. It needs what you have to offer. It needs your fresh ideas and observations. It needs your leadership, motivation, talents, and abilities. By considering the issues mentioned in questions 15 and 16, you can set goals for your postgraduation involvement.

Perhaps you have already written a research paper, constructed an exhibit, or participated in a scholar bowl competition. Do not stop now. You have momentum working in your favor. Consider how these projects may have brought you satisfaction and served to motivate you further. Think about how you may set goals for doing additional projects or presentations as a radiographer for state or national presentations.

Local, state, and national professional organizations in radiologic technology need the involvement of motivated, committed professionals. Gauge your interest in becoming involved. Do not let fear of the unknown deter you. Remember, individuals who are currently active were at one time attending their first meeting, serving on a committee for the first time, or holding their first office. Think about how such involvement may add to your career and personal satisfaction.

In the space provided, write your thoughts and feelings about pursuing these activities. Describe how you would feel if you became involved at this level of the profession.

The special projects that brought me the most satisfaction were:

_____

_____

_____

I wish to become involved in the following organization(s) in this capacity:

_____

_____

_____

17. Do I believe I will have an interest in working with students when I am employed?

Rationale: You will need to assess your interest in working with students. Many of us truly enjoy helping students acquire skills, whereas some would prefer to avoid educating others. If you believe you would enjoy teaching, seeking employment in an academic environment is a reasonable goal. If you would prefer not to work with students, it would be better for you and for the students if you seek employment in another setting. Many otherwise excellent radiographers find frustration on the job because they are not suited to the clinical teaching role. Do not take this issue lightly. Having a student assigned to you every day of work can be exhilarating or burdensome, depending on your professional preferences.

In the space provided, state whether you prefer to work with students or to find employment in a nonteaching institution.

I would or would not like to work with students after graduation. Here are my reasons:

_____

_____

_____

18. In what type of clinical setting am I most comfortable (e.g., hospital, small clinic, physician's office, urgent care)?

Rationale: Health care assumes many forms, depending in part on the environment in which it is delivered. If you have had the opportunity to spend clinical time in more than one of the settings mentioned, decide which you enjoyed most. If you have not had this opportunity, check with your program director about the availability of clinical rotations. If none are available in the program, consider spending time outside of school in one or more of these clinical settings to get some idea of how they operate and to observe the radiographer at work.

Each clinical setting has qualities that may appeal to you as a radiographer and others that may make it a less attractive choice. You may also be guided by a strong personal preference about where you would like to work. Consider these factors carefully when setting goals for employment.

I have had experience in the following clinical settings. Here is what I liked and disliked:

_____

_____

_____

_____

19. What particular talents do I possess about which I feel proud?

Rationale: Identify your talents and all you have to offer a potential employer. Consider how you may use these talents to pursue your personal and professional goals. Think of how your strengths may benefit the patients you serve. Understand the impact you may have on coworkers. It is important to be proud of your talents and use them. It is not conceited to list them. You must concentrate on being the best you can be by developing your abilities and acquiring others. Use them to enhance your practice of radiography and your personal life.

My particular talents and positive attributes follow. Here is how I have used them and why I am excited about them:

_____

_____

_____

_____

KEY POINTS
Career Planning Inventory

- Examine your motivation for seeking employment and establishing a career in radiologic technology.
- Adjust your goals regularly.
- Being passionate about what you do is key to your longevity in the field.
- Identify people who have been particularly helpful to you in clinical education.
- Concentrate on positive people who enjoy working with patients and students.
- A true professional has the ability to summon the highest level of performance even during difficult times.
- Consider what your needs will be for employment when you graduate.
- It is important to ascertain your financial needs.
- Determine whether you will remain where you are or if you wish to, or will need to, relocate.
- Balancing high tech with high touch is key to quality patient care. Knowing your preference leads to your success.
- A thorough understanding of options in radiologic technology can assist with career goals.

- This profession needs your fresh ideas, observations, leadership, motivation, talents, and abilities.
- Consider professional involvement such as presenting at conferences, writing a research paper, constructing a scientific exhibit, or holding office in a professional organization.
- Assess your interest in working with students and seek employment accordingly.
- Consider the numerous venues in which you may practice radiography, such as hospitals, clinics, physician offices, and prompt care sites.
- Identify the talents you have to offer a potential employer and how you may use these talents to pursue your personal and professional goals.
- Examine how your strengths may benefit the patients you serve and how they may have a positive impact on your coworkers.

GOAL SETTING

By carefully answering the previous questions, you should develop a good idea of the things that motivate you in this field. The choice of a career is important, and you should be intent on doing the things you particularly enjoy.

Individuals who have been successful in the field of radiologic technology have set goals for themselves and worked hard to achieve them. Goal setting is not an easy task, particularly because it is seldom taught in school. However, all of the great motivational speakers and career planners indicate that goal setting should be a priority, not only when beginning a career, but throughout your working lifetime.

Goals are not meant to be etched in granite and never changed or updated. Goal statements should be flexible and fluid. They should be realistic, measurable, and achievable. If you are the type of person who needs to see immediate or short-term progress, break down your goals into smaller events. Approach these goals incrementally and celebrate each achievement. As mentioned previously, goals should be updated as needed and at least annually.

The wording of goal statements can be as important as setting the goals themselves. Statements such as "I want to be a nuclear medicine technologist within 3 years" are not powerful enough. "I will be a registered nuclear medicine technologist by the end of (specify year)" is more specific. It is action oriented. It says you will do something, and you will direct your energies toward achieving that goal within a specific time frame. It is more than a wish; it is a statement of a goal that you expect to realize.

Post your goals where you can see them daily, and share them with the people who are significant in your life. Encouragement and moral support of loved ones can help you achieve your goals. Shared goals are more likely to be met because of the increased sense of accountability to others who are aware of them.

Following is a series of questions to consider as you write your goal statements. Sample goal statements are provided. Note that they are specific, have time frames, and use the words "I will." You may be thinking that you lack some of the information needed to write your goal statements. However, recognize that by writing goals and planning your future, you are in the process of making that future a reality. This helps you direct your energies toward pursuing and accomplishing your goals.

Setting goals should not be taken lightly, but it should not be so arduous a task that it becomes a burden. Be excited about setting your goals and beginning to map out your future. Do not get discouraged if your goals seem simple at first. They are there to provide you with direction. It will be up to you to adjust them and to direct the course you plan to follow.

1. What deadline have I set for completion of my goal statements?

GOAL: I will list my goals along with a timetable by the following date:

_____

2. What kind of review schedule have I established to prepare for the radiography certification exam?

GOAL: I will review the subjects included on the exam according to the following schedule:

Radiation protection:

_____

Equipment acquistion and quality control:

_____

Image production and evaluation:

_____

Imaging procedures:

_____

Patient care and education:

_____

3. Do I want to pursue additional education in radiologic technology or seek an advanced degree?

GOAL: I will visit college or university websites to examine baccalaureate degree options by the following date: _____

GOAL: I will take _____ number of credit hours per semester beginning on _____ so that I will complete my degree on _____.

GOAL: I will visit websites regarding educational programs in _____ (e.g., sonography, nuclear medicine, radiation therapy, CT, MRI) by _____.

GOAL: I will attend an educational program in _____ (e.g., sonography, nuclear medicine, radiation therapy, CT, MRI) beginning _____ and will graduate from the program in _____.

4. Do my regular study habits need to be examined and fine-tuned?

GOAL: I will examine my current study habits on _____.

GOAL: I am modifying my current study habits as follows:

_____

GOAL: I will begin my new study habits on _____.

5. Do I need to examine my lifestyle choices regarding diet, exercise, and sleep requirements?

GOAL: I will evaluate my lifestyle choices in diet, exercise, sleep, and recreation on _____.

GOAL: I am modifying my diet as follows (be specific):

_____

_____

_____

GOAL: I am modifying my exercise routine as follows (be specific):

_____

_____

_____

_____

GOAL: I am modifying my sleep routine as follows:

_____

_____

_____

_____

GOAL: I am taking time for recreation as follows:

_____

_____

_____

_____

6. Have I taken into account the needs of my family or significant others?

GOAL: I will consult with my significant others regarding these goals on _____.

GOAL: I will list here the needs of my significant others in view of the goals I have set on:

_____

_____

_____

_____

7. What do I want to accomplish in the next 30, 60, and 90 days related to my career?

GOAL: By 30 days from now, on _____, I will have accomplished the following to advance my career goals:

_____

_____

_____

_____

GOAL: By 60 days from now, on _____, I will have accomplished the following to advance my career goals (built on my 30-day objectives):

_____

_____

_____

_____

GOAL: By 90 days from now, on _____, I will have accomplished the following to advance my career goals (built on my 30-day and 60-day objectives):

_____

_____

_____

_____

8. To reinforce my positive attitude, I will need to obtain access to motivational materials.

GOAL: By _____ I will read the following motivational books:

_____

_____

_____

_____

9. I must consider postgraduation needs.

GOAL: I will begin work by _____.

GOAL: I will make the following hourly salary to maintain the lifestyle I have chosen:

GOAL: I will live in the following type of housing:

GOAL: I will live in the following city or geographic area:

10. What are my preferences regarding high-tech versus high-touch aspects of radiography?

GOAL: I will work in the following direct patient care area of medical radiography:

GOAL: I will work in the following patient care support area:

11. I need to consider continuing education in radiography.

GOAL: I will follow this schedule for remaining current in my chosen field:
Type of meetings or conferences I will attend regularly:

Local:

State:

National:

12. What other radiologic specialties should I explore?

GOAL: I will do extra reading and clinical observation in the following radiologic technology specialties (e.g., angiography, mammography, CT, MRI, sonography, nuclear medicine, radiation therapy, quality control) by the dates I have listed:

13. I will pursue special projects after graduation.

GOAL: I will write a research paper and submit it for competition at the state or national level on _____. The possible subjects for this paper are:

GOAL: I will prepare a scientific exhibit for presentation at a state or national meeting on _____. The possible subjects for this exhibit are:

GOAL: I will assist with planning the following local or state meeting: _____ on _____.

GOAL: I will run for the office of my local, state, or national professional organization on _____.

14. What is my attitude toward working with students?

GOAL: I will work in a department that (is/is not) in a teaching institution.

15. I will explore different work settings.

GOAL: I will work in the following type of institution: hospital, clinic, imaging center, physician's office, urgent care.

16. What professional attributes do I consider important?

GOAL: I will work to maintain the attributes that I admire most in the professionals who have helped me in my clinical education. Those attributes are:

17. What other goals will I set for myself?

GOAL:

GOAL:

_____

_____

_____

_____

GOAL:

_____

_____

_____

_____

GOAL:

_____

_____

_____

_____

By now you have had considerable experience in describing the aspects of this field that you find motivating. You have also listed specific career goals that you have the ability to achieve. Performing this type of personal inventory has gotten you off to a great start. In addition to reading your goal statements daily, reexamine these goals at regular intervals over the coming months. There will be no stopping you now!

KEY POINTS
Goal Setting

- A career choice is significant; focus on doing the things you particularly enjoy.
- Success in radiologic technology is based on setting goals and working hard to achieve them.
- Goal setting must be a priority throughout your working lifetime.
- Goals are not meant to be rigid and inflexible but alive and fluid.
- Goals should be realistic, measurable, and achievable.
- Approach goals incrementally; celebrate each achievement.
- Goals should be updated as needed and examined at least annually.
- Make goal statements specific and action oriented.
- Direct your energy toward achieving your goal within a specific time frame.
- Goals must be more than wishes; they must be a visualization of what you expect to achieve.
- Post your goals where you can see them daily, and share them with the people who are significant in your life.
- Shared goals are more likely to be met.
- Goal statements use the words "I will."
- Setting goals should not be taken lightly, but it should not be a difficult task

CONTINUING EDUCATION REQUIREMENTS

The quality of a person's life is in direct proportion to their commitment to excellence regardless of their chosen field of endeavor.
Vince Lombardi

MEETING PROFESSIONAL AND GOVERNMENTAL REQUIREMENTS

The purpose of certification is to assure the public that you are competent to practice in your chosen field. However, passing a certification exam to enter the profession is no assurance that you will remain competent. It is of critical importance that you have the most current knowledge and skills needed to practice radiologic technology.

Mandatory continuing education has been established in an attempt to ensure the continued competence of clinicians. Although research indicates that mandatory continuing education in any field of study is not a guarantee of competence, it is the route that has been chosen for many health professions, including radiologic technology, to maintain credibility with the public.

After you successfully pass the certification exam and receive your initial registration, the American Registry of Radiologic Technologists (ARRT) requires documentation of continuing education for you to renew your registration. Participating in continuing education and documenting your participation are your responsibility as a registered technologist. Although acquiring continuing education credits is not difficult for most technologists, knowledge of the applicable rules and regulations is of paramount importance.

In addition to certification, many states require individuals practicing medical radiography to hold licensure or accreditation issued by the state. Because legislation regulating state licensure may be subject to the addition or revision of statutes at any time, the requirements specific to each state are not listed here. Many states accept ARRT certification as proof of the applicant's competency. In those states, you need to apply to the appropriate agency, supply a copy of your ARRT credentials, and pay the proper fee. Be sure to obtain the rules and regulations pertaining to licensure in the state or states in which you will be employed. Such rules advise you of the application process, any testing or fees involved, continuing education requirements, and the status of any reciprocity with the ARRT. Visit the ARRT website at www.arrt.org to obtain a complete list of state agencies responsible for credentialing and requirements.

Because state and national continuing education requirements may differ, it is the responsibility of the individual technologist to keep abreast of the current requirements for continuing education. Neither state nor national agencies accept a lack of knowledge of the rules and regulations as an excuse for failure to meet the requirements. An insufficient number of continuing education credits may result in the issuance of probationary status, the levy of fines by the state, or loss of the ability to work.

You need to renew your certification with the ARRT each year, and you will need to submit proof of continuing education activities every 2 years (known as a biennium). There are three ways to satisfy the requirement of 24 hours of continuing education for a biennium. The first is to participate in 24 hours of continuing education activities that have met the criteria established by the ARRT. The second is to pass a primary examination in an area of radiologic technology in which you were not previously credentialed (e.g., radiation therapy, nuclear medicine, sonography). The third way is to pass one of the post primary exams offered by the ARRT.

You must comply with the ARRT rules governing continuing education beginning with the first day of your birth month after you pass the radiography examination. Your subsequent bienniums then occur in your birth month. State continuing education requirements may, and probably will, differ on their due dates. Be sure to keep the two sets of requirements clear. You should choose continuing education activities based on the area of practice that would meet your needs and the needs of your patients. Remember, this is *your* practice of radiography. What activities would help you be a better caregiver and imaging technologist?

State requirements may differ on the type of activities that satisfy their continuing education requirements. Know the law in your state, and keep files on both state and ARRT requirements, as applicable.

As a registered technologist, it is your responsibility to know whether the continuing education program you are attending has been approved and to obtain the necessary documentation proving your participation in the activity. As an attendee, you are not responsible for submitting a program for approval to obtain credit. The sponsor of the event seeks approval before the date of the presentation. The coordinator of a continuing education program can answer questions concerning the approval of the event.

At the end of each biennium, you must provide proof that you have satisfied the continuing education requirement. Keep the original attendance documents for at least 1 year beyond the 2-year period. The ARRT may conduct random audits to verify such documentation. The documentation must show the date of the program; title and content; number of contact hours; and signature of an individual associated with the program, such as the speaker, instructor, or coordinator. The documentation should also include a continuing education reference number provided by the Recognized Continuing Education Evaluation Mechanism (RCEEM). It is a good idea to set up your own file for continuing education for both the ARRT and the state requirements before you graduate so that it will be in place and ready for immediate use as soon as you are registered. Be certain to keep copies of all documents for audit purposes.

Technologists who fail to meet the ARRT continuing education requirements are placed on probationary status by the ARRT. This means the technologist must make up continuing education credits by a specific date and keep up with credits in the current biennium. Failure to satisfy probationary requirements can lead to further sanctions up to and including a requirement for reexamination. Inquiries submitted to ARRT by employers receive a response that includes a notation of probationary status or revocation; this could result in your rejection as a job applicant or loss of employment.

Penalties regarding noncompliance with state continuing education requirements vary by state. Be certain you are aware of the statutory requirements and regulations.

It is your responsibility to learn about modifications to the continuing education requirements. Be sure to read all of the information sent to you from the ARRT, particularly the "Annual Report to Technologists," published every spring. You should also remain alert for changes to such requirements in your state.

Take time to review the ARRT's "Continuing Education Requirements for Renewal of Certification" at www.arrt.org. This is your best source for complete up-to-date information on continuing education requirements along with frequently asked questions (FAQs). Your instructors can assist you with questions, or you may contact the ARRT office by telephone at 651-687-0048.

CONTINUING EDUCATION OPPORTUNITIES

There are many opportunities to obtain continuing education credits. The primary mission of your professional societies is continuing education. Become an active member of the American Society of Radiologic Technologists (ASRT). Through its sponsorship of conference events, numerous online programs, and its Directed Readings in the journal *Radiologic Technology*, you can obtain a considerable portion of your continuing education credits. The ASRT may be visited at www.asrt.org.

The various state affiliate societies of the ASRT provide many continuing education opportunities every year. Ask your instructors or radiologic technologists in clinical settings for membership information. As part of the state society, your local professional society may have monthly or quarterly meetings that stress continuing education. Take advantage of these meetings.

If you choose a career in any of the radiologic specialties, education, or management, there are many other professional organizations you may join. Each organization offers approved continuing education as part of its mission. Being an active member of a professional society helps ensure that you are informed about the continuing education programs that will contribute most to your skill development.

Continuing education is a vital part of your medical radiography practice. View it as an opportunity to learn and enhance your skills rather than as an imposed obligation. Attend programs that you know will help you become a better technologist. Take an active part in these events, both as an attendee and as a coordinator. Conduct your own presentation for a more complete learning experience. You will find that such activities enhance your professional image and gain you the respect and admiration of your colleagues. Stay in regular contact via www. arrt.org and www.asrt.org.

CONTINUING QUALIFICATION REQUIREMENTS (CQR)

Continuing Qualification Requirements (CQR) are required every 10 years for technologists who have become certified in any area of radiologic technology since January 1, 2011. This is in addition to the continuing education requirement. Certificates earned before 2011 are exempt from CQR.

Documenting continued qualifications through the use of time-limited certificates is the next logical step beyond testing and certification (entry-level knowledge), registration (annual renewal and compliance with ethical requirements), and continuing education (biennially). Before the end of the 10-year period from the original date of certification, technologists will have to demonstrate, choosing from a choice of ARRT-approved activities, that they have kept up with changes in their specific field and the core knowledge required to practice.

Requirements may include an assessment of your practice area, choice of several activities to demonstrate competence, and verification of being current. These requirements are congruent with the mission of the ARRT regarding high patient care standards. Note that re-taking the entry-level certification exam will NOT be a requirement.

> ARRT has been considering for several years what it means to be qualified at points *beyond* entry into the profession. Although at one time the shelf life of knowledge was sufficiently long that the "once certified, forever qualified" approach was reasonable, this proposition can no longer be defended. The reality is that the rate of technological change is so rapid that knowledge has a limited shelf life, and we want consumers to know that ARRT certification means that the individual has relevant current knowledge that enhances his or her ability to provide high-quality patient care.

Regulatory agencies are placing more emphasis on accountability for individuals practicing in the health care professions. CQR is an integral part of your practice. Be certain to remain current on the requirements by visiting www.arrt.org often and consulting the "Annual Report to Technologists."

KEY POINTS
Continuing Education

- Quality patient care dictates that you have the most current knowledge and skills needed to practice radiologic technology.
- Mandatory continuing education was established to ensure the continued competence of clinicians.
- States may have their own continuing education requirements.
- ARRT requires proof of 24 hours continuing education activities every 2 years (known as a biennium).
- There are three ways to satisfy the requirement of 24 hours of continuing education: 24 hours of continuing education activities, pass a primary exam in an area of radiologic technology, or pass a post primary exam offered by the ARRT.
- The continuing education requirement begins the first day of your birth month after you pass the radiography examination.
- Keep continuing education documents for at least 1 year beyond the biennium for possible ARRT audit.
- Consult "Continuing Education Requirements for Renewal of Certification" at www.arrt.org.
- Continuing education opportunities include ASRT (sponsored programs and Directed Readings), state and local radiologic technology conferences, and employer-sponsored approved activities.

RADIOLOGIC SPECIALTIES

> *No one can predict to what height you can soar. Even you will not know until you spread your wings.*

As demand increases for radiologic technologists with multispecialty capabilities, many radiography students, graduates, and practicing technologists are considering furthering their education in imaging, therapy, education, or management. The radiologic clinical specialties requiring formal advanced level education at the present time are diagnostic medical sonography, nuclear medicine technology, and radiation therapy technology. Other radiologic specialties such as CT, angiography, MRI, quality management, interventional technology, mammography, and bone densitometry do not have specific formal additional educational requirements for credentialing, although clinical requirements are being established. Numerous education programs are offered in those areas, and an online search of such opportunities is recommended.

In many cases, the education for specialty areas is provided on the job or through extensive study programs set up between the employer and the employee. Formal classes should be attended whenever possible. However, medical imaging is advancing at such a rapid pace that often the responsibility for obtaining education in a certain modality falls completely on the imaging technologist. Information concerning advanced level, or post primary, examinations in these areas is available from the ARRT. The requirements for all specialty areas could change at any time; the appropriate credentialing agencies listed in this chapter should be contacted when the technologist is pursuing a specialty.

Information about the specialties presented in this chapter provides you with access to the website of the professional organization associated with each specialty. The websites give you access to the most current and accurate listings of all educational programs in the United States accredited by that organization and the certification requirements. Because certification requirements and educational programs are subject to change for various reasons, the interested professional should use the websites for such information.

For each examination and specialty listed in this chapter, it is important to contact the certifying organization for details regarding specific clinical requirements that may have to be documented as part of the application process. This chapter is meant to be informational only and does not attempt to take the place of the formal and comprehensive handbooks published by the respective organizations.

DIAGNOSTIC MEDICAL SONOGRAPHY

Educational programs in sonography may be 1½, 2, or 4 years in length, depending on the curriculum offered and the inclusion of earned credit hours for an academic degree. The course of study involves biology, sectional anatomy, patient care, physics and equipment of sonography, diagnostic procedures, imaging, and image evaluation. Clinical education also constitutes a major portion of the program. Use of the following websites will ensure that you obtain the most accurate, current information available.

For information on a career as a diagnostic medical sonographer, contact the following organization:

Society of Diagnostic Medical Sonography
Plano, TX
www.sdms.org

For a listing of accredited educational programs in sonography, contact:

The Committee on Accreditation of Allied Health Education Programs
www.caahep.org

For information on certification exams in sonography, contact either:

American Registry of Diagnostic Medical Sonographers
Rockville, MD
www.ardms.org
Exams offered for sonographers:
   Abdomen
   Adult echocardiography
   Breast
   Fetal echocardiography
   Neurosonography
   Obstetrics and gynecology
   Pediatric echocardiography
   Physicians' vascular interpretation
   Sonography principles and instrumentation
   Vascular technology

or

American Registry of Radiologic Technologists
St. Paul, MN
www.arrt.org
Exams offered for sonographers:
   Sonography (primary and post primary exam)
   Vascular sonography (post primary exam)
   Breast sonography (post primary exam)

NUCLEAR MEDICINE

Educational programs in nuclear medicine technology may be 1, 2, or 4 years in length, depending on the curriculum offered and the inclusion of earned credit hours for an academic degree. The course of study involves biology, anatomy, patient care, nuclear physics and instrumentation, computer technology, biochemistry, radiopharmacology, radiation biology and health physics, radiation protection, immunology, radionuclide therapy, and statistics. Diagnostic procedures, imaging, and image evaluation, including extensive clinical education, also constitute a major portion of the program. Use of the following websites will ensure that you obtain the most accurate, current information available.

For information on a career as a nuclear medicine technologist, contact the following organizations:

American Society of Radiologic Technologists
Albuquerque, NM
www.asrt.org
Society of Nuclear Medicine
Reston, VA
www.snm.org

For a listing of accredited educational programs in nuclear medicine technology, contact:

Joint Review Committee on Education in Radiologic Technology
Chicago, IL
www.jrcert.org

For information on certification exams in nuclear medicine technology, contact either:

American Registry of Radiologic Technologists
St. Paul, MN
www.arrt.org
Nuclear medicine exam offered:
   Nuclear medicine

or

Nuclear Medicine Technology Certification Board
Tucker, GA
www.nmtcb.org
Nuclear medicine exams offered:
   Nuclear medicine
   Cardiology
   Positron emission tomography (PET)

For further information, contact:

American Registry of Radiologic Technologists
St. Paul, MN
www.arrt.org

RADIATION THERAPY TECHNOLOGY

Educational programs in radiation therapy technology may be 1, 2, or 4 years in length depending on the curriculum offered and the inclusion of earned credit hours for an academic degree. The course of study involves biology, radiation oncology, pathology, radiation biology, physics and equipment of radiation therapy, intensity modulated radiation therapy, dosimetry, computer technology, and quality assurance. Use of the following websites will ensure that you obtain the most accurate, current information available.

For information on a career as a radiation therapist, contact the following organization:

American Society of Radiologic Technologists
Albuquerque, NM
www.asrt.org

For a listing of accredited educational programs in radiation therapy technology, contact:

Joint Review Committee on Education in Radiologic
  Technology
Chicago, IL
www.jrcert.org

For information on the certification exam in radiation therapy technology, contact:

American Registry of Radiologic Technologists
St. Paul, MN
www.arrt.org
Radiation therapy exam offered:
  Radiation therapy

OTHER IMAGING SPECIALTIES

Education in other imaging specialties may be provided on the job or in courses that are one semester or one academic year in length depending on the curriculum offered, the current credentials of the radiologic technologist, and the inclusion of earned credit hours for an academic degree. The course of study should provide educational opportunities specific to the imaging modality, including pathology, radiation biology, anatomy, patient care, physics and instrumentation, computer technology, radiation protection, diagnostic procedures, imaging, image evaluation, quality assurance, and clinical education. The imaging specialties that might be included are:

Angiography (all types)
Bone densitometry
CT
Fusion imaging
MRI
Mammography
Quality management

Use of the following websites will ensure that you obtain the most accurate, current information available.

For information on a career in these specialty areas, contact:

American Society of Radiologic Technologists
Albuquerque, NM
www.asrt.org (search by topic)

Alternatively, use any comprehensive Internet search engine, such as Google (search by topic).

For a listing of educational programs for these imaging specialties, use any comprehensive Internet search engine, such as Google (search by topic).

For information on certification exams in these specialties, contact:

American Registry of Radiologic Technologists
St. Paul, MN
www.arrt.org
Post primary exams offered:
  CT
  MRI (also a primary exam)
  Cardiac interventional radiography
  Vascular interventional radiography
  Mammography
  Quality management
  Bone densitometry

RADIOLOGIST ASSISTANT

As structured by the ASRT, a radiologist assistant is "an advanced-level radiologic technologist who works under the supervision of a radiologist to enhance patient care by assisting the radiologist in the diagnostic imaging environment."* Radiologist assistants are ARRT-certified radiographers who have "successfully completed an advanced academic program encompassing a nationally recognized radiologist assistant curriculum and a radiologist directed clinical preceptorship."* Working under the supervision of a radiologist, "the Radiologist Assistant performs patient assessment, patient management and selected exams."*

Education of radiologist assistants is based at the baccalaureate and postbaccalaureate levels. The ASRT has written a core curriculum for a bachelor of science in radiologic sciences (B.S.R.S.) degree. The ASRT states that the radiologist assistant has the following areas of responsibility:

1. Participate in patient assessment, patient management, and patient education
2. Perform selected radiology procedures including, but not limited to, fluoroscopy
3. Evaluate image quality and perform initial image observations*

---

*American Society of Radiologic Technologists, www.asrt.org, 2011.

For information on a career as a radiologist assistant, contact either:

American Society of Radiologic Technologists
Albuquerque, NM
www.asrt.org

American College of Radiology
www.acr.org

For a listing of educational programs for radiologist assistants, contact:

American Society of Radiologic Technologists
Albuquerque, NM
www.asrt.org

For information on the certification exam for radiologist assistant, contact:

American Registry of Radiologic Technologists
St. Paul, MN
www.arrt.org

RADIOGRAPHY EDUCATOR

One of the fastest growing specialties in radiologic technology over the next 10 to 15 years will be in the area of radiography education. There are currently nearly 800 radiography programs in the United States. They are staffed, depending on size and enrollment, with directors, clinical coordinators, instructors, and laboratory assistants. Similar to a large percentage of the population as a whole, radiography educators are nearing retirement in unprecedented numbers. For registered technologists who enjoy working with students and teaching, countless opportunities for career advancement and great satisfaction will be available. The profession will need a steady supply of educators to keep its programs functioning and to graduate the record numbers of radiographers who will be needed in the coming decades. The need for educators in all of the medical imaging and therapy professions will be great. Radiography education is highlighted here because the need will be greatest in that field.

If you are interested in a career specialty in radiography education, prepare by earning degrees as follows, in addition to RT (R) credentials:

- Program director: Master's degree (consider radiologic technology, education, adult education, curriculum design)
- Clinical coordinator: Baccalaureate degree or master's degree (consider radiologic technology, education, adult education, curriculum design)
- Instructor or laboratory assistant: Baccalaureate degree (for full-time instructors), with strong clinical experience, a great interest in teaching, and proven expertise in radiography

For information on requirements for becoming a radiography program official or instructor, contact the following organization:

Joint Review Committee on Education in Radiologic Technology
Chicago, IL
www.jrcert.org

For information specific to radiography educators, contact the following organizations:

Association of Collegiate Educators in Radiologic Technology (ACERT)
www.acert.org

Association of Educators in Imaging and Radiological Sciences (AEIRS)
www.aeirs.org

IMAGING MANAGER

In many clinical environments, individuals advance into management, shift supervisor, or radiology administrative positions by promotion. In such situations, promotion occurs because an individual has proved to be exemplary in some field of clinical work. If you are planning a career in radiology management, seriously consider college degrees that provide you with the managerial and legal foundation to be effective in management. Managing the human and physical resources in an imaging or therapy department requires mastery of an entirely different set of skills. Consider a master's degree in radiologic technology, management, communication, human resources, or business administration.

For information on degrees in these areas, use any comprehensive Internet search engine, such as Google (search by degree).

For information on a career as an imaging manager and for the examination for a certified radiology administrator, contact:

American Healthcare Radiology Administrators (AHRA)
Sudbury, MA
www.ahra.com

ACADEMIC DEGREES

You cannot discover new oceans unless you have the courage to lose sight of the shore.

An increasing number of radiography students and technologists are interested in pursuing higher level academic degrees. This is particularly true for individuals seeking a career in radiology management or education. Master's degrees are required of radiography program directors. Baccalaureate degrees are required of clinical coordinators and full-time instructors. Others would like to pursue degrees because they enjoy learning or would find the achievement fulfilling. Some hope to expand their earning potential or raise the level of their professional status. The baccalaureate degree is considered the professional level for radiologic technologists.

The U.S. Departments of Education and Labor possess ample data to support the contention that earnings and employment opportunities are greater for individuals with higher levels of education. Regardless of the motivation, career planning and goal setting must be based on accurate information.

Individuals interested in pursuing advanced degrees should visit the institution's website and request the latest edition of the college or university catalog to determine what curriculum is offered. Information available on the Internet also provides listings of degree programs as they become available.

As with many other health professions, an advanced degree in radiologic technology is not required for career advancement. However, baccalaureate and master's degrees in business, management, and education have become increasingly important. You should carefully define your career goals and pursue advanced education opportunities that are specific enough to provide skills in certain areas but broad enough to allow flexibility. Advancing to higher levels of responsibility in radiologic technology no longer depends entirely on moving up through the ranks; a solid college education is required.

If an advanced degree is among your career goals, begin planning now. Requests for information take time. The use of websites greatly expedites the process. The sooner you acquire the needed information, the sooner you will be able to establish your plans for further education and achieve your desired goals.

Consider interviewing radiologic technologists at your clinical sites who are currently enrolled in degree completion programs. They can provide helpful information about the college or university in which they are enrolled.

For specific college and university information, visit the institution's website or use major search engines, such as Google, typing in keywords such as "radiologic technology," "radiography," and "radiologic technology degree."

As you begin planning for an advanced degree, inquire about advanced standing or credit for previous radiologic technology education. Many institutions award up to 2 full years of college credit. Your program director may have advice about writing a portfolio of educational and work experiences to help you receive additional college credit for what you already know and have accomplished.

The work environment of the twenty-first century requires that you have as much knowledge and as many credentials as possible to advance in your career. Now is a good time to begin planning and setting goals for a lifetime of learning and achievement!

KEY POINTS
Radiologic Specialties and Academic Degrees

- Demand is increasing for radiologic technologists with multispecialty capabilities.
- Specialties requiring formal advanced level education include diagnostic medical sonography, nuclear medicine technology, and radiation therapy technology.
- Specialties without a formal education requirement include CT, angiography, MRI, quality management, interventional technology, mammography, and bone densitometry.
- Formal classes should be attended whenever possible.
- Information concerning advanced level, or post primary, examinations is available from the ARRT.
- Visit the website of the professional organization associated with each specialty for specific educational, clinical, and credentialing requirements.
- Other specialties to be considered include radiography educator and imaging department administrator or manager.
- Academic degrees enhance career opportunities in every aspect of radiologic technology.

Writing a Professional Resume

PURPOSE OF A RESUME

Your resume serves as your professional calling card. It is a summary of your academic and work history and relevant accomplishments and credentials. It should be brief (i.e., one to two pages). It is essentially a snapshot of your career to date. In addition to offering samples of resumes, this chapter describes ways to use the resume and provides the rationale for including or excluding certain information.

There are probably as many different styles and formats for resumes as there are instructors attempting to describe them. Take advantage of your radiography instructor's expertise in this area. In addition, if you are enrolled in a collegiate radiography program, the college may have a learning resource center, a writing center, or a career counseling center from which you can obtain additional guidance. There are many books available on the subject of writing resumes. In addition, numerous software packages provide guidance on writing resumes. With all of these resources to choose from, writing a resume can become a dizzying experience. The material presented in this chapter was developed for courses taught by a radiographer and has been used by students and graduates.

The resume may be used in three ways. It may be (1) sent as part of a mailing to prospective employers and followed with a telephone call, (2) left with an interviewer after an appointment, or (3) included with the job application form submitted to the human resources department.

Often the student or graduate radiographer wishes to indicate availability to numerous prospective employers in a certain geographic area. The resume, accompanied by a cover letter, may be mailed to the directors of radiology at all facilities in the area where the student is interested in working. Although this is the least effective method to use in a job search, a well-constructed resume with an appropriate cover letter can produce results. Figure 9-1 shows a sample cover letter to accompany the resume in these situations. Such a mailing should always be followed by a personal telephone call to the radiology manager, as promised in the cover letter. Following up in this way can be time-consuming, but it is one method for reaching a large number of prospective employers.

In certain situations, the student or graduate radiographer may have an informal interview with a radiology manager who is considering filling a position. This often occurs when students or graduates are told about a job opening. In these circumstances, there may be insufficient time to mail a resume in advance. In this situation, the interviewee should take a copy of the resume and give it to the radiology manager at the interview. Similar to appropriate attire and grooming, a professional resume can make a powerful first impression during an interview.

CONTENTS OF A RESUME

In addition to ensuring that you have the appropriate writing tools available, you should spend time thinking about what to include in the resume and what to exclude. Include all postsecondary (i.e., after high school) education. You should account for all of your time since high school. Include all professional society memberships, credential numbers, awards, and accomplishments on the resume.

The resume should contain only information that is relevant to your accomplishments and goals as a professional. Information of a personal nature (beyond that presented in the next section) or data that could be used to discriminate should be excluded from the resume. Your resume is an opportunity to advertise yourself in your absence. Construct it wisely.

WRITING THE RESUME

Figures 9-2 and 9-3 show two resumes that could have been written by a student and a graduate radiographer. The resumes present applicants with slightly different backgrounds and so include different information. Your resume is likely to be a variant of these. Remember, brevity is the rule when constructing your resume. However, do not use abbreviations. Keep your resume polished and proper.

PERSONAL DATA

The first section should include your name, followed by the address and telephone number (and e-mail address; this is optional) at which you may be reached during your current job search. If your address and telephone number change during the course of your job search, a prospective

Date

Director of Radiology
XYZ Hospital
Main Street
Anytown, USA 01234

Dear Director:

Enclosed please find my professional resume
outlining my education and work experiences. I am
very interested in being considered for
employment in your department of radiology in the
position of staff radiographer. I appreciate
whatever time and attention you are able to give to
this inquiry.

I will call you in a few days to see what
employment opportunities you may have available.

Sincerely,

Enclosure

FIGURE 9-1 Sample cover letter, general mailing.

employer would be unable to contact you, possibly eliminating you as a candidate for the position. If you must change your address and telephone number after submitting the resume, inform prospective employers in writing.

No additional personal information should be included on the resume. Specific items to be excluded are date of birth, gender, race, marital status, church affiliation, number of children, disabilities, hobbies, and any other data that are irrelevant to your status as a job seeker. Although a prospective employer may not use such information, including it on your resume places you in the position of having raised it as an issue.

GOAL STATEMENT

As shown in the examples, the next section of the resume should include your goal statement. The goal statement can be as simple as "To obtain a position as an entry-level radiographer," or it may include your desire to cross-train in another specialty, such as "To obtain a position as an entry-level radiographer; desire to cross-train in computed tomography." Careful consideration should be given to the goal statement. If the wording suggests that you absolutely must have the opportunity to cross-train in other modalities, you would be eliminated from consideration if the prospective employer is looking for a staff radiographer only. Wording such as "To obtain a position as an entry-level radiographer; willing to be cross-trained in other modalities" indicates your desire to expand your horizons but without the sense of urgency conveyed by the previous statement.

The goal statement may also be altered depending on where you are seeking employment. If you know the prospective employer is seeking radiographers who definitely want to cross-train, that interest should be included in your goal statement. In addition, if one of your goals is to cross-train and you are unwilling to accept a position that does not offer that opportunity, you should include it in your goal statement, realizing that you may be excluded from consideration if such a position is unavailable. Words in the goal statement that identify the strength of your interest are "desire to cross-train" or "willing to cross-train."

As you prepare to write your resume and begin setting your professional goals, give them serious consideration. The goal statement may include you in the final group of candidates for a position, or it may exclude you immediately, depending on how it is worded. As a final example, consider the goal statement of an applicant to a clinic or urgent care setting. The responsibilities in these positions often are multifaceted. A goal statement such as "To obtain a position as a radiographer; willing to perform venipuncture, simple laboratory procedures, and electrocardiograms, and take patient histories and vital signs" indicates not only a willingness to learn new procedures but also an ability to be flexible and work as a team member in a small clinic setting. Conversely, if you have no desire to perform these other functions, you should not include such places in your job search.

EMPLOYMENT EXPERIENCES

Beginning with your most recent employment and working backward, you should list all employment experiences related either to health care or to working with the public. Indicate the month and year that each position began and ended, the name of the employer, the location of the employer, and a simple phrase describing your responsibilities. It is unnecessary to list the names of supervisors or the salary you received. It is also unnecessary to account for every job held since high school. The resume is your statement of professional experience. Include the positions that demonstrate your ability to work with people. Try to avoid lapses in dates whenever possible. Your work experience and education should blend into a seamless timeline.

EDUCATION

Your resume should include all of the formal education you have acquired since high school, listed in reverse chronological order (i.e., beginning with the most recent). It is unnecessary to provide a detailed list of the courses studied. Rather, you may wish to indicate a broad area of study (e.g., liberal arts and sciences). Some entries in this section are self-explanatory. A radiology manager would not require explanation of an entry such as "Radiography Program." In each of your educational

Personal Data

Name
Address
City, State, Zip Code
Telephone Number
Email Address

Goal

To obtain a position as an entry-level radiographer; willing to cross-train in computed tomography.

Employment Experience

September 20___-Present

Front Office Clerk
Medical Imaging Department
City Medical Center
This Town, State
Duties: Greet patients arriving for radiographic exams; update electronic medical record

November 20___-August 20___
Certified Nursing Assistant
Extended Care Unit
County Rehabilitation Center
Our Town, State
Duties: Provided care to patients such as bathing, grooming, basic exercise, and assistance with meals

Education

June 20___-Present
Radiography Program Name
Our Community College (or) Our Hospital
This City, State
Graduation scheduled for May 20___

Fall 20___-Spring 20___
Radiography program prerequisites
Our Community College
This Town, State
Earned 48 semester hours in liberal arts and sciences

Professional Accomplishments, Associations, and Credentials

• Taking American Registry of Radiologic Technologists radiography exam, May 20___
• Student member, American Society of Radiologic Technologists
• Student member, This State Society of Radiologic Technologists
• Awarded First Place for scientific exhibit entitled "Osteogenesis Imperfecta" at State Society
   Radiologic Technologists Annual Conference
• Participant, Scholar Bowl, State Society of Radiologic Technologists Annual Conference
• Certified Nursing Assistant, credentialed by Our State

References available upon request.

FIGURE 9-2 Sample resume, second-year student.

Personal Data

Name

Address

City, State, Zip Code

Telephone Number

Email Address

Goal

To obtain a position as an entry-level radiographer; desire to cross-train in mammography.

Employment Experience

December 20__-Present

Patient Transporter

Department of Imaging

XYZ Area Hospital

This Town, State

Duties: Transport inpatients to and from imaging department

May 20__-November 20__

Great Food Restaurant

This Town, State

Duties: Greeted customers at their table; took order, served food

Education

August 20__-July 20__

Radiography Program Name

Our Medical Center (or) Our College

That City, State

Graduated July 20__

Awarded Diploma in Medical Radiography (or) Associate in Applied Sciences Degree

Spring 20__-Spring 20__

Liberal Arts Coursework

Community College

This Town, State

Earned 36 semester hours

Professional Accomplishments, Associations, and Credentials

• Took Registry exam in August; passed; awaiting credentials

  (or) Registered by the American Registry of Radiologic Technologists, #123456 through January 20__

• Credentialed by the State of __, #987654, through July 20__

• Active member, American Society of Radiologic Technologists

• Active member, This State Society of Radiologic Technologists

• Member of student team winning first place in radiography scholar bowl at This State Society of Radiologic Technologists Annual Conference, 20__

• Awarded first place for scientific paper presentation entitled "Cervical Spine injuries" at This State Society of Radiologic Technologists Annual Conference, 20__

References available upon request.

FIGURE 9-3 Sample resume, recent graduate.

experience entries, indicate whether you graduated or received some form of certificate, diploma, or degree. The dates in this section, along with the dates accompanying your employment history, should account for most of your time since high school.

PROFESSIONAL ACCOMPLISHMENTS, ASSOCIATIONS, AND CREDENTIALS

In this section, you should list all professional organizations to which you belong. Include any offices or other positions of responsibility you have held, such as being a member or chair of a committee. Examples of information for this section include membership in local, state, or national professional societies; membership in student radiographer associations; and any professional licenses already held. Awards for academic excellence such as honors listings should be included and participation in competitions, such as research paper writing, scientific exhibits, and scholar bowls. You may also wish to include a list of your attendance at state or national professional society meetings.

If you have not yet taken the ARRT exam, you should describe your status such as "Taking ARRT exam in May." If you have taken the exam but have not yet received your credentials, describe your status such as "Took Registry exam on August 20; passed; waiting for credentials." Note there is no such status as "Registry eligible"; do not use the term. Radiology managers encounter this situation routinely and are not dissuaded from considering your application because of your transitional status. If you have received your credentials, you should indicate your ARRT number and expiration date. Do not include your test score.

REFERENCES

References are not listed on the professional resume. A prospective employer provides space on the job application form for listing both work and personal references. For the resume itself, the statement "References available upon request" suffices. Be sure you have obtained the permission of the individuals you wish to use as references so that they will be expecting inquiries from prospective employers.

COVER LETTER

If mailed in response to an actual job posting or advertisement, the resume should always be accompanied by a concise cover letter. Figure 9-4 shows a sample of a cover letter that you can adapt for your use.

APPEARANCE OF THE RESUME AND COVER LETTER

As you compose your resume, it is a foregone conclusion that you will do so on a computer. Handwritten resumes are unacceptable. You will be able to work

Date

Director of Radiology
XYZ Hospital
Main Street
Anytown, USA 01234

Dear Director:

It was with great interest that I read your hospital's advertisement for the position of staff radiographer. Enclosed please find my professional resume outlining the experiences and education that I believe qualify me for this position.

I wish to notify you of my interest in being employed in your department. I am also completing an application for employment in your Department of Human Resources and am including a copy of my resume with it. I look forward to hearing from you regarding a personal interview so that we may discuss our mutual needs and interests.

Sincerely,

Enclosure

FIGURE 9-4 Sample cover letter, response to job posting.

through a rough draft and then refine the resume fairly easily. Use the "spell check" feature in your software. Print your resume using a high-quality laser or ink-jet printer. After printing, make certain there is no smeared ink or partially printed lines caused by a faulty printer.

Be aware that others who are competing with you for the same positions are preparing and printing their resumes in the same fashion. If you do not own such equipment, computers are available in college writing centers, in many copy center retail stores, and in some state employment centers. Use of these facilities and equipment, which typically are available free or at a modest price, is a wise investment.

There are as many different types of paper available as there are resume formats. The resume and cover letter should be printed on 60- to 75-lb text paper that is preferably white or ivory, which provides a positive image for your resume. Because this paper has a heavier weight, it should not be folded. You should use a large manila envelope so that the resume and cover letter are flat and unfolded. If you are unfamiliar with paper types and weights, your writing center or retail copy shop can provide you with information.

Avoid using copier-type paper; it is an inexpensive grade of paper and does not make a positive impression on the reader. In addition, many papers of this type produce a poorer printed image when used with a laser printer.

JOB APPLICATION

Students are often dismayed that after investing much time and effort in writing a resume, they must still complete a job application form. This is a standard practice for many employers and is required by institutional accrediting agencies. Regardless of whether you are applying at several radiology facilities or just one, you should always bring a copy of the resume and ensure it is attached to the job application form. You should never indicate on the application form that the resume is attached and leave blanks on the application; by bringing the resume to the human resources office, however, you will have most of the information you need to fill in the job application form. Make certain you bring all needed information with you (e.g., names and addresses of former employers; names, addresses, and telephone numbers of references), especially if it is not included on the resume.

You may request that former or current employers not be contacted. In addition, a detailed employment and reference check cannot be conducted without your signed authorization. Carefully read the statement at the bottom of the application form before you sign it. Remember, although you have provided all of the information requested on the application form, it is still important to attach the resume.

Many individuals apply for professional positions online. This may be accomplished by going to a prospective employer's website, filling out an on-screen application form, and attaching your resume electronically. Job search websites permit you to post your resume for employers to examine. In either case, a professional resume, clearly indicating your professional experience and goals, will go a long way toward securing the position you desire.

Proper preparation of a professional resume is not a task to be taken lightly. Spend the time needed to construct your resume carefully, and be aware of its impact on potential employers. Your resume is a statement of your professionalism that speaks for you in your absence.

KEY POINTS
Writing a Professional Resume

- Your resume is a summary of your academic and work history and relevant accomplishments and credentials.
- Keep resume length to one or two pages, as a snapshot of your career to date.
- Include your name, address, phone number, and email address.
- Exclude date of birth, gender, race, marital status, church affiliation, number of children, disabilities, hobbies, and any other data that are irrelevant to your status as a job seeker.
- Include only information that is relevant to your accomplishments and goals as a professional.
- Brevity is the rule.
- Do not use abbreviations of any kind.
- Resumes may be used as part of a mailing to prospective employers, left with an interviewer after an appointment, or included with the job application form.
- Prepare a cover letter to accompany your resume if doing a mailing.
- Include a simple goal statement.
- List all jobs held since high school, oldest first; include all jobs that dealt with the public; emphasize jobs in health care.
- List all postsecondary education; high school should be left off.
- Indicate whether you graduated and whether you received a certificate, diploma, or degree.
- List offices or other positions of responsibility you have held, such as membership in local, state, or national professional societies and membership in student radiographer associations; any professional licenses already held; awards for academic excellence such as honors listings; and participation in competitions such as research paper writing, scientific exhibits, and scholar bowls and attendance at state or national professional society meetings.
- References are not listed on the professional resume.
- Use spell check.
- Print on high-quality, 60- to 75-lb paper, white or ivory, using a good printer.
- If applying in person, bring a copy of the resume, and make sure it is included with the job application form.
- If applying online, attach the resume electronically if possible.
- Your resume is a statement of your professionalism that speaks for you in your absence.

Interviewing Techniques

Don't wait for your ship to come in. Swim out to it.

PURPOSE OF AN INTERVIEW

If your resume is your detailed calling card, your personal interview is your house call. It is your only opportunity to make a strong, lasting first impression with your possible future employer. Because of the legalities surrounding the issue of discrimination, the personal interview may not be as detailed as it has been in the past. However, this does not diminish its significance or the importance of proper preparation.

The employer can use the personal interview to verify information submitted on the resume or job application. It can serve as an opportunity for the employer to show you the facilities in which you may be working, familiarize you with the equipment, and determine your experience with such equipment. The interviewer may also be interested in your career goals and plans for establishing a career.

Another purpose of an interview is for you to become acquainted with your prospective employer. It is also a time for you to decide whether you want to work for that department or organization if offered a job. As you prepare for the interview, always remember it is a two-way street.

PERSONAL APPEARANCE

There is no substitute for making a strong first impression with the person or persons who will be conducting your interview. Like it or not, we are visual creatures, and your physical appearance during your initial contact with the receptionist and the interviewers has a profound effect on their perception of you as a potential employee.

How you choose to present yourself for your interview says a lot about your professional self-image. Regardless of where you work, you represent that department or organization to the patient or customer. Appropriate professional attire begins with the interview and continues every day once the job begins.

Dressing for social occasions varies by age group and geographic region. However, dressing for a professional job interview is fairly standard regardless of age or location. What you choose *not* to wear is as important as what you do wear. For the interview, do not wear your professional uniform. Casual attire and trendy clothing, such as blue jeans, casual slacks, shorts, T-shirts, and athletic shoes, are also inappropriate. Be careful not to overapply cologne or arrive at the interview smelling of smoke. Pay attention to details. It does little good to wear a clean, pressed business suit only to have the interviewer see dirty fingernails. Similarly, proper grooming loses its impact when your cologne precedes you to the interview by 5 minutes.

Conservative clothing is a must. Men should always wear a business suit or blazer, tie (optional), and dress slacks. Women should wear a business suit. Clothing must be clean and free of wrinkles. Shoes (polished), socks, and belt should complement the clothing. Hose must be free of runs. Hair should be neatly styled and pulled back if shoulder length or longer. Jewelry should be conservative and kept to a minimum, including visible piercings.

Because you will undoubtedly be nervous, your mouth will likely be dry. Until the interview begins, use a breath mint to keep your mouth moist and your breath fresh. Gum chewing is never acceptable in a professional setting. Be certain your cell phone is turned off (not just on vibrate).

As your attire varies from these suggestions, the likelihood of a favorable impression on the interviewer decreases. Applying for a professional position requires that you dress and present yourself professionally.

By taking the time to prepare your personal appearance and dress professionally, you are telling the interviewers you respect their time and appreciate their serious consideration of you as a job candidate. You are also making a statement about how you believe a professional should appear, not only to potential employers but also to your peers. The interviewers will assume that although you would be wearing a professional uniform or even scrubs at work, you would appear as neat and clean when caring for patients as your appearance during the interview suggests.

PREPARING FOR THE INTERVIEW

To prepare for the interview, you should attempt to find out as much about your potential employer as possible. If you cannot ascertain this information ahead of time, be prepared with questions about the employer you can ask during the interview.

Before the interview, you may wish to examine the organization's most recent annual report (which is normally found on the organization's website). The overall reputation in the community and the financial stability of your prospective employer are factors you should consider before accepting a job offer.

It should not be necessary to bring anything to the interview unless you have not previously submitted your resume to the interviewer; if you have not, bring a clean copy inside a manila folder or large envelope. All the facts pertaining to your professional preparation are on the resume. If documentation is required for any item, it may be submitted at a later time to the department of human resources. Similarly, your list of references is probably already entered on the job application form. If not, these may also be furnished later to the human resources department. In most cases, individual department directors do not perform reference checks because of the legalities involved.

If you are unsure where the interview will be held, you should find the building and the office several days ahead of time. You do not want to spend time searching for the site on the day the interview is scheduled. You should allow plenty of time to get to your destination. If you arrive early, there is always a waiting area. Arriving late for an interview is inexcusable.

When you arrive at the interview site, you may want to visit the restroom. Anxiety about the interview may make this necessary, but it also gives you the opportunity to make sure your hair and attire are presentable. When arriving at the appropriate office, greet everyone as if they were going to conduct the interview. Many radiology managers ask receptionists their impressions of the interviewee.

Feeling nervous and apprehensive about an interview is normal, especially if you greatly desire the position. Try to convert your nervous energy into enthusiasm when speaking with others throughout the course of the interview.

INTERVIEW PROCESS

When the interviewer approaches, stand and shake hands firmly. Make eye contact. A smile and an enthusiastic (although not excessively demonstrative) attitude create a positive first impression. As the interview begins, try to appear as calm, comfortable, and professional as possible. Maintain appropriate eye contact and smile. Maintain good posture and remain alert. Be pleasant, avoid joking, and be attentive. Speak distinctly, and use appropriate terminology. Be a good listener. You may wish to bring up your career goals as summarized in the goal statement on your resume. Carefully indicate how you may be an asset to the department without sounding as though you are bossy or demanding. Answer the interviewer's questions clearly, avoiding very short or very long answers. Be prepared to discuss any items you have included on your resume.

There have been numerous legal challenges in recent years to what are alleged to be discriminatory interview questions and techniques. Although the emphasis of such legal rulings has been to require the interviewer to ask only questions that reveal your job qualifications, it is wise for you to know what can and cannot be asked in a job interview. This knowledge assists you in preparing for the interview. It also makes you aware of your rights so you may recognize potentially discriminatory situations.

Be prepared for behavioral interviews. Such interviews probe your responses to various interpersonal and professional situations. Don't attempt to outwit the interviewer. It is best to answer the questions honestly and professionally.

The following box lists topics that may be addressed during an interview. They are relevant to the job and are legitimate areas of inquiry. You may wish to write out your answers ahead of time in anticipation of the interview. Other interview questions not included in this list may also be appropriate and within current legal guidelines.

- Whether you were promoted and on what criteria the promotion was based (e.g., merit, length of service)
- How much you expect an employer to communicate with you and to keep you involved in workplace activities
- Which mode of communication you prefer

The interviewer will probably provide you with information about the salary structure, benefits package, sick leave, and vacation time allowed. Although this information is important to you, try to wait until the interviewer brings it up. In this way, you will not appear to be interested only in money and benefits.

In any interviewing situation, you should be aware of the types of questions that may not be asked. Although it is not likely to occur in a truly professional organization, it is always possible that you may be asked an inappropriate question. If you are asked an inappropriate question relating to the subjects listed in the following box, you may wish to ask the interviewer, "Can you explain to me how this question relates to the requirements of this position?" Most likely, the interviewer will retract the question. However, if a series of improper questions is asked, and you realize it is intentional, you may not wish to continue pursuing the position. If blatant harassment or violation of ethical interviewing guidelines occurs, you must ask yourself whether you wish to work in such an environment, regardless of how much you might desire the position. If either of these situations develops, you may decide to conclude the interview with a statement such as, "Thank you for your time, but I feel you are asking irrelevant questions in violation of my rights. Please remove my name from consideration for this position," or you may opt to finish the interview and remove your name from consideration in a follow-up letter.

Be careful not to answer questions on the topics in the accompanying box. You are not required to answer them and should not volunteer such information. If you believe you have been discriminated against based on questionable interview practices, you may wish to seek private legal counsel or remedy through the Equal Employment Opportunity Commission (EEOC) as a last resort. Recommendations concerning legal issues that may arise during the interview are beyond the scope of this text. A personal attorney is best equipped to answer such questions.

KEY POINTS
Questions You May Be Asked That Are Not Appropriate and That You Should Not Answer

- Your age
- Your birth date
- How long you have resided at your present address
- Your previous address
- The church you choose to attend (if any) or the name of your priest, minister, or rabbi
- Your father's surname
- Your maiden name, if you are female

- Whether you are married, divorced, separated, widowed, or single
- Who lives with you
- How many children you have or intend to have
- The ages of your children
- Who will care for your children while you are working
- How you will get to work (unless owning a car is a job requirement)
- Where a spouse or parent works or lives
- Whether you own or rent your place of residence
- The name of your bank or any information concerning outstanding loan amounts
- Whether you have ever had your wages garnished or filed bankruptcy
- Whether you have ever been arrested
- Whether you have ever served in the armed forces of another country
- How you spend your spare time or to which clubs or organizations you belong
- Your position on labor unions or whether you have ever been a member of a union
- The nationality of your name

Do not allow the interviewer to take advantage of your friendly nature to ask questions that should not be asked or to pry into personal aspects of your life. This is not a conversation between friends; it is a professional job interview. If you conduct yourself professionally, a competent interviewer will respect you and your position.

INTERVIEW OUTCOMES AND FOLLOW-UP

Even after a good interview, you may not be hired or take the job offer. The following box lists some of the appropriate reasons.

KEY POINTS
Why You May Not Be Hired

- You are unable to work the required hours.
- You choose to reject the job offer because you are not interested in the position.
- You are not qualified for the position, or other candidates were better qualified.
- You were obviously under the influence of drugs or alcohol during the interview, or you did not pass the preemployment drug screening or background check.
- Inconsistent, inaccurate, or fraudulent statements were made on your application form.
- You are physically unable to perform the job duties; however, the Americans with Disabilities Act guidelines must be considered.
- Your references were unsatisfactory.
- Your interview created a poor impression; you did not seem interested; you used poor grammar or other unacceptable communication skills.
- There was not a good match between what you had to offer and this employer's needs.

The last impression can be as important as the first. At the conclusion of the interview, shake hands firmly, make eye contact, and thank the interviewer for the time spent with you. The interviewer will probably give some indication of when the hiring decision will be made based on the number of applicants and the date by which the position must be filled. As you leave, say good-bye to the receptionists you pass and thank them for their assistance.

Immediately send a follow-up letter to the interviewer. A sample letter is shown in Figure 10-1. Be sure it is printed on good-quality paper and reinforces the positive impression you have sought to make. Keep in mind this is basically a thank-you letter and is not meant to provide additional information about yourself. Most important, be sure to send it. Many individuals fail to follow up with a letter, and consequently, you will stand out from the rest!

Following the guidelines and suggestions in this chapter will not guarantee employment. However, it will guarantee that you will present yourself as the true professional you have worked so hard to become.

Radiology Manager's Name
Imaging Center
Shepherd Road
My Town, VA 12345-9876

Dear Radiology Manager's Name:

Thank you for the opportunity to interview for the position of staff radiographer. I appreciate the time you spent with me yesterday. It was a pleasure meeting you and seeing your imaging department.

I look forward to hearing from you regarding this position.

Sincerely,

Applicant, R.T. (R)

FIGURE 10-1 Sample interview follow-up letter.

CHAPTER 11

Employment Expectations

Excellence can be attained if you care more than others think is wise, risk more than others think is safe, dream more than others think is practical, expect more than others think is possible.

ENTERING THE HEALTH CARE WORKFORCE

As you enter the workforce in medical radiography, the individuals in charge of the facility in which you will work will have expectations of you as a professional. From their standpoint, it is reasonable to expect you will be able to fulfill the requirements of your job description. You are being hired because you have the abilities to function as an entry-level radiographer. Ultimately, the most important expectations you must exceed are those of the patient.

The task inventory conducted by the American Registry of Radiologic Technologists (ARRT) lists the skills expected of an entry-level radiographer. Although these should coincide with the terminal competencies of your educational program, your new employer will have these expectations regardless of where you attended school. The task inventory is provided here so that you can understand the technical skills expected of you as you enter the workforce.

TASK INVENTORY*

Completion of your educational program should enable you to carry out the following tasks.

1. Confirm patient's identity.
2. Evaluate patient's ability to understand and comply with requirements for the requested examination.
3. Explain and confirm patient's preparation (e.g., diet restrictions, preparatory medications) prior to imaging examinations.
4. Examine imaging examination requisition to verify accuracy and completeness of information (e.g., patient history, clinical diagnosis).
5. Sequence imaging procedures to avoid residual contrast material affecting future exams.
6. Responsible for medical equipment attached to patients (e.g., IVs, oxygen) during the imaging procedures.
7. Provide for patient safety, comfort, and modesty.

8. Communicate scheduling delays to waiting patients.
9. Verify or obtain patient consent as necessary (e.g., contrast studies).
10. Explain procedure instructions to patient or patient's family.
11. Practice standard precautions.
12. Follow appropriate procedures when in contact with patient in isolation.
13. Select immobilization devices, when indicated, to prevent patient's movement and/or ensure patient's safety.
14. Use proper body mechanics and/or mechanical transfer devices when assisting patient.
15. Prior to administration of contrast agent, gather information to determine appropriate dosage.
16. Prior to administration of contrast agent determine if patient is at increased risk of adverse reaction (preparatory medication reconciliation).
17. Confirm type of contrast media and prepare for administration.
18. Use sterile or aseptic technique when indicated.
19. Perform venipuncture for contrast administration.
20. Administer IV contrast media.
21. Observe patient after administration of contrast media to detect adverse reactions.
22. Obtain vital signs.
23. Recognize need for prompt medical attention and administer emergency care.
24. Explain postprocedural instructions to patient or patient's family.
25. Maintain confidentiality of patient's information.
26. Clean, disinfect, or sterilize facilities and equipment, and dispose of contaminated items in preparation for next examination.
27. Document required information on patient's medical record (e.g., imaging procedure documentation, images).
    a. On paper
    b. Electronically
28. Evaluate the need for and use of protective shielding.
29. Take appropriate precautions to minimize radiation exposure to patient.
30. Question female patient of child-bearing age about possible pregnancy and take appropriate action (i.e., document response, contact physician).

---

*From American Registry of Radiologic Technologists: *Task inventory for radiography*, St Paul, Minn, 2010, ARRT.

31. Restrict beam to limit exposure area, improve image quality, and reduce radiation dose.
32. Set kVp, mA, and time or automatic exposure system to achieve optimum image quality, safe operating conditions, and minimum radiation dose.
    a. Use pulse fluoroscopy
    b. Document fluoroscopy time
33. Prevent all unnecessary persons from remaining in area during x-ray exposure.
34. Take appropriate precautions to minimize occupational radiation exposure.
35. Wear a personnel monitoring device while on duty.
36. Evaluate individual occupational exposure reports to determine if values for the reporting period are within established limits.
37. Determine appropriate exposure factors using:
    a. Fixed kVp technique chart
    b. Variable kVp technique chart
    c. Calipers (to determine patient thickness for exposure)
38. Select radiographic exposure factors.
    a. Automatic Exposure Control (AEC)
    b. kVp and mAs (manual)
    c. Pre-programmed techniques (Anatomically Programmed Radiography)
39. Operate radiographic unit and accessories.
    a. Fixed unit
    b. Mobile unit (portable)
40. Operate fluoroscopic unit and accessories.
    a. Fixed fluoroscopic unit
    b. Mobile fluoroscopic unit (C-arm)
41. Operate electronic imaging and record keeping devices.
    a. Computerized Radiography (CR)
    b. Direct Digital Radiography (DR)
    c. Picture Archival and Communication System (PACS)
    d. Hospital Information System (HIS)
    e. Radiology Information System (RIS)
42. Prepare and operate specialized units.
    a. Chest unit
    b. Tomography unit
43. Remove all radiopaque materials from patient or table that could interfere with the image.
44. Perform post-processing on digital images in preparation for interpretation (e.g., exposure indicator, brightness/contrast, window and level.
45. Use radiopaque markers to indicate anatomical side, position, or other relevant information (e.g., time, upright, decubitus, post-void).
46. Add electronic annotations on digital images to indicate position, or other relevant information (e.g., time, upright, decubitus, post-void)
47. Use film-screen cassettes and automatic film processing.
48. Select equipment and accessories (e.g., grid, compensating filter, shielding) for the examination requested.
49. Explain breathing instructions prior to making the exposure.
50. Position patient to demonstrate the desired anatomy using body landmarks.
51. Modify exposure factors for such circumstances as involuntary motion, casts and splints, pathological conditions, or patient's inability to cooperate.
52. Verify accuracy of patient identification on image.
53. Evaluate radiographs for diagnostic quality.
54. Determine corrective measures if image is not of diagnostic quality and take appropriate action.
55. Store and handle image receptor in a manner which will reduce the possibility of artifact production.
56. Visually inspect, recognize, and report malfunctions in the imaging unit and accessories.
57. Recognize the need for basic evaluations of radiographic equipment and accessories.
    a. Light field to radiation field alignment
    b. Central-ray alignment
    c. Shielding accessories (lead aprons and gloves)
58. Perform routine maintenance on digital equipment.
    a. Perform start-up or shut-down
    b. Erase CR plate
    c. Equipment cleanliness (e.g., imaging plates, CR cassettes)
    d. Recognize and report malfunctions

Position patient, x-ray tube, and image receptor to produce the following diagnostic images:
59. Chest
60. Ribs
61. Sternum
62. Soft tissue neck
63. Abdomen
64. Esophagus
65. Swallowing dysfunction study
66. Upper GI series, single or double contrast
67. Small bowel series
68. Barium enema, single or double contrast
69. Surgical cholangiography
70. Endoscopic retrograde cholangiopancreatography
71. Cystography
72. Cystourethrography
73. Intravenous urography
74. Retrograde pyelography
75. Cervical spine
76. Thoracic spine
77. Scoliosis series
78. Lumbar spine
79. Sacrum and coccyx
80. Sacroiliac joints
81. Pelvis and hip
82. Skull
83. Facial bones
84. Mandible
85. Zygomatic arch
86. Temporomandibular joints

87. Nasal bones
88. Orbits
89. Paranasal sinuses
90. Toes
91. Foot
92. Calcaneus (os calcis)
93. Ankle
94. Tibia, fibula
95. Knee
96. Patella
97. Femur
98. Fingers
99. Hand
100. Wrist
101. Forearm
102. Elbow
103. Humerus
104. Shoulder
105. Scapula
106. Clavicle
107. Acromioclavicular joints
108. Bone survey
109. Long bone measurement
110. Bone age
111. Soft tissue/foreign body
112. Arthrography
113. Myelography

ORGANIZATIONAL STRUCTURE AND YOUR PROFESSIONAL RESPONSIBILITY

The employer has a right to expect you to use your knowledge and abilities in radiography efficiently and provide high-quality service to the patient. In return, you have a right to expect the salary and benefits to which you and your employer agreed. You should also expect to perform your job in an environment that is in compliance with safety and public health requirements and free of all forms of harassment and discrimination.

You are entering a dynamic and fluid sector of the national economy. Health care advances in diagnosis, treatment, and delivery are in a constant state of flux. Funding of health care services is a matter of national debate. This is the nature of the industry in which you have chosen to work and build a career. You should expect to stay abreast of changes in the delivery of health care and remain alert to how such changes affect your employer. Remember, issues affecting your employer also affect you and your coworkers.

Your employer will expect you to function as part of a team, all of the members of which will be dedicated to the cost-effective provision of efficient, accurate, and compassionate care to the patient. At the same time, the employer is the coach of the team and has an obligation to maintain the provision of high-quality service to patients and proper accountability to payers. An examination of the expectations of your employer will reveal your professional responsibilities are accountable to the four distinct groups described in this chapter.

Two primary expectations are common to each of the four groups. The first expectation is you will provide the highest quality patient care of which you are capable in congruence with what your employer and your profession require. Such patient care is all-encompassing, from providing quality service to the patient, to supporting the patient's physical needs, to creating the most diagnostic images possible. The second expectation is you will respect and accommodate diversity in all of its forms. Such diversity may be linked to culture, language, gender, age, ethnicity, socioeconomics, and the multitude of other unique characteristics that are an integral part of each person. In health care, we serve patients as they are, not as we may wish them to be. Our practice of radiography must be blind to differences while being caring and compassionate to all.

EXPECTATIONS OF ADMINISTRATORS

The administrators of the facility in which you will be employed expect you are going to fulfill the job description associated with an entry-level radiographer. They expect you to be honest and straightforward with them while providing excellent care and service to the patient or customer. High-quality customer service is paramount to your success. It is vital that the patient knows true professionals are providing care.

Administrators trust you will speak highly of the facility and be supportive of its efforts to provide high-quality patient care. You are expected to arrive for work on time and keep absenteeism to an absolute minimum. There may be times when you are expected to work extra hours, such as when another employee is on vacation or is sick. Administrators are looking for employees who are willing to be strong, supportive team players.

Administrators also expect you will be willing to contribute new ideas for more efficient operation. They assume you will work in harmony with other departments in the facility. They may request you serve on committees or perform other tasks not directly related to radiography. Be the type of employee who exceeds the expectations of administrators, and you will be well on your way toward establishing the type of reputation that will ensure your success.

EXPECTATIONS OF PHYSICIANS

Physicians are customers, too. The physicians with whom you will be working, including radiologists and referring physicians, have their own particular set of expectations. Referring physicians expect their orders for radiologic examinations will be carried out as indicated. They expect good-quality radiographs will be made by the radiographers and interpreted properly by the radiologists. Although your interactions with these physicians may be minimal, they are nevertheless important.

Referring physicians often come to the radiology department to view radiographs themselves or consult with the radiologist. They may be unfamiliar with the department and where supplies are kept. They may be there to perform a procedure. They expect to be treated as professionals. They expect to be shown where supplies are kept and be assisted as needed. As a professional radiographer, it will be your responsibility to meet or exceed expectations and provide high-quality service to the physician as well as the patient.

The physicians with whom you will interact most frequently are the radiologists, and most of this exchange will occur during fluoroscopy. The radiologists expect to receive the highest quality radiographs you are capable of producing. They will be providing the diagnosis from your radiographs. Radiologists do not expect to have to ask you to reacquire an image you already know is unacceptable. They do not want to hear excuses for poor radiographs. Radiologists insist you keep them informed about variations from protocol. They expect you to take an adequate but concise patient history for their use during the interpretation of the images.

As a student, you may have had radiographers facilitate your interactions with the radiologists. As a new, entry-level radiographer, you now have the responsibility to be straightforward and professional during interactions with the radiologists. This includes not only providing the highest quality radiographs of which you are capable but also demonstrating a willingness to resolve personality and work-related conflicts.

It is important to determine ahead of time how you wish to be regarded by the physicians. You have a right to be treated respectfully and should take immediate steps to rectify a situation in which you are being mistreated. At the same time, the physicians have a right to expect you will reciprocate in your professional conduct.

EXPECTATIONS OF THE RADIOLOGY MANAGER

The person who is hiring you, the radiology manager, also has a particular set of expectations. This individual is directly responsible for your on-the-job performance and overall value to the patient or customer and the administration. In research I conducted, radiology managers responded to a survey regarding their expectations of new radiography graduates. Of particular interest are the traits the radiology managers considered most important in an applicant and the areas in which radiology managers have had the most difficulty with employees after they were hired.

When hiring a new graduate radiographer, 43% of radiology managers said knowledge of the technical aspects of radiography was the most important factor they considered; this is a given because the new employee must be able to perform the job. However, 33% responded customer service skills and interpersonal communication skills were the factors they most considered when hiring a recent graduate. These individuals are assuming you know how to perform the job and expect you will provide excellent service to the patient while performing it. This research shows radiology managers have high expectations of you. They expect you to know the practice of radiography, deliver quality service to patients, and be capable of establishing positive relationships with your coworkers.

A second question inquired about problems radiology managers encountered with radiographers on the job. Poor communication skills were identified by 37% as the most significant problem and usual cause for a reprimand or termination. Lack of knowledge of the technical aspects of the job was cited as the primary reason for a reprimand or termination by 36%. In handwritten comments on the survey forms, many radiology managers mentioned attendance problems, tardiness, lack of dependability, and substance abuse as problems in the workplace that led to reprimands and terminations. The need for balance between the high-touch and high-tech aspects of radiography is evident. Radiology managers have high expectations of new employees. Be prepared to exceed those expectations.

Another survey question asked the managers which areas should be most strongly emphasized with student radiographers as they prepare to enter the workforce. They stressed the following:

1. Ongoing technical training
2. Knowledge of basic nursing skills, such as using IV pumps, taking vital signs, and performing venipuncture
3. Ability to work alone without constant supervision
4. Awareness of the customer's or patient's viewpoint
5. Strong communication skills
6. Provision of high-quality service with a smile
7. Professionalism in dealing with the public
8. Loyalty to the employer
9. Maintenance of clinical skills

Because you are ready to enter the workforce, you must determine how many of these traits are present in your practice already and which ones need additional attention. The managers have carefully described what they need and expect. Are you prepared to enter their workplace?

The radiology managers were asked to rank the factors they considered to have the most positive effect on customer service in their department. The most important factor (according to 60% of the respondents) was a pleasant and courteous staff.

Similar to the administrators to whom they report, radiology managers expect you to be ready to begin work on time and to keep absenteeism to a minimum. They are counting on you to show up—on time—and provide the highest quality patient care each day you are assigned to work. Such patient care is expected to be delivered within the scope of practice determined by the profession and in full compliance with the standards of ethics and confidentiality of radiologic technology.

The radiology manager also expects you to conduct yourself as a professional in your dealings with the patient or customer, the physicians, and your coworkers. You are expected to be a reliable member of the radiology team. You must be flexible and have a positive attitude about handling all the different assignments you may be given in a typical workday.

Other areas of concern raised by the radiology managers included bringing personal problems to work, substance abuse by employees, and overall lack of initiative. These are problems you should keep out of your radiography practice. Should any of these issues become matters of personal concern for you, seek counseling immediately so that you can bring such problems under control. Your employer and your patients deserve no less.

Your radiology manager will expect you to remain busy throughout the day. In addition to performing your primary job duties, you may be asked to complete assignments that do not involve patient care. Quality control testing or the routine cleaning of imaging equipment or lead aprons may be a part of your job responsibility. If you think of your work area as an integral part of your practice, that sense of ownership will motivate you to care for it. Slow periods at work may be few and far between; you should take advantage of them whenever they occur. Your attitude toward the aspects of your work that do not involve patient care may determine whether the radiology manager gives you other assignments you may be seeking. If you consider lounge areas off limits and keep busy throughout the day, you will find great fulfillment in your work and will likely exceed the radiology manager's expectations.

In a field that changes as rapidly as medical imaging, your radiology manager will expect you to be knowledgeable about the newest types of equipment and advances in imaging techniques. You are also expected to keep your skills at a level that allows you to perform all of the different types of radiographic procedures required in your radiology department. On a regular basis, you should review your favorite text on radiographic positioning and procedures to refresh your memory and maintain your skills.

You have become accustomed to studying, and throughout the course of your radiography program, you have had to learn how to learn. This process does not end with graduation or passing the certification exam. It is important to keep abreast of events in the field by reading the latest radiologic technology journals and textbooks. Textbooks are not written solely for students. As a practicing radiographer, you will want to keep your personal library updated with the best resources available.

Another way to be aware of current developments in the field and exceed your manager's expectations is to become an active member of your national and state professional organizations. Both have publications that will bring you the latest news in the profession. In addition, these organizations need your talents to be successful. As a student, you have acquired a store of information and have developed skill in communicating this knowledge. Take advantage of that momentum, and continue to do research in the field.

Most radiology managers will expect you to give something back to your profession, which will increase your level of knowledge. Present research papers at state or national meetings, hold an office in one of the organizations, or offer to help out in planning and conducting a continuing education meeting. Organizing and conducting an in-service education program for your department is a great place to begin. If you have never taken part in such activities, this is a perfect time to begin. It does not matter whether you are sure about what you are doing; just offer to help or do that first research paper as a graduate.

Meeting and exceeding the radiology manager's expectations are sure ways to set a course for success in your chosen field. Individuals who follow this path derive the most satisfaction from their job and are held in the highest esteem by their employers. Most important, a commitment to excellence in your profession results in healthy self-esteem, which is reflected in the care and service provided to the patients.

EXPECTATIONS OF STUDENTS UNDER YOUR SUPERVISION

Your new employer may have students present as part of an educational program in radiologic technology. The employer may be the sponsor of the program or may serve as a clinical site for a program sponsored by another institution.

It may seem ironic that although you are probably reading this as a student still in school, it is already time to consider the aspect of future expectations for students. Should you choose to work in an imaging department that serves as a clinical site, you will be working with students shortly after graduation. This is an awesome responsibility, especially because you will still be in learning mode yourself, mastering the requirements of a staff radiographer in your new position.

Working with students is a task to be taken seriously. As you already know from your experiences, the students will expect you to share with them your knowledge of the art and science of imaging and patient care. They will want fair and honest evaluations of their performance. They will want to be treated with the respect due an adult in college, not as another worker, an inexpensive laborer, or someone to perform menial tasks. The students under your supervision will rely on you to help them through the learning process.

Whether or not it is part of the orientation to your new job, seek out the clinical instructor for students in your department. Find out what is expected of you from the educational program. Become thoroughly familiar with the evaluation forms and competency testing forms and system you may be expected to use. As a new graduate yourself, determine whether there is a limit to what role you can play. Learn the specific requirements of direct and indirect supervision of students performing examinations and repeat radiographs. Consider carefully the legal ramifications of following such supervisory requirements.

As you work with students, remember you are shaping the next generation of radiographers. These individuals will be your coworkers after their graduation. This is a key role to play as you become acclimated to the role of radiographer as well. You have the ability to be a strong influence on future professionals in your field. Take the responsibility seriously, and take pride in the impact you will have on these radiographers who will follow you into the field.

EXPECTATIONS OF YOUR NEW COWORKERS

At the same time you are becoming oriented to a new job, possibly working with students, taking and passing the credentialing exam, and learning your new employer's expectations, there will be another very important set of expectations to consider. This area includes your employer's expectations of your relationship with your new coworkers.

As a new graduate, you will, in some respects, be like a new student all over again. Learning the technical aspects of a new job, even in your chosen field, will take much time and energy. At the same time, becoming part of a work group such as a department of radiology, urgent care center, cardiac catheterization laboratory, or physician's office will probably take more energy than you might expect. Establishing your professional relationships will make a world of difference in the satisfaction you receive from your work and your ability to provide the level of care you expect of yourself.

Approach your new position as a learner, eager to find out all you can regarding routines, protocols, professional relationships within the work setting, and how the group functions together. Determine everyone's level of responsibility and where you fit in. Your new employer expects you will establish professional working relationships and conduct yourself with everyone as a member of a tight work unit. You will be expected to avoid gossip, cliques, and any other behavior that inhibits the delivery of high-quality patient care and service. Your employer will expect you are ready to learn all you can from your coworkers regarding the technical aspects of imaging and

operation of the imaging department or clinic. You and your coworkers will need to work out personal problems as professionals and not allow them to enter the flow of the workplace.

Your coworkers will expect you to come up to speed quickly and to ask questions when necessary. They will expect you conduct yourself as a new graduate, still in learning mode but ready to assume a high level of responsibility and take on your share of patient care. They will expect you to establish a positive, uplifting relationship with them. They can assist you as you enter the field as a professional. Use their experience and knowledge to your benefit as you deliver patient care. Respond to their help by working with them cooperatively, as a new colleague and as a professional who is eager to assume a key role in their work unit. Exceed your new employer's expectations by working cooperatively and learning all you can from your new coworkers.

There will be expectations from everyone associated with your new position as a graduate radiographer. Meeting and exceeding those expectations while learning your new position will create the need to balance all aspects of your radiography practice. In doing so, you will then exceed the expectations of your program's instructors, who first guided you on your road to success.

KEY POINTS
Employment Expectations

- Skills expected of an entry-level radiographer are outlined in the ARRT Task Inventory.
- Advances in diagnosis and treatment are in a constant state of change.
- Be honest and straightforward while providing excellent care and service to the patient.
- Speak highly of the facility and be supportive of its efforts to provide high-quality patient care.
- Arrive for work on time; keep absenteeism to a minimum.
- Be a strong, supportive team player.
- Work in harmony with other departments in the facility.
- Carry out referring physicians' orders for radiologic examinations as written.
- Interact professionally with physicians visiting the imaging department.
- Work with radiologists as fellow team members, providing them the finest diagnostic images possible.
- Make knowledge of technical aspects of radiography, customer service, and communication skills the foundation of your practice.
- Maintain knowledge and skills as imaging procedures change.
- Share knowledge and provide direction to students assigned to you.
- Come up to speed quickly and ask questions of coworkers to assimilate into the department.

Students: Welcome to my classroom!

Below are the answers to the review questions in the book. I have provided rationales where appropriate. The explanations are written for you in the same way I go over exams in my own classes. In most cases, I provide key points regarding the answer, study suggestions, or both. For other questions, such as labeled drawings or radiographs, the answers may be obvious and don't require a detailed explanation.

You will also encounter facts asked in multiple ways, challenging you to think about information from several different directions. This will help prepare you for whatever way the questions may be asked on the certification exam and will also reinforce the material by causing you to interact with it more than once. In any case, be sure to return to the chapter and use the study outline for detailed review and to reinforce concepts, facts, and illustrations that need extra attention.

Now let's see if you really know the material...

CHAPTER 2

1. B. Of this 82%, most comes from radon gas.
2. D. Radon gas is part of humans' natural background exposure, which totals 50% of humans' total exposure.
3. D. Earth's atmosphere and magnetic fields help shield us from cosmic radiation, a source of approximately 30 mrem annually.
4. A. Radon gas may be present in homes, particularly basements. Special kits should be used to determine its presence.
5. C. Artificial, or human-made, radiation represents 48% of the total human exposure.
6. C. The OSL dosimeter is extremely sensitive. The thermoluminescent dosimeter is accurate as low as 5 mrem, whereas the film badge is sensitive to 10 mrem.
7. B. Diagnostic procedures account for approximately 3 mSv per year.
8. B. Microwave ovens do not emit ionizing radiation.
9. D. Pair production does not occur at diagnostic levels.
10. C. This form of scatter has no effect on the image below 70 kVp and does not cause ionization. It is negligible above 70 kVp.
11. D. Pair production occurs above 1.02 million electron volts.
12. A. Photoelectric interaction results in absorption of the incident, or incoming, x-ray photon. The difference between this interaction and the rays that pass through the body unaltered to strike the image receptor is what provides contrast. Compton scatter, with its resultant fog, certainly affects contrast, but it does not produce contrast itself.

13. B. Compton scatter that is not absorbed by a grid may strike the image receptor and reduce contrast.
14. C. This is also known as classical or Thompson's scattering. It has no effect on the image below 70 kVp. It is negligible above 70 kVp.
15. A. This complete deposition of energy results in contrast being produced on the image.
16. C. No electrons are removed from the atoms being struck.
17. D. Pair production occurs at megavoltage levels.
18. A. Photoelectric effect occurs as incident photons deposit their energy in the K-shell.
19. B. Compton interaction primarily involves outer shell electrons, wherein both the electron and the photon scatter, causing the atom to become ionized.
20. A. The inner-shell electron is ejected, becoming a photoelectron. The atom becomes ionized.
21. B. Because Compton interaction causes the production of scatter, a grid is needed to attempt to absorb the scatter before it reaches the image receptor.
22. B. Compton produces scatter, which during fluoroscopy or mobile procedures may expose the radiographer. Hence a lead apron is required when either one is performed.
23. B. *Rad* stands for *radiation absorbed dose*. In a case such as this, the key word "deposited" in the stem of the question will lead you to the correct answer.
24. C. Rem is the unit of equi-valent dose, which takes into account biologic effects caused by different forms of radiation. The equation is Rem=Rad ´ WR (radiation weighting factor).
25. A. Roentgen is the unit of in-air exposure.
26. A. Actually, choice B is a good choice as well, but A is more complete. Remember, *LET* stands for *linear energy transfer*. Choice C is incorrect because particulate radiations deposit more energy than wave radiations. Choice D is incorrect because a radiation weighting factor is used in the calculation of equivalent dose, not absorbed dose. Keep in mind that the certification exam will require you to choose the one best answer.
27. C. NCRP reports are the standards on which radiation protection practices are based.
28. A. The NRC has the authority to enforce radiation protection standards relating to radioactive material.
29. D. Choice A is not as complete. Choices B and C are incorrect because they imply that there is no risk of damage to the individual.
30. D. *ALARA* stands for *as low as reasonably achievable*.
31. D. The effects mentioned in choices A and B are graphically demonstrated on dose-response curves. H & D curves demonstrate the relationship between exposure and density on a sheet of film.

32. B. It is assumed that for every dose of radiation there is some response in the organism. This does not mean there is damage, just a response.

33. A. Be sure to refer to the illustrations in Chapter 2.

34. B. This forms the basis for all radiation protection standards. Be sure to review the dose-response curves in Chapter 2 and be able to recognize them both from a diagram and from a written description.

35. C. The presence of a threshold means that exposures below that level will not cause a response resulting in certain conditions. For example, certain doses will not cause cataracts. Those doses are below the threshold dose.

36. D. Be sure to review the dose-response curves in Chapter 2 and be able to recognize them both from a diagram and from a written description.

37. B. Increased dose equals increased probability of effects, although it does not increase severity of effects.

38. B. Deterministic effects have threshold doses below which the effects do not occur.

39. D. The total equivalent dose limit for gestation is 0.5 rem.

40. D. For example, a 29-year-old radiographer could have a cumulative exposure of 29 rem.

41. A. This is the dose to remember when you are asked about radiographers' annual exposure limit.

42. B. Students age 18 years and older are measured using the annual limit of 5 rem or 5000 mrem.

43. C. This is 500 mrem, one-tenth the occupational limit.

44. C. This the same as the annual general public dose for infrequent exposure.

45. B. This is 100 mrem. The dose for the general public for infrequent exposure is 500 mrem.

46. A. Be sure to master all of the effective dose limits for occupational exposure and exposure of the general public.

47. C. The radiation weighting factor takes into account the source of exposure, which may be wave or particulate, and the actual amount of energy deposited per unit length of tissue—the LET (linear energy transfer).

48. A. The amount of energy deposited in tissues is directly responsible for any biologic damage that may occur.

49. C. Relative biologic effectiveness.

50. D. Remember that the cellular life cycle always begins with interphase. The reason D is the correct answer is because the three steps in interphase are listed in their proper order. This makes choice D a better answer than choice B.

51. D. Choice A defines cell division for somatic cells only.

52. C. The DNA in the cell's nucleus has been directly struck by the photons.

53. B. The master molecule is the DNA in the cell's nucleus.

54. C. The doubling dose in humans ranges from 50 to 250 rads.

55. A. The energy is deposited in the cytoplasm, causing radiolysis to occur, which poisons the cell. This indirectly causes the damage to the cell's nucleus.

56. A. Radiolysis causes the production of hydrogen peroxide in the cytoplasm, a poison to the cell.

57. D. Most radiation-induced mutations are recessive.

58. A. Free radicals are produced as a result of radiolysis.

59. C. The master molecule is DNA, located in the cellular nucleus.

60. A. This is a result of radiolysis.

61. D. Because the cellular cytoplasm is so much larger than a cell's nucleus, it is more likely to be struck by an incoming x-ray photon. Therefore, statistically speaking, more damage will occur to cells because of indirect effect than from the less probable occurrence of direct effect.

62. B. The Law of Bergonié and Tribondeau states that cells are most radiosensitive when they are immature, undifferentiated, and rapidly dividing.

63. B. This law describes cell radiosensitivity.

64. A. This is known as oxygen enhancement ratio (OER).

65. A. Although the numerical portion of this answer, 25, is correct for both A and B, the unit of measurement must also be correct.

66. A. The least radiosensitive cells are nerve and muscle cells.

67. C. Epithelial cells are very radiosensitive.

68. B. Ova are more radiosensitive in young girls and after middle age.

69. B. It is important to remember that most somatic effects of exposure to ionizing radiation do not occur at doses used during diagnostic procedures, unless repeated procedures are performed at high dose levels. It is always important to practice ALARA.

70. A. Genetic effects may occur in the next generation as mutations.

71. A. Alzheimer's disease and Parkinson's disease have not been linked to radiation exposure.

72. C.

73. A. Gonadal shields may reduce exposure to males by up to 95%.

74. B. Use of low-mAs, high-kVp techniques always results in a lower patient dose. In this case it is coupled with a 400-speed system. Choice A would result in a higher dose because it is a high-mAs, low-kVp technique. Choices C and D have slower speed systems. Focal-spot size is not related to patient dose.

75. C. The other choices all result in increased dose to the patient.

76. C. These are the three basic methods for providing optimal radiation protection.

77. C. TLDs and film badges are used for personnel measurement, whereas a Geiger-Mueller detector is used to detect the location of a specific source of radiation such as a radio-nuclide.

78. B. The TLD is accurate down to 5 mrem. The hand-held ionization chamber and Geiger-Mueller Detector do not read in mrem.

79. B. Metal and plastic filters are incorporated into the film badge case.

80. C. This is the monitor of choice to be used when surveying radiation dose in a fluoroscopic installation. The TLD and film badge are used for personal monitoring, and the Geiger-Mueller detector surveys for radioactive particles.

81. D.

82. A. The film badge is accurate as low as 10 mrem.

83. D. The TLD and film badge are not digital and are used to measure personal dose.

84. A. The optically stimulated luminescent dosimeter may also be used up to 3 months.

85. B. The film badge is sensitive to extremes in temperature and humidity. It is being phased out of use.

86. C. *MMD* stands for *mean marrow dose*.

87. A. *GSD* stands for *genetically significant dose*.

88. D. Choice A is incorrect because the timer must sound an alarm after 300 seconds (5 minutes). Choice B is incorrect because the purpose of the alarm is to sound an alert. Choice C is incorrect because the alarm sounds after 5 minutes.

89. D. This is one of the three cardinal principles of radiation protection; the others are time and shielding.

90. B. This problem is different from many you have been asked: you are being given the new dose and asked to figure out what the new distance should be. You should not need to use an equation on paper or a calculator to solve this problem. The question wants you to reduce your dose to ¹/4 the amount you receive at a distance of 2 feet. Keeping in mind the inverse square law, you may recall that doubling distance causes the dose to drop to ¹/4. Therefore the correct answer would be to step back to a distance of 4 feet from the table. Choice A implies that you need to qu-ad-ru-ple your distance from the table to reduce the dose to ¹/4. Choice D would result in a decrease in dose because of shielding but not the specific reduction in dose mentioned in the problem.

91. D. This thickness is the minimum that *must* be worn; 0.5-mm lead equivalent *should* be worn. This is tricky and is used here to make the point that careful reading of the question is very important.

92. C. Choice A is incorrect because holding patients should never be routine. Choice B is incorrect because a radio-grapher should be the last choice to hold the patient. Choice D is incorrect because routinely using student radiographers is unacceptable in practice.

93. A.

94. B. Hence this is the best place to stand whenever possible, when necessary.

95. A. Film badges are sensitive to a reading as low as 10 mrem.

96. A. Handheld ionization chambers are digital, so the dose indicated is accurate. Choice C is incorrect because it indicates millirads.

97. C. The OSL dosimeter is sensitive as low as 1 mrem. The TLD is sensitive as low as 5 mrem, and the film badge is sensitive as low as 10 mrem.

98. B.

99. D. It is also known by its abbreviation of PBL.

100. D. Choices A, B, and C are all reasons filtration is used; however, filtration should never be adjusted by the radiographer. A qualified radiation physicist should be the only person adjusting x-ray beam filtration.

CHAPTER 3

1. B. Most views required by the radiologist are acquired digitally during fluoroscopy.

2. B. The atom may be broken down into subatomic particles but they would not have the characteristics of the element.

3. C. The information acquired by scanning the imaging plate must be converted from its analog form to digital for further manipulation. This is an extra step when compared with direct digital radiography (DR).

4. D. Photons may also be called *quanta*.

5. A. Atomic number is the number of protons. Protons and neutrons are contained in the atomic nucleus.

6. C. The AEC is calibrated to provide the images most preferred by the radiologists.

7. D. Hence, the exposure time when using an AEC is very dependent upon the kVp.

8. D. The falling load generator makes use of the maximum heat storage capacity at every mA and time combination. This allows for the shortest exposure time possible.

9. A. This necessitates the using of a rectifier to change AC to DC.

10. B. The octet rule states that no more than eight electrons can be in the outer shell. It does not stipulate that there must be eight electrons in the outer shell.

11. B. Particulate radiations are highly ionizing.

12. A. Because it has mass, particulate radiation may travel along different paths.

13. D. X-rays exit the x-ray tube in bursts of energy called *photons*.

14. C. Don't be fooled by choices that use different units of measurement. Light speed is expressed in miles per second, not miles per hour.

15. A. Wavelength and frequency are inverse to one another.

16. D. Wavelength can be measured from crest to crest or trough to trough.

17. B. Higher-frequency waves have shorter wavelengths, lower-frequency waves have longer wavelengths.

18. D. The speed of x-ray travel is constant, regardless of the factors used to produce them.

19. B. Higher-frequency waves have shorter wavelengths, lower-frequency waves have longer wavelengths.

20. B. Attenuation means that the x-rays may be absorbed or scattered.

21. C. Be certain to review the inverse square law; always remember the inverse square relationship. For example, if the dose of radiation is 10 R at a distance of 3 feet, the dose at a distance of 6 feet is only 2.5 R. It is one fourth, not half, which is a common mistake.

22. C. Energy cannot be created or destroyed, only changed in form. The energy is merely transferred.

23. B. Choice 2 cannot be the answer because the movement of electrons from one object to another is called *electrification*. Choice 3 cannot be the answer because like charges repel and unlike charges attract. Choice 5 cannot be the answer because friction, contact, and induction are methods of electrification. You may encounter some questions in this format. Simply make each possible choice a true-false statement, then choose the one answer that includes the true choices. These are not difficult questions, just challenging.

24. A. Keep in mind that the question asks for which statements are false. Choice 4 is false because the ampere is the unit of electric current. Choice 6 is false because the volt is the unit of electromotive force, and choice 9 is false because Ohm's law is calculated by use of the equation $V = IR$. This question is a bit long, and you probably won't encounter one this complex. However, it is one more practice with a question of this type. Again, just treat it like a long true-false question.

25. D. Electromagnetic induction does not require that two conductors touch each other.

26. B. Self-induction occurs in the autotransformer; mutual induction occurs in the step-up and step-down transformers.

27. B. Mutual induction occurs in the step-up and step-down transformers.

28. B. This intensifies the magnetic fields, making the transformers more efficient.

29. C. A generator at the power company converts mechanical energy to electrical energy. A motor converts electrical energy to mechanical energy.

30. C. 60 Hertz means 60 cycles per second. The voltage may be 110 or 220.

31. A. 60 cycles per second results in 120 pulses per second, because it cycles back and forth 120 times per second.

32. B. Such a low ripple means higher average photon energy. High frequency is very efficient.

33. C. Three-phase power produces higher average photon energy than single-phase power.

34. B. The autotransformer is a variable transformer that operates on the principle of self-induction.

35. A. Voltage is stepped up while current is stepped down in the same proportion. A transformer is named for what it does to voltage.

36. C. The voltage is varied at the autotransformer, then boosted to kilovoltage levels by the step-up transformer.

37. D. Older x-ray machines require that the line voltage compensator be adjusted manually, whereas newer equipment lets the machine do the adjustment itself.

38. A. A transformer is named for what it does to voltage.

39. C. Thermionic emission is the boiling off of electrons from the filament wire.

40. D. The kVp meter indicates what the voltage will be after being stepped up. Hence it is prereading.

41. A. The step-down transformer is located in the filament circuit.

42. D. The timer is accurate as low as $^1/1000$ of a second (which is 1 ms or 0.001 second).

43. B. The rectifier changes incoming alternating current from the power company into direct current for use by the x-ray tube.

44. C. The filament and focusing cup are part of the cathode assembly. The focusing cup has a negative charge at the moment of exposure so as to repel the electrons from the cathode.

45. B. The rectifier changes AC to DC.

46. D. Most equipment uses an electronic timer.

47. B. At this point, AC is changed to DC so that current is flowing in only one direction through the x-ray tube.

48. B. Current is the flow of electrons, as measured in milliamperes (mA). Hence the mA meter provides the reading.

49. A. High-speed anodes spin from 10,000 to 12,000 rotations per minute (rpm).

50. D. This type of generator allows extremely short exposure times.

51. A. These are the x-rays produced by two types of interactions that occur between incident electrons from the cathode and the tungsten atoms of the anode.

52. D. This is where voltage is boosted to kilovoltage levels.

53. C. The ionization chamber is located between the patient and the image receptor. Phototimers are seldom used.

54. D. Coupled with an electronic timer, this results in times as short as $^1/1000$ second.

55. A. Pressing the rotor button activates a motor that turns the anode. It also begins thermionic emission at the cathode.

56. C. The ionization chamber is a wafer-thin chamber containing gas that is ionized by the x-rays passing through it. At a predetermined level of ionization, current flows that terminates the exposure.

57. A. The machine keeps the filament warm between exposures.

58. B. Each time the rotor is ac-tivated, thermionic emission begins to occur at the filament. This heating of the filament causes tungsten to evaporate, thus slowly deteriorating the filament.

59. B. Choice C is incorrect, although many first-year students experience this activity when technologists try to hurry them from the room! Choices A and D are incorrect because unnecessarily heating the filament actually reduces x-ray tube life.

60. D. This causes a space charge or electron cloud to form around the filament.

61. A. This is the flow of electrons, as a result of AC being changed to DC in the rectifier.

62. B. This is primarily a result of bremsstrahlung interactions at the anode.

63. C. X-rays and heat are produced at the anode. This is the result of a massive energy conversion in which more than 99% of the incident electrons' kinetic energy is converted to heat energy, while less than 1% is converted to x-ray energy. This is a clear example of the law of conservation of energy. No light is produced in the x-ray tube.

64. C. As incident electrons fly past the atomic nuclei, they are slowed, causing the production of heat and x-rays by bremsstrahlung. X-rays are also produced by the characteristic interaction.

65. A. As incident electrons dislodge K-shell electrons in the target material, outer-shell electrons fall inward to fill the holes. This causes the release of energy in the form of x-rays, with energy characteristic of the difference in energy levels between the K-shell and L-shell.

66. C. More than 99% of the energy is converted to heat.

67. B. Choice 1 is incorrect because x-rays do not carry electrical charges. Choice 5 is incorrect because the speed of light is 186,000 miles per second. Choice 6 is incorrect because the wavelengths of x-rays are between 0.1 and 0.5 angstroms. Choice 9 is incorrect because x-rays cannot be focused by any means. Collimation merely restricts the area being irradiated. Again, you are not likely to encounter such a long question on the exam, but this question provides a good review of the properties of x-rays. Don't be intimidated by slight changes in question format. Always read the question carefully, determine what is being asked, and read each choice carefully to determine the correct answer. When you have mastered that, you can answer any qu-estion that pops up on the screen.

68. D. Choice A is correct in stating that the x-ray beam is heterogeneous, but the second half of choice A is incorrect.

69. C. We don't often discuss the x-ray beam in this detail, but be sure to review *discrete* and *continuous* in Chapter 3.

70. A. Choice B is incorrect because soft rays have long wavelengths. Choice C is true, but it is not the primary purpose of filtration. Choice D is incorrect because long-wavelength rays are called *soft rays*.

71. B. We more commonly discuss beam quality using the term *half-value layer*. Regardless of the fraction, it is always the amount of material needed to reduce beam intensity to that level.

72. D. These are detailed statements attempting to define the amount of filtration required. D is the most complete and accurate of all the choices. A is incorrect as to amount, B is incorrect because we cannot remove all soft rays from the beam, and C is incorrect because compensating filtration is added only for certain examinations.

73. D. Fill-in questions may be used on the certification exam, although they probably won't have three blanks like this one. Although we don't often deal with heat units, be sure to review the constants used in heat unit production.

74. D. kVp must be within plus or minus 4 of what is set.

75. D.

76. A. This is where the electronic image again becomes visible.

77. B. The electrons are then concentrated and accelerated toward the output phosphor.

78. C. This is the point where the rays exiting the patient strike the input phosphor and it glows with visible light, releasing electrons from the photocathode.

79. A. This is the equation used to calculate total brightness gain.

80. D. Although A, B, and C are all good answers, remember that we need to choose the one best answer, which is D. You are not likely to encounter this type of wording, but this question is a good exercise to remind you to look for the one best answer.

81. A. 13% ripple direct current, not alternating current. Three-phase, 12-pulse produces ripple as low as 4%. Single-phase ripple is 100%.

82. B. Three-phase, six-pulse produces ripple as low as 13%. Single-phase ripple is 100%.

83. D. This is why the formula for heat units for three-phase, six-pulse equipment is multiplied by 1.35.

84. B. This is why the formula for calculating heat units for three-phase, 12-pulse equipment is multiplied by 1.41.

85. C. This question asks for two answers; be sure you know what is meant by each term.

86. D. Just a quick question to see if you understand dedicated equipment. "All of the above" and "None of the above" type questions are not used on the certification exam.

87. C. Be sure to review these quality control standards before you take the certification exam.

88. A. Be sure to review these quality control standards before you take the certification exam.

89. D. Be sure to review these quality control standards before you take the certification exam.

90. B. Be sure to review these quality control standards before you take the certification exam.

91. C. An exposure of 1 second would demonstrate 120 dots, because single-phase, full-rectified units pulse every $^1/120$ second. An exposure of $^1/30$ second should demonstrate 4 dots (120 times $^1/30$) if it is working properly.

92. C. Keep in mind that because the current never falls to zero when three-phase equipment is used, a spinning top test will not show dots but will show arcs. A 1-second exposure would be expected to produce a full circle, which would be an arc of 360 degrees. A timer setting of $^1/60$ second would be expected to produce a $^1/60$-degree arc, which is a 6-degree arc (360 times $^1/60$). Choices A and B would be incorrect because they indicate dots. Choice D is incorrect.

93. D. Be sure to review these quality control standards before you take the certification exam.

94. A. Be sure to review these quality control standards before you take the certification exam.

95. D. Be sure to review these quality control standards before you take the certification exam. Though 'all of the above' is not used on the ARRT exam review questions like this can assess if you really know the various equipment used.

96. C. Be sure to review these quality control standards before you take the certification exam.

97. A. This provides for actually radiographing an object.

98. B. Note that this question is asking the amount of mA actually used and not the setting of the mA on the control panel.

99. C. Choices A, B, and D are also marks on the focal track, but they are caused by malfunctions.

100. A. Representatives of The Joint Commission (TJC) regularly visit health care facilities to examine documentation of compliance with quality control and quality assurance standards.

CHAPTER 4

1. A.

2. A.

3. B. mAs controls the electrons flowing through the x-ray tube and striking the anode. Therefore it directly controls the number of x-rays produced. In digital imaging, brightness may be manipulated using window level.

4. A. Whatever is changed in mAs directly impacts density.

5. C. mAs controls the electrons flowing through the x-ray tube and striking the anode. Therefore it directly controls the number of x-rays produced.

6. C. Sometimes written as mAs=mAs.

7. B. Photostimulable phosphor.

8. D. mAs is a quantitative factor.

9. D.

10. D. kVp controls the wavelength and penetrating ability of the beam. In digital imaging window width can be used to manipulate contrast.

11. B. It is governed by the 15% rule.

12. A.

13. A. Think about each answer individually before answer this question.

14. B. The use of the 15% rule to increase kVp results in double the density.

15. C.

16. D. This is another way of asking about the inverse square law.

17. A. This is the density maintenance formula. Note the question asks what needs to be done to maintain density, not what happens to density if nothing is changed.

18. A. These factors all impact the geometry of the image.

19. B. The monitor must be high resolution, but can be plasma, LCD, LED, etc.

20. A.

21. B. This necessitates the use of grid conversion factors.

22. D. Overall the beam is harder so contrast may be lower.

23. C.

24. B. Due to a change in SID resulting from the tube angle.

25. C. The intensity of the x-ray beam is actually a little higher toward the cathode side of the tube.

26. B. Anode heel effect.

27. D. Without contrast, produced by differential absorption of the x-ray beam, detail cannot be visible.

28. A.

29. D. This is the space from center to center of adjacent pixels.

30. B. The shorter wavelength beam more uniformly penetrates the various anatomic structures.

31. A. This is the opposite of question 30.

32. B.

33. D. Photoelectric interaction results in absorption of incoming photons. It is also very influenced by the atomic number, not atomic mass, of anatomical structures.

34. D. Compton interactions produce scatter, which causes contrast to decrease.

35. D. Rays that have been removed from the beam must be restored by increasing mAs. The area being irradiated still remains smaller.

36. B. Many of the scatter photons are being absorbed by the grid resulting in higher contrast.

37. C. The overall wavelength of the beam is shorter, resulting in lower contrast.

38. D.

39. D. Controlled by SID, OID, and focal spot size.

40. B. This is a rather involved question that you're not likely to see on the Registry exam, but it is a good review of factors related to recorded detail. Remember, this is also a study guide, not just practice tests. Be sure to review these factors in Chapter 4 if any of the answers don't seem right to you.

41. B. Pixel pitch is very important to detail in digital imaging.

42. C.

43. A. Choices b, c, and d are all examples of distortion.

44. B.

45. B. The optimum conditions are longer SID and shorter OID.

46. D. This results in the part appearing shorter than it really is.

47. A. This results in the part appearing longer than it really is.

48. B. Digital imaging takes into account the total dose to the patient.

49. C.

50. B. But erasing daily is better and preferred.

51. A.

52. A. However, smoothing may negatively impact resolution.

53. A. Detection of collimated edges is crucial to obtaining an accurate histogram.

54. D. This is in congruence with ALARA.

55. A.

56. D.

57. C. Technologists' monitors are not usually high definition (HD).

58. D. Total exposure reaching the IR.

59. D.

60. B. This enhances visibility of detail.

61. A. This may allow for higher kVp and lower mAs, which causes an increase in quantum mottle or noise.

62. C. More total exposure is required to produce a useable image.

63. C.

64. A. The more the image is processed the greater the opportunity for image degradation.

65. B. There is a greater difference between the signal and any noise that may be present.

66. A.

67. D.

68. C. Expressed as H/D. Did you notice how choice B tried to get your attention? Be sure to read the entire answer.

69. D.

70. A. Keep in mind that grids are used over part thickness of 10 cm; the grid conversion factors are used to change mAs, not kVp; and grids don't prevent the production of scatter, they just try to absorb it after it's been produced.

71. B. These grids can be used only within a certain range of SIDs, as stated on the label on the grid.

72. D. Using a focused grid outside of its grid radius will result in grid cutoff.

73. C. But crosshatch grids prevent angling of the tube and are extremely susceptible to grid cutoff.

74. B. Choice A is incorrect because decreased density in the middle would not be caused by use of an inverted parallel grid. Choice C is incorrect because density would decrease in the middle of this radiograph. Choice D is incorrect because density could decrease across the entire radiograph, depending on how the grid has been positioned.

75. A. The grid conversion factor or Bucky factor for a 12:1 grid is 5 times the original mAs.

76. D. Even though not used much anymore, it is particularly effective on lateral cervical spine radiographs.

77. D. Technique charts are generally not needed for exams when AECs are used.

78. D. Automatic exposure controls are set to terminate the exposure after a certain amount of radiation has passed through the ionization chamber. Consequently, changes in kVp will have no effect on density. Some effect on contrast may occur if the change in kVp is substantial.

The following answers relate to terminology used in digital imaging. Be certain to review these basic concepts. Keep in mind the ARRT exam will not ask questions related to specific brands of equipment made by various manufacturers. Therefore the concepts tested will be broad in nature, similar to these questions.

79. B.

80. C.

81. B

82. D

83. B

84. B.

85. B. DEL.

86. C.

87. B.

88. D.

89. B.

90. B.

91. A. Modulation transfer function.

92. D.

93. D.

94. B. Picture element.

95. A.

96. C.

97. B.

98. A.

99. B.

100. A.

CHAPTER 5

1. D. Be sure you can identify each body habitus by word description and by diagram. Review them in Chapter 5.

2. A. Be sure you can identify each body habitus by word description and by diagram. Review them in Chapter 5.

3. D. Be sure you can identify each body habitus by word description and by diagram. Review them in Chapter 5.

4. C. Be sure you can identify each body habitus by word description and by diagram. Review them in Chapter 5.

5. B. Be sure you can identify each body habitus by word description and by diagram. Review them in Chapter 5.

6. A. Be sure you can identify each body habitus by word description and by diagram. Review them in Chapter 5.

7. D. Be sure you can identify each body habitus by word description and by diagram. Review them in Chapter 5.

8. A. Be sure you can identify each body habitus by word description and by diagram. Review them in Chapter 5.

9. B. Reread each of the other choices carefully, and you will see that this is the one best answer. Other choices have certain valid points, but only this one covers the most important aspects of pediatric radiography.

10. C. Although choices A and B are certainly valid, choice C takes precedence over all the others. Choice D is incorrect because the radiographer may take additional projections as needed.

11. D. Choice A is incorrect because it does not mention that a physician has approved such removal. Choice B is incorrect because it is not necessary for a radiologist to provide the order. Choice C is incorrect because the patient's attending physician may direct that the collar be removed.

12. A. This plane divides the body into superior and inferior portions.

13. C. This plane divides the body into equal right and left portions.

14. A. A transverse plane passes crosswise through the body at right angles to its longitudinal axis.

15. B. This plane divides the body into anterior and posterior portions.

16. D. This plane would still divide the body into right and left portions, but they would be unequal.

17. A. A ball-and-socket joint has a rounded head of one base moving in a cuplike cavity; it is capable of movement in an in-finite number of axes.

18. A. The primary example is the hip. Do you see how questions can be worded differently to ask for basically the same information? Reread questions 17 and 18. Be sure to really know what you are studying, so you can choose the correct answer no matter how the question is worded.

19. C. An example of a hinge joint is the elbow. Do you see why patients with elbow injuries are in so much pain? Any movement whatsoever causes great discomfort.

20. D. Motions can be flexion, extension, adduction, and abduction; an example is the carpometacarpal joint of the thumb.

21. B. An example of this type of joint is the proximal radioulnar articulation.

22. B. Pregnancy would be a contraindication to performing hysterosalpingography.

23. B. AP and lateral projections are not required. AP and AP with internal rotation films may suffice. Choice 3 is incorrect because deep veins can be imaged.

24. A. All of the answers are valid. Be sure to know at least the basic points regarding arthrography, even though it is gradually being replaced by MRI.

25. D. Choice 1 is incorrect when cervical myelography is performed. Choice 2 is incorrect because contrast agents used in myelography are water soluble. Choice 4 is incorrect because gravity is used to distribute the contrast medium. Choice 5 is incorrect when lumbar myelography is performed. Be sure to know at least the basic points regarding myelography, even though it is gradually being replaced by MRI.

26. C. Be familiar with tomography primarily because of its use in excretory urography.

27. B. Notice how similar are choices A and B? Read carefully, and then choose only the correct answer.

28. A. Choice B is incorrect because the ulnar surface is in contact with the film. Choice C is incomplete; parallel with what? Choice D is incorrect, because using the fastest imaging system is not imperative. In fact, many film-screen departments would stipulate the slowest imaging system.

29. C. Choice 2 is incorrect because the thumb should be up. Choice 4 is incorrect because the elbow should be flexed 90 degrees. Choice 5 is incorrect because the central ray should be directed to the midpoint of the forearm.

30. B. Choice 1 is incorrect because the forearm and humerus should be in the same plane. Choice 4 is incorrect because the hand must be supinated.

31. A. Choice 1 is incorrect because the hand is not pronated. Choice 4 is incorrect because the arm may be slightly abducted. Notice the difference one letter can make in a me-dical term (adducted vs. abducted). Read carefully.

32. C. Choice 2 is incorrect because no angle is put on the central ray. Choice 4 is incorrect because respiration should be suspended.

33. B. Choice A is incorrect because it would not be appropriate to double-expose the film. You may put both joints on one film, but not both joints with and without weights. Choice C is incorrect because both joints may not necessarily be placed on the same film. Choice D is incorrect because the patient should be standing, if possible, and respiration must be suspended.

34. D. Choice 1 is incorrect because an AP projection is commonly used to radiograph the clavicle. PA may be used, but it is not mandatory. Choice 2 is incorrect because the direction of tube angle in the PA axial projection should be caudad.

35. A. Choice 2 is incorrect because the affected scapula should be centered to the cassette.

36. D. Be sure to review all of the fractures listed in the chapter.
37. A. Be sure to review all of the fractures listed in the chapter.
38. C. This is characterized by degeneration of one or several joints. The patient is likely to be in great discomfort.
39. B. A giant cell myeloma is a type of tumor that is easy to penetrate.
40. C. These patients require slow and careful handling.
41. D. Choice 1 is incorrect because a trough filter is used for chest radiography. A wedge filter would be used for the foot. Choice 2 is incorrect because the plantar surface rests on the cassette. Choice 3 is incorrect because the central ray would be directed toward the heel. Choice 4 is incorrect because the central ray is directed at the base of the third metatarsal.
42. A. Choice 2 is incorrect because the plantar surface of the foot should be perpendicular to the cassette. Choice 4 is incorrect because the central ray enters the foot at the base of the fifth metatarsal.
43. B. Choice 2 is incorrect because this rotates the ankle too far. Choice 3 is incorrect because rotation should be adjusted 15 to 20 degrees for the mortise joint. Choice 4 is incorrect because rotation should be at 45 degrees for the bony stru-cture.
44. D. Choice 3 is incorrect because the patient should be rolled toward the affected side. Choice 6 is incorrect because the fibula should appear po-sterior to the tibia on the radiograph.
45. C. Choice 3 is incorrect because the patella must be perpendicular to the film. Choice 4 is incorrect because the central ray should be directed 5 degrees cephalad.
46. A. All of these conditions are needed for an accurate examination of the patella in the tangential projection.
47. D. Choice A is the opposite of the correct answer. Choice B is incorrect; both joints should be included. Choice C is incorrect; the patient should be supine.
48. D. Direction of the central ray for some projections can be very specific. Notice how similar the choices are for this question. Be sure to know central ray directions for all major projections.
49. B. Hangman's fracture is caused by acute hyperextension of the head on the neck; the arch of C2 is fractured and there is anterior subluxation of C2 onto C3.
50. B. Note the opposite way of asking question 49. Be prepared for questions to be asked either way.
51. D. Such patients require special care and handling while positioning. Let them take it at their own speed.
52. C. The pars articularis is between the superior and inferior articular processes of a vertebra.
53. A. Any cervical injury must be handled with the utmost care.
54. B. Choice 4 is incorrect because the lateral projection of the cervical spine is always taken with the cervical collar in place until the finished radiograph has been cleared by a physician. Choice 5 is incorrect because it would distort the image.
55. C. Choice 2 is incorrect because no angulation is placed on the central ray. Why not a falling load generator? It is not possible on such a machine to get long exposure times, which you want to have for the "breathing technique" used for a lateral projection of the thoracic spine. If all generators in a department are the falling load type, you must do the best you can. Little blurring will occur, however, because the exposure time is so short.
56. D. Choice 2 is incorrect because the hips and knees should be flexed.
57. C. Choice A is the opposite of the correct answer. Choice B is incorrect; the part should be elevated 25 to 30 degrees from the table. Choice D is incorrect; there is no angle on the central ray.
58. A. Be sure to keep the central ray paths clear among all the projections you've learned.
59. D. Emphysema is a condition in which air is trapped in the alveoli, which hyperinflates the lungs and makes them much easier for x-rays to penetrate.
60. A. There is a fine line between just learning medical terminology and knowing something about pathologic conditions. Be sure to review the major pathologic conditions presented in this chapter. Pathology is on the ARRT exam.
61. D. This is another way to ask about emphysema.
62. D. Because emphysema makes the lungs so easy to penetrate, automatic exposure controls sometimes cannot shut off fast enough, which causes the film to be too dense.
63. B. Even if you're not sure about an answer, this one is a good example of how to narrow your choices. Notice the similarity between the word "bronchial" in the stem of the question and the word "bronchogenic" in choice B. If you encounter questions about which you are not totally sure, look for such similarities. In many cases they will lead you to the correct answer.
64. C. These letters stand for *chronic obstructive pulmonary disease.*
65. A. Choice 2 is incorrect because the shoulders should be rotated anteriorly, moving the scapulae out of the field of the ribs. Choice 4 is incorrect because respiration should be on full inspiration.
66. C. Choice A is incorrect because the body should be rotated only 15 to 20 degrees. Choice B is incorrect because this is an anterior oblique. Choice D is incorrect because breathing causes a blurring of lung detail. A falling load generator should not be used because it inhibits the ability to use long exposure times that run several seconds.
67. B. Choice A is incorrect because a PA projection causes superimposition of the spine and a lateral

projection is not possible. Choice C is incorrect because respiration should be suspended. Choice D is incorrect because an AP projection would increase magnification.

68. D. Rickets is easy to penetrate.

69. B. Paget's disease is a nonmetabolic bone disease.

70. C. Osteoporosis is very easy to penetrate. Manual technique should be used if possible. An AEC often cannot terminate the exposure fast enough, resulting in an overexposed image. Be knowledgeable about manual techniques you may use in these types of situations.

71. A. Hydrocephalus is harder to penetrate.

72. C. These patients may be frail and brittle. Be sure to take your time with them.

73. D. D is the more complete answer when compared with choice C. There is no angle on the central ray.

74. B. Be sure to read carefully and distinguish between parallel and perpendicular. Even though head radiography has been largely replaced by computed tomography, basic skull positioning may still appear on the Registry exam.

75. D. Choice A is incorrect because it describes the wrong three-point landing. Choice B is incorrect because it describes angulation from the perpendicular. Choice C is incorrect because the central ray exits the affected orbit.

76. C. Choice B is incorrect because of the degree of angulation. Choice D is incorrect because it indicates that the head is resting on the nose.

77. A. Read choices B, C, and D carefully and note that only one or two words are different from those in the correct answer. It is not likely that the questions on the certification exam will have answers this similar. The question is worded this way to help you really sort out the specific details of this projection. How did you do? Do you see why choice A is correct?

78. D. Choices A and B are clearly incorrect, because this is a submentovertical projection. Choices C and D differ only in the perpendicular versus parallel placement of the IOML.

79. C. Whereas the Waters projection also shows all of the paranasal sinuses, the upright projection will best indicate fluid levels.

80. C. This will be demonstrated during an upper GI series.

81. D. Intestinal obstructions are sometimes difficult to image properly, because the obstruction may be more difficult to penetrate while the backed-up gas may be quite easy to penetrate. Again, using a manual technique may be beneficial.

82. B. Other portions of the bowel may be perfectly normal. These patients are usually in some degree of discomfort.

83. D. Bowel obstructions make the patient extremely ill and uncomfortable. Consider using a manual technique.

84. A. This form of cancer requires immediate intervention. Being familiar with the various pathologic conditions you will encounter makes radiography that much more interesting. Look up any conditions with which you are unfamiliar.

85. C. The other conditions are all in the bowel.

86. D. This condition is characterized by large amounts of gas; use care when choosing the exposure technique.

87. A. Patients with diverticula may be nearly asymptomatic or in great discomfort.

88. C. This condition may be characterized by projectile vomiting. Have emesis basins at hand.

89. B. This is a very painful condition for the patient. Work quickly.

90. B. Take careful note of the degree and direction of rotation.

91. D. This is the most accurate and complete answer. The others are incomplete.

92. C. Because this is an LPO, the patient must be supine. That rules out choices A and D.

93. A. Choices B and D can immediately be eliminated because they place the patient prone. A lateral decubitus position requires the patient to be lying on the side.

94. C. This stands for *endoscopic retrograde cholangiopancreatography.*

95. D. These are harder to penetrate.

96. C. Wilms' tumor is seen primarily in children.

97. A. PKD is harder to penetrate.

98. C. Wilms' tumor is harder to penetrate.

99. B. Patients are typically in extreme pain.

100. C. Questions on RPO and LPO kidneys tend to be confusing because it is hard to remember which kidney ends up perpendicular or parallel. Be sure to review these projections.

CHAPTER 6

1. D. Be sure to know all of these.

2. C. Material Safety Data Sheets.

3. C. Elderly patients tend to be stronger earlier in the day.

4. B. Patients who have been held without food should be imaged first.

5. C. The need for insulin means diabetic patients should be imaged early.

6. B. It is important that either the stomach or the colon be empty, with nothing interfering from a previous procedure.

7. D. Be sure to know these basic legal concepts.

8. D. All are considered a form of striking the patient.

9. A. Keep in mind that assault does not have to involve touching the patient.

10. B. Notice that the question asks which item is false concerning invasion of privacy. Choice B could be considered false imprisonment.

11. A. Although unintentional, it still carries with it penalties. Something that should have been done was not done.

12. B. The defendant is compared with individuals having similar experience.

13. D. The employer is always responsible for the actions of the employees.

14. C. Choice B actually involves loss of life or limb; gross negligence does not have to involve an actual loss.

15. D. Be familiar with these facts concerning malpractice.

16. D. This means "the thing speaks for itself." It is something that could not have occurred by natural means.

17. A. Choice 2 is incorrect because a brochure does not have to be given to the patient. Choice 5 is incorrect because patients are unlikely to completely understand all aspects of a procedure.

18. B. Choice A is incorrect because a patient who is ambulatory would not be on a cart. Choice C is incorrect because patient care must never be compromised because of short staffing. Choice D is incorrect because safety is of paramount importance.

19. D. There are several very important reasons for obtaining an accurate patient history.

20. B. Be sure to review the principles of infection control.

21. D.

22. D.

23. A. Vectors involve animals.

24. B. This differs from vectorborne transmission and does not involve motor vehicles.

25. B. Choice C would be vectorborne and choice D would be direct contact.

26. B. Choice A would be droplet transmission, choice C would be vectorborne transmission, and choice D would be direct contact.

27. B. Standard Precautions were formerly called *Universal Precautions*.

28. A. Standard Precautions are used because we can never know for sure what each patient may carry.

29. D. Handwashing is always the first defense. However, it does not replace any other methods.

30. A. This is the ideal apparel for these procedures. Head and shoe coverings do little, and a regular uniform may carry organisms after the exam is over.

31. C. This precaution is very important to observe.

32. A. This greatly increases the chance for a needlestick injury and the transmission of pathogens.

33. A. Health care workers must always assume that pathogens are present. Washing per protocol is mandatory.

34. B. Handwashing is the best protection against transmission of pathogens.

35. C. Surgical asepsis is the complete removal of organisms.

36. A. This is much more complete than medical asepsis.

37. B. Always wash hands before beginning any procedure.

38. D. Underarms (because of perspiration), sides, and back are considered nonsterile.

39. D. These are all key points to remember.

40. B. Droplet transmission involves coughs and sneezes, direct contact involves a person, and airborne transmission involves droplets and dust. Radiographers must be constantly aware of the methods of transmission.

41. D. Standard Precautions must be practiced at all times.

42. D. Note the constant emphasis on handwashing. None of the other choices must be followed in every circumstance.

43. B. Gloves need not be worn with respiratory isolation. All of the other choices involve body fluids.

44. D. This prevents the patient from contracting something from the health care worker or the equipment.

45. A. This is the most restrictive form of isolation.

46. C. Enteric refers to the gastrointestinal system.

47. B. The risk here is with coughs and sneezes.

48. C. The risk here is from fluids in the GI system and any needles that have entered the GI system.

49. B. Coughs and sneezes could transmit disease.

50. D. This assumes the patient may have something that the health care worker does not want transmitted.

51. D. The radiographer should be constantly observing the patient for any such signs.

52. D. Choice A is incorrect because it indicates degrees centigrade. Choice B is incorrect because it indicates a range of normal temperature in degrees centigrade.

53. C.

54. B.

55. C. This is the real name for a "blood pressure cuff."

56. D. The numerator indicates the blood pressure when the heart is pumping, the systolic pressure. The denominator indicates the blood pressure when the heart is at rest, the diastolic pressure. The symbol "Hg" stands for mercury.

57. C. Be certain to flow the oxygen at the proper rate, which is per minute.

58. C. The Heimlich maneuver is performed by a person, CPR is for cardiac/respiratory arrest, and a nasogastric (NG) tube is for introducing substances directly into the stomach.

59. A. The radiographer must always be familiar with the contents of the crash cart and what each item does.

60. C. Anaphylaxis is an allergic reaction to foreign proteins, cardiogenic shock results from cardiac failure, septic shock occurs when toxins produced during infection cause a dramatic drop in blood pressure.

61. D. Anaphylaxis is an allergic reaction to foreign proteins, cardiogenic shock results from cardiac failure, hypovolemic shock occurs following loss of a large amount of blood or plasma.

62. A. Cardiogenic shock results from cardiac failure, hypovolemic shock occurs following loss of a large amount of blood or plasma, septic shock occurs when toxins produced during infection cause a dramatic drop in blood pressure.

63. D. Anaphylaxis is an allergic reaction to foreign proteins, cardiogenic shock results from cardiac failure, hypovolemic shock occurs following loss of a large amount of blood or plasma.

64. B. Anaphylaxis is an allergic reaction to foreign proteins, cardiogenic shock results from cardiac failure, hypovolemic shock occurs following loss of a large amount of blood or plasma.

65. A. Anaphylaxis is an allergic reaction to foreign proteins. Cardiogenic shock results from cardiac failure, hypovolemic shock occurs following loss of a large amount of blood or plasma, septic shock occurs when toxins produced during infection cause a dramatic drop in blood pressure.

66. D. The radiographer must be able to recognize all of these. These types of questions may be on the certification exam because patient care in imaging is the responsibility of the radiographer.

67. B. Keep blood flowing to the brain by placing the patient in the Trendelenburg position, head lower than the hips.

68. C. Choice 2 is incorrect because the patient should never be left alone under any circumstances. Choice 3 is incorrect because of potentially devastating consequences; a spinal injury should always be assumed.

69. D. Be sure to be familiar with these various devices that may be present in a patient.

70. D. Be sure to be familiar with these various devices that may be present in a patient.

71. A. Nosocomial infections are those acquired in the health care setting. Most of these infections are the result of use of the urinary catheter.

72. C. The radiographer must be careful working around the ventilator so as to not affect its operation.

73. D. Air is a negative contrast agent. Hence chest x-ray exams are contrast studies.

74. A. Choice 1 is incorrect because air is a negative contrast agent. Choice 3 is incorrect because barium should be mixed with warm water. Choice 4 is incorrect because nonionic contrast media do contain iodine.

75. D. This is the first and most important issue that must be taken into consideration. Be sure to read the package inserts that come with contrast agents and review the contraindications and side effects.

76. A. Extravasation involves escape of the contrast agent into the tissues surrounding the injection site.

77. D. The radiographer must be aware of all possible symptoms and know what to do immediately.

78. B. It is important to remain with the patient and observe for symptoms of a possible reaction.

79. B. Maintain composure, yet react quickly.

80. D. This is sometimes confusing, so be sure to review and be familiar with it.

81. A. Special care must be taken when venipuncture is performed. Review all of the steps in venipuncture.

82. B. Butterfly sets are used in some circumstances.

83. D. Be familiar with all the items used for venipuncture.

84. C. You already know that any list of steps for a procedure will begin with washing hands. That immediately rules out choices A and D. As soon as hands are washed, the next step must be gloving. That points directly to choice C, which is the only possible answer to this question. Always evaluate the question and read all of the possible answers. Many times you will recognize a shortcut such as this.

85. A. Venipuncture is part of a radiographer's scope of practice. It is tested on the ARRT exam. It may, however, be regulated by state law in some circumstances. Be sure to know what you can and cannot do on the job.

86. D. All relevant history and blood values must be present on the chart and consulted before the exam is begun.

87. A.

88. C.

89. A. This may indicate that a reaction is starting.

90. B. The radiographer must respond quickly and be aware that more reaction may be imminent.

91. B. Understanding of diversity is a prime part of every radiographer's practice.

92. B. The radiographer should be calling for assistance.

93. A. While the other choices may be part of a radiographer's practice in various venues, patient education is always part of practice.

94. B. A code blue should be called; CPR should be initiated.

95. B.

96. C.

97. D. The Rules are enforceable by the ARRT. Be certain to understand these for the ARRT exam.

98. B. The Code of Ethics is aspirational, goals for radiographers' practice.

99. A. Contrast agent reactions can begin with very benign symptoms. Never leave the patient alone.

100. B.

CHAPTER 7

Answers to Challenge Test Number 1

1. B. These changes may include absorption and scatter radiation. Radiation that emerges from the patient is called *exit radiation.*

2. C. Photoelectric interaction produces contrast as a result of the differential absorption of the incoming x-ray photons in the body's tissues. Rays are completely absorbed in some areas of the patient. Choices A and B are types of scattering. Pair production does not occur in radiography.

3. A. Compton interaction produces scattered photons that emerge from the patient in divergent paths and may expose the radiographer or radiologist. The photoelectric effect is responsible for total absorption of the incoming x-ray photon during attenuation. Coherent scattering and pair production occur when x-ray energies are beyond the moderate range used in radiography.

4. D. *Rad* stands for *radiation absorbed dose*. The gray is the SI, not the traditional, unit of absorbed dose. The coulombs/kilogram is the SI unit of radiation exposure in the air. The curie is the traditional unit of radioactivity.

5. D. The curie, used primarily in nuclear medicine, is the traditional unit of radioactivity. The becquerel is the SI unit of radioactivity. The gray is the SI unit of absorbed dose. The radiation weighting factor is a value used to adjust the absorbed dose amount to compensate for the greater damage caused by some ionizing radiation.

6. C. The roentgen is the traditional measure of in-air exposure. The curie is the traditional unit of radioactivity. The becquerel measures radioactivity, and the gray measures absorbed dose.

7. D. LET varies because of different levels of ionization. It occurs with high-ionization radiations such as neutrons and alpha particles, as well as during x-ray and gamma-ray procedures.

8. D. The curie measures the quantity of radioactive material.

9. C. This describes a dose-response curve, such as linear-nonthreshold. The H & D, or characteristic, curve represents the relationship between radiation exposure and optical density. Study tip: When two or more choices are similar, such as choices A and C, one of them is often the correct answer.

10. B. Medical x-rays are an artificial source of ionizing radiation; diagnostic procedures account for the largest source of artificial radiation exposure to humans. Natural background radiation is that contained in the environment.

11. A. There is a definite safe, or threshold, dose at which cataractogenesis does not occur. Choice C does not make logical sense, because the question states that cataractogenesis does not occur at low levels of radiation exposure. Occupational dose is the amount of radiation to which radiographers are exposed. Study tip: When there are opposite choices (e.g., threshold and nonthreshold), one of them is usually the correct answer.

12. A. Be sure to review stochastic and nonstochastic, deterministic and probabalistic. The severity, not the probability, of nonstochastic effects increases with increased dose. Direct effect and indirect effect differentiate whether the initial ionizing event occurs on the most radiosensitive molecule (direct effect) or on another molecule (indirect effect).

13. D. Occupational cumulative exposure is determined by multiplying years of age times 1 rem. Study tip: Be sure to read each choice carefully and entirely before choosing an answer. Choice A may appear correct at first glance, but according to the equation, the correct answer is 22 rem, not 22 mrem. An mrem, or millirem, is one-thousandth of a rem.

14. D. This limit is important to keep in mind when considering ALARA.

15. D. Lead, not aluminum, equivalent will absorb most of the scatter radiation energy. Because the secondary barrier is located where only scatter or leakage occur, $1/32$-inch lead equivalent is sufficient. Primary barriers require $1/16$-inch lead equivalent.

16. C. Photons lose considerable energy after scattering.

17. A. The dose is determined by the inverse square law. The distance was halved; therefore the dose went up 4 times (not 2 times).

18. A. The minimum source-to-skin distance for fixed fluoroscopes is 15 inches; for portable fluoroscopes, 12 inches (although 15 inches is preferred). Be sure to review these required distances.

19. A. Gonadal shielding is even more effective for males, reducing the gonad dose by up to 95%.

20. D. Target theory states that for a cell to die after radiation exposure, its master, or target, molecule (DNA) must be inactivated. Direct effect occurs when radiation transfers its energy directly to the DNA. The doubling dose is the dose of radiation necessary to produce twice the frequency of genetic mutations as would have occurred in the absence of the radiation. Be sure to review these concepts.

21. B. The dose equivalent at which blood count is depressed is much higher than diagnostic levels but may occur during radiation therapy.

22. D. This is the definition of free radicals, which can cause biologic damage to the cell. Some free radicals may chemically combine to form hydrogen peroxide. Radiolysis results in an ion pair in the cell: a positively charged water molecule and a free electron.

23. D. According to target theory, substantial research indicates that DNA, contained in the cellular nucleus, is the master molecule. Hydrogen peroxide is a poison that can cause damage to the cell. A free radical is a highly reactive ion with unpaired electrons in the outer shell. RNA transmits genetic instructions from the nucleus to the cytoplasm of the cell.

24. A. *Cytogenesis* refers to the origin and development of cells. *Spermatogenesis* is the development of spermatozoa. *Organogenesis* refers to the formation and differentiation of organs during embryonic development. Germ cell division is called *meiosis*.

25. D. Although all of these effects may occur, the most common result of LET is no effect. However, ALARA must still be practiced.

26. C. Adult nerve tissue and even immature cells, which are very radiosensitive, require doses of radiation

higher than those used in medical diagnostic procedures, although ALARA must still be practiced.

27. D. Doses lower than 15 to 20 still pose low risk to the embryo-fetus, so ALARA must still be practiced.

28. D. *As low as reasonably achievable* is a concept used in radiography to protect both the patient and the radiographer.

29. A. Epithelial tissue and reproductive cells, including immature sperm cells, are highly radiosensitive. On the other hand, adult nerve tissue requires very high doses to cause damage, although ALARA must still be practiced because once cells are damaged, repair may not take place.

30. B. In general, these take large doses to manifest themselves.

31. D. Repeats double the dose to the patient for each exposure.

32. C. This is what may cause harmful effects.

33. D. Ionization is multifaceted. Study tip: Be sure to read all choices before choosing an answer. Choice A is true, but you must read all the choices to see that choice D is the correct answer.

34. A. Cell damage may be exhibited as loss of function or abnormal function.

35. C. Damage from somatic effects is evident in the organism being irradiated. Most of the time these effects are benign. Genetic damage is passed to the next generation.

36. A. Somatic effects are evident in the organism being irradiated.

37. C. There is no control over natural background radiation, which has been present in the environment since the formation of the universe. Choices A, B, and D all refer to artificially produced radiation, that made by humans. Study tip: Choices A, B, and D are basically the same; they are too similar for one of them to be the correct answer. Choice C is the only unique answer.

38. B. Natural background radiation, which has been present since the formation of the universe, accounts for 50% of human exposure. The greatest single source is radon.

39. B. You can safely assume that natural background radiation would be below the annual recommended limits of exposure from diagnostic imaging. Although all choices are below this limit, choice B is correct. Background exposure is not high but is always present.

40. C. Radon, which exists as a gas, accounts for 55% of human exposure to natural background radiation.

41. D. The huge increase in the use of CT since the 1980's has primarily caused this increase.

42. C.

43. A.

44. B.

45. A.

46. B.

47. A. Don't confuse atomic mass with atomic number.

48. D. X-rays exit the anode as burst of energy knows as photons.

49. C. We usually focus on frequency and wavelength due to their relevance in imaging.

50. D. Frequency is inverse to wavelength.

51. D. Other transformers operate on the principle of mutual induction.

52. B. One millisecond is the shortest time possible.

53. C. Automatic exposure control (usually an ionization chamber) is the only choice that has to do with consistency of radiographic quality.

54. D. Choice A does not make sense because if a predetermined level of ionization is reached, the unit could not be malfunctioning because it reached that predetermined level.

55. D. A falling load generator has the advantage of adjusting to the shortest exposure time and highest mA allowed by the high-voltage generator, but it is not capable of long exposure times.

56. D. A falling load generator allows very short exposure times by taking advantage of tube heat loading potential. When the tube's maximum heat load has been reached for a set mA, the generator drops the mA to the next lower level that the tube can handle (falling heat load).

57. D. Transformers operate on the principle of mutual induction. They are either step-up (increases voltage) or step-down (decreases voltage) transformers.

58. A. The step-up transformer, also called a *high-voltage transformer,* increases or steps up the voltage to kilovoltage levels.

59. C. DC is needed for the x-ray tube, and a rectifier changes alternating current (AC) to direct current (DC).

60. A. The x-ray tube requires a direct current (DC) to operate properly. The rectifier changes AC to DC. Choices B and D do not describe a type of current and can be eliminated immediately.

61. D. If two very similar choices are presented, one of them is usually the correct answer. Silicon is the nonmetallic chemical element often used in the manufacture of rectifiers. Silicon-based semiconductors are solid-state diodes.

62. B. Thermionic emission occurs when one filament is heated to a level that causes the electrons to be "boiled off" or emitted, creating a cloud of electrons at the cathode. *Therm* refers to heat, *ion* refers to a charged particle, and *emit* means "to give off."

63. A. The focusing cup is part of the cathode assembly; it keeps the electron stream narrow.

64. A. This is a description of characteristic radiation. Although both characteristic and brems radiation produce x-rays at the anode, brems radiation occurs when a projectile electron misses the outer-shell target electrons and moves close to the nucleus. Photoelectric interaction does involve outer-shell electrons

filling holes in the K-shell, but it does not produce x-rays at the anode. Both photoelectric effect and Compton interaction, which produces scatter radiation, occur in the body. Study tip: Be sure to differentiate brems/characteristic from photoelectric/ Compton.

65. C. Adjacent mA stations should be within 10% of one another. Be sure you know these QC standards.
66. D. When exposure reproducibility is tested, variation in measured radiation intensity should not be more than 5%. Be sure you know these QC standards.
67. A. The collimator must be accurate to within 2% of the SID.
68. B.
69. A. Postprocessing provides for maximum manipulation of the image.
70. B.
71. D. This occurs in the reader unit.
72. C.
73. B.
74. C.
75. B.
76. B. Window width adjusts contrast.
77. C.
78. B. Window level adjusts brightness.
79. D.
80. A. The image prior to processing is called the latent image.
81. D.
82. D. This is governed by the 15% rule.
83. C. mAs has been doubled.
84. D. This is governed by the inverse square law.
85. B
86. D. There is no minification.
87. C. These are the two types of shape distortion.
88. D. An increase in OID will cause magnification.
89. A. This is a recommendation. They must be erased at least every 48 hours.
90. C. Height of the lead strips divided by the distance between them.
91. A.
92. B. Fewer x-rays are required to produce the image. This causes an increase in noise or quantum mottle.
93. A.
94. A. If the grid is placed in this position, rays can only get through the middle of the grid.
95. C.
96. A.
97. B. Generally, diagnostic stations have higher resolution monitors.
98. C.
99. B. The overall noise is evened out by this process.
100. B. It is important that proper algorithms be used for each projection.
101. D. There is an increase in photoelectric interactions.
102. D. There is more uniform penetration of the part.
103. C. It has the shortest SID.

104. D. It has the highest kVp.
105. C. It reduces the amount of scatter produced by reducing the number of Compton interactions.
106. C. The beam is more penetrating.
107. C. Density is directly proportional to mAs.
108. C. These grids can be used only within a range of SIDs.
109. B.
110. C. The grid also absorbs image-forming rays, so mAs must be increased to restore them.
111. B. Such as trough and wedge filters.
112. D. Distortion includes elongation and foreshortening and magnification.
113. C.
114. D.
115. A. Be sure to know all of the major anatomy of the urinary system and be able to identify it on radiographs and drawings.
116. B.
117. C.
118. A.
119. D. Be sure to know all of the major anatomy of the colon and be able to identify it on radiographs and drawings.
120. D.
121. C.
122. A.
123. B. Be sure to know all of the major anatomy of the stomach and be able to identify it on radiographs and drawings.
124. B.
125. D.
126. A.
127. C. Be sure to know all of the major anatomy of the lumbar spine and be able to identify it on radiographs and drawings.
128. A.
129. C. Be sure to know all of the major anatomy of the cervical spine and be able to identify it on radiographs and drawings.
130. D.
131. C.
132. B. Be sure to know all of the major anatomy of the hip and be able to identify it on radiographs and drawings.
133. B.
134. C.
135. D.
136. A. Be sure to know all of the major anatomy of the knee and be able to identify it on radiographs and drawings.
137. B.
138. D.
139. A.
140. C. Be sure to know all of the major anatomy of the hand and be able to identify it on radiographs and drawings.

141. D.
142. B.
143. C.
144. A.
145. B.
146. C.
147. D.
148. A. Be sure to know all of the major anatomy of the wrist and be able to identify it on radiographs and drawings.
149. D.
150. B.
151. C.
152. A. Be sure to know all of the major anatomy of the shoulder girdle and be able to identify it on radiographs and drawings.
153. D.
154. B.
155. A.
156. B.
157. C.
158. D. Be sure to know all of the major anatomy of the foot and be able to identify it on radiographs and drawings.
159. D.
160. C.
161. A.
162. B. Be sure to know all of the major anatomy of the elbow and be able to identify it on radiographs and drawings.
163. B.
164. C.
165. D.
166. A. Be sure to know all of the major anatomy of the skull and be able to identify it on radiographs and drawings.
167. D.
168. C.
169. B.
170. A. Be sure to know all of the major anatomy of the facial bones and be able to identify it on radiographs and drawings.
171. C.
172. D.
173. B. Infectious waste containers are usually made of plastic, but not always. The best answer contains the most detail relevant to the radiographer: You should place infectious waste in containers or bags properly labeled as to the type of waste therein. Study tip: Look out for words like "always" and "never." Choices containing these words are usually not the best answer.
174. C. Sharps should never be recapped.
175. A. Assault, battery, false imprisonment, and invasion of privacy are all types of intentional misconduct, but assault can be defined as anything the radiographer does that causes fear in a patient.

Assault can be verbal as well as physical. A remark that causes a patient to feel apprehensive about being injured is considered assault.

176. D. Assault, battery, false imprisonment, and invasion of privacy are all types of intentional misconduct. Invasion of privacy is a violation of confidentiality of any patient information.
177. D. Negligence, the neglect or omission of reasonable care, is a kind of unintentional misconduct. This kind of misconduct is considered unintentional because it arises from an indirect action (not providing care), rather than an overt action (doing harm). Gross negligence is the kind that demonstrates reckless disregard for life or limb. *Respondeat superior* is the legal doctrine that states that an employer is liable for an employee's negligent act. *Res ipsa loquitur* is the legal doctrine that states that the cause of negligence is obvious.
178. B. Pulse is an important vital sign. To detect the presence of bradycardia, the pulse must be taken accurately. Tachycardia is defined as more than 100 beats per minute. Study tip: When two choices are similar (e.g., "More than 100 beats per minute" and "Fewer than 60 beats per minute"), one of them is often the correct answer.
179. A. All the choices except choice A are pieces of equipment, so they wouldn't contain all equipment and drugs needed for respiratory or cardiac arrest. Be sure to know the location of the crash cart and its contents. Study tip: Be sure to read the questions carefully. Common sense can sometimes help you eliminate incorrect choices.
180. D. A sphygmomanometer is also called a *blood pressure cuff.*
181. D. Aqueous iodine compound may be used if surgery is imminent, for example, in the case of perforated ulcers or a ruptured appendix, where barium could be a surgical contaminant.
182. C. Most symptoms of contrast media reactions are observable, so patients must be carefully watched when contrast agents are used.
183. A. The difference between medical and surgical asepsis is that surgical asepsis removes all microorganisms. Study tip: When two choices are similar (e.g., "Medical asepsis" and "Surgical asepsis"), one of them is often the correct answer.
184. A. Always take a history of the patient! *MI* stands for *myocardial infarction.* Bx and hs are not medical abbreviations.
185. D. *MI* stands for *myocardial infarction. Hx* stands for *history,* and *CVA* stands for *cerebrovascular accident.* HA is not a medical abbreviation.
186. C. Because residual barium could compromise any exams that follow barium studies, barium studies should be scheduled last.
187. C. The Centers for Disease Control and Prevention has specific guidelines that must be followed.

188. A. No special equipment is needed to measure respirations.
189. D. The word *nasal* in the answer helps lead you to the correct response.
190. D. These are items commonly encountered throughout the day. Contact transmission is person to person. Airborne transmission involves such things as droplets and dust. Droplet transmission is a result of coughs and sneezes.
191. C. The activity of the heart is electrical. Therefore stimulating the heart with current commonly jolts it back into proper rhythm.
192. D. Blood pressure is not expressed in "beats," which rules out choices A and B.
193. D. *Health Insurance Portability and Accountability Act (HIPAA). CDC stands for Centers for Disease Control and Prevention. HHS stands for the Department of Health and Human Services. ALARA stands for as low as reasonably achievable.*
194. D. *Cardio* refers to the heart. Hypovolemic shock is a result of loss of great amounts of blood. Septic shock occurs when toxins produced during an infection cause a dramatic drop in blood pressure. Neurogenic shock causes blood to pool in the peripheral vessels.
195. B.
196. B.
197. A.
198. B.
199. B.
200. A.

CHAPTER 7

Answers to Challenge Test Number 2
1. C. More energy is deposited by particulate forms of radiation than by waveforms of radiation.
2. D. All are examples of radiation effects on the individual being exposed.
3. D. Choice A is incorrect because photoelectric interaction produces contrast.
4. D. The correct equation would be rads multiplied by a radiation weighting factor equals rem.
5. A. Choice B is incorrect because no level of radiation is considered completely safe. Choice C is incorrect because no such immunity has been proved. Choice D is incorrect because the effective dose limit for the general public is 500 mrem per year.
6. B. High-LET radiation is depositing a lot of energy in the tissues, causing much ionization.
7. C. It is assumed that for every dose of radiation, a response occurs in the atoms of the person being irradiated.
8. B. Cells such as epithelial, ovarian, and sperm cells.
9. D. Because the cellular cytoplasm is substantially larger than the cellular nucleus, it is more likely to be struck by incoming x-ray photons. Thus most of the cellular response to radiation is indirect. The direct effect results from x-ray photons directly striking the cellular nucleus.
10. A. Indirect effect occurs when radiation strikes the cytoplasm of the cell. Target theory states there is a master molecule that governs cellular activities, that is, DNA.
11. B. This is 50 to 250 rads in humans.
12. C. Be sure to review the units of radiation measurement.
13. B. This is human-produced radiation.
14. A. This is the same as the general public's annual limit for infrequent exposure.
15. A. Choices B and D refer to electrons and brems radiation, which apply to action inside the x-ray tube; the photoelectric effect is a photon-tissue interaction.
16. C. Be sure to get the amount and unit of measurement correct!
17. D. This is the definition of mean marrow dose (MMD). It is not called the bone dose. The doubling dose is the amount of radiation that causes the number of mutations in a population to double. The GSD is the genetically significant dose.
18. A. This describes the GSD, or genetically significant dose (not called genetic dose). The doubling dose is the amount of radiation that causes the number of mutations in a population to double. Mean marrow dose is the average dose to active bone marrow as an indicator of somatic effects on population.
19. B. Shielding of lead (Pb) equivalent, not aluminum (Al) equivalent, is used to protect from scatter radiation. The requirement for a lead apron is at least 0.25-mm Pb equivalent; it should be 0.5-mm Pb equivalent, which is what the question asks. There is a difference between "shall" and "should."
20. B. The requirement for a thyroid shield, if used, during fluoroscopy is 0.5-mm lead, not aluminum, equivalent.
21. D. Primary protective barriers consist of 1/16-inch lead equivalent, not aluminum equivalent. Secondary protective barriers consist of 1/32-inch lead equivalent.
22. C. Primary protective barriers in the wall must extend to a height of at least 7 feet, because this height is taller than most people.
23. C. The secondary protective barrier extends from where the primary protective barrier ends to the ceiling with a 1/2-inch overlap.
24. D. The protective curtain hanging from the fluoroscopy tower must be at least 0.25-mm Pb, not Al, equivalent. Be sure to remember all the shielding requirements.
25. D. Be sure to remember all the shielding requirements.
26. C. Filters made of aluminum and copper are placed in the film badge to measure the x-ray energy striking the film badge. This is a measure of the beam's

quality, not quantity. Film badges do not measure the source or type of x-ray beam.

27. D. A film badge should not be worn longer than 1 month, at which time a film badge report with readings is returned to the institution.

28. B. Lithium fluoride crystals, which release energy as visible light when heated, are used to record dose in TLDs.

29. B. TLDs are heated and release visible light energy to indicate dose. This energy is read by a photomultiplier tube.

30. A. OSL dosimeters are sen-sitive to exposures as low as 1 mrem, which makes them 5 times as sensitive as TLDs. This feature, along with their wide dynamic range, greater accuracy, and long-term stability, make them ideal for personnel monitoring.

31. C. The recording material in an OSL dosimeter is aluminum oxide, which is then scanned by a laser beam. Film badges use film as the recording material; TLDs use lithium fluoride. Silver halide is the active ingredient in radiographic film emulsion.

32. C. The energy stored in an OSL dosimeter is released by exposure to a laser. The energy is then released as visible light. The energy stored in a TLD is released by heat.

33. C. OSL dosimeters can be worn for up to a quarter, although in many cases they may be changed monthly.

34. D. One of the key advantages of OSL dosimeters is the capability of reanalysis for confirmation of dose, which is especially important if a dose is in question.

35. C. The flat contact shield, which consists of a piece of lead placed over the gonads, is most commonly used. It may be as simple as a lead apron properly placed. The shadow shield, which is suspended from the x-ray housing and does not come in contact with the patient, is used when sterile technique is required. A collimator is not considered a gonadal shielding device.

36. D. Low mAs reduces the amount of radiation striking the patient. Choosing the optimum kVp for the part being radiographed increases the quality of the x-ray beam. Low kVp, high mAs would result in the opposite.

37. D. The fastest practical speed for the part being radiographed should be used to reduce patient dose. Slow speed increases patient dose.

38. A. Be sure to review the source-to-skin distance requirements.

39. D. Filtration is adjusted by a medical radiation physicist, not by the radiographer. Compensating filtration such as wedge filters are manipulated by the radiographer.

40. D. The personal dosimetry report usually reads in units of mrem, the unit of equivalent dose and effective dose, which uses a radiation weighting factor to modify the absorbed dose amount to account for greater damage inflicted by some forms of radiation

(rad ´ WR = rem). Rads measure the absorbed dose, which does not take into account the different biologic effects caused by different types of radiation. Roentgens measure the amount of in-air radiation. Curies measure the quantity of radioactive material.

41. A. The current alternates 120 times per second.

42. D. As wavelength increases, frequency decreases, and vice versa.

43. C. The smallest particle of an element that retains the characteristics of the element is an atom.

44. A. This question asks which of the choices does not define matter. According to Einstein, matter cannot travel at or beyond the speed of light.

45. B. A step-up transformer steps up voltage and steps down current.

46. D. The ionization chamber is the most common form of automatic exposure control.

47. D. Choice B looks tempting, but silicone is a substance that is sometimes used in plastic surgery.

48. C. Hence the use of the constant 1.41 when calculating heat units for this type of equipment.

49. D. This is where you should place the thicker part being radiographed.

50. B. During this time, the exposure is still taking place.

51. A. Although seldom used, this is based on heat units that would be produced for a given exposure.

52. B. Electron focusing lenses.

53. D. Photocathode.

54. A. Output phosphor.

55. C. Input phosphor. Be sure to review the parts of the image intensifier and know what occurs at each.

56. D. Exposure linearity tests the accuracy of the mA stations.

57. D. Exposure reproducibility tests the accuracy of successive exposures when the same technique is used.

58. A. It will be visualized as a blurry pattern on the image of the mesh.

59. A. Half-value layer is the amount of absorbing material that reduces the intensity of the beam by half.

60. B. The accuracy of collimation must be within 2% of the SID.

61. C. The accuracy of kVp must be within 4 kVp.

62. D. The actual focal spot is the physical area on the anode from which the x-rays emanate.

63. D. The rays appear to be coming from a smaller area. This results in a sharper image.

64. B. X-rays are also produced by the characteristic interaction at the anode.

65. D. This technique has the highest mAs and the highest kVp.

66. D. This technique has the highest mAs and the highest kVp.

67. C. Be sure to keep lead and aluminum in their proper places.

68. D. The primary beam does not contain scatter, contrast goes up when a grid is used, and the dose to the patient actually goes up, not down.

69. D. Choice A is nearly correct, but choice D includes tooth enamel. Read all the answers carefully.
70. A. Bit depth is equal to $2n$, where n is the number of bits.
71. C. kVp is governed by the 15% rule.
72. A.
73. D.
74. A.
75. B.
76. A.
77. A.
78. B.
79. B. It is critical to choose the correct algorithm for each projection.
80. D. This is currently the fastest way to obtain the image.
81. B.
82. A. See figure 4-18.
83. D. Picture Archiving and Communication System.
84. A.
85. C.
86. B. Violation of the grid radius will cause grid cutoff.
87. D.
88. B.
89. B.
90. A. A smaller effective focal spot is produced.
91. B. Although kVp is the controlling factor of contrast, a change in mAs of this magnitude would bury the contrast under excessive density.
92. B. Density decreases as distance is increased, with no changes in exposure factors.
93. A. A decrease in OID results in less magnification of the image.
94. B.
95. B. Higher kVp results in more Compton interactions and a more uniform penetration of the part.
96. C. However, this technology is evolving rapidly.
97. A. The grid absorbs scatter radiation. In addition, because no compensation has been made in mAs, the absorption of image-forming rays will be quite noticeable.
98. A. A shorter SID will result in greater magnification.
99. C. There is no correlation between kVp and recorded detail. kVp, and the contrast it provides, does control visibility of detail.
100. B. This results in an increase in OID. The point could be made that such a small change (approximately 2 inches) would cause little appreciable effect. It is not likely that the certification exam would attempt to examine such a fine point. However, the single best answer is B, because there is an increase in OID.
101. B. This results in magnification of the image.
102. A.
103. B. The beam wavelength becomes predominantly shorter, which makes it more penetrating. Therefore, contrast will go down.

104. B. As collimation is tightened without technique compensa-tion, fewer rays strike the patient.
105. A. There is a decrease in the number of Compton int-eractions as the area being ir-radiated is limited. This is true regardless of whether co-mpensation is made by adjustment of mAs.
106. C. Focal-spot size controls recorded detail, not density.
107. C. Changing kVp while using automatic exposure controls has no effect on density.
108. D. This causes the production of x-rays and heat at the anode.
109. D. This occurs in the patient and produces scatter.
110. A. This causes the production of x-rays and heat at the anode.
111. A.
112. C.
113. D.
114. C.
115. A. Be sure to review the placement of the carpal bones.
116. D. Two similar answers such as A and D usually that indicate one of them is the correct answer.
117. D. The Jefferson fracture is a comminuted fracture of the ring of the atlas.
118. C. A boxer's fracture is a transverse fracture of the neck of the fifth metacarpal.
119. B. A Colles' fracture is a transverse fracture through the distal radius.
120. A. Talipes is another term for clubfoot.
121. D. Ankylosing spondylitis is an inflammatory disease of the spine that causes fusion of the joints involved.
122. D.
123. D.
124. A.
125. D.
126. C.
127. C. Be sure to know all of the major anatomy of the hand and wrist and be able to identify it on radiographs and drawings.
128. B.
129. A.
130. D.
131. B.
132. A. Be sure to know all of the major anatomy of the elbow and be able to identify it on radiographs and drawings.
133. D.
134. A.
135. B.
136. B.
137. D. Be sure to know all of the major anatomy of the vertebrae and be able to identify it on radiographs and drawings.
138. C.
139. B.

140. D

141. C. Be sure to know all of the major anatomy of the lower leg and be able to identify it on radiographs and drawings.

142. D.

143. B.

144. A.

145. C.

146. A.

147. D. Be sure to know all of the major anatomy of the shoulder girdle and be able to identify it on radiographs and drawings.

148. D. Choice A is incorrect because this is a radiograph of a lower leg. Choice B is in-correct because the tibia and fibula cannot be superimposed. Choice C is incorrect because both joints should be included.

149. C. Although it is seldom performed, this T-tube cholangiogram shows the hepatobiliary ductwork.

150. B. Be sure to review the anatomy visualized on the elbow obliques.

151. C. This is the only choice that places the skull in a true lateral.

152. A. Note the placement of the petrous ridge.

153. B.

154. D.

155. B.

156. D.

157. C. Be sure to know all of the major anatomy of the "Scotty dog" and be able to identify it on radiographs and drawings.

158. C. Autotomography involves placing superimposing structures in motion while the x-ray tube and IR remain stationary.

159. B. Knowing the effect of injuries helps with positioning of the patient and prevents further injury.

160. D. This is a PA axial projection of the clavicle, so the tube angulation is caudad. The tube angulation is cephalad for the AP axial projection.

161. C. Note the use of a range in the answer. This is what you will probably encounter on the ARRT exam.

162. D.

163. B. Place the proximal femur (the thicker part of the thigh) under the cathode portion of the x-ray beam. A trough filter is used for chest radiography.

164. A. Know those exact centering points.

165. D. If this were a PA oblique projection, choice B would be correct.

166. B. This is an AP oblique.

167. B. This is a PA oblique.

168. C. The second inspiration would be deeper than just a single inspiration. This is a more complete and descriptive answer than choice A.

169. A. Be sure you know why certain projections are used.

170. B. Choice 3 is incorrect because the central ray exits at the nasion when the frontal bone is being examined. Choice 4 is incorrect because the MSP is perpendicular to the cassette.

171. C.

172. B.

173. D.

174. C. Another correct answer would be "if the OML formed a 53-degree angle from the perpendicular."

175. D. The key word is *must*, although radiographers should also be proficient in taking blood pressure. As radiographers' scope of practice expands, so will the need to be proficient in the use of a wide range of medical instruments. Be aware that in some states oxygen is considered a medication.

176. C. Be familiar with all tubes you may encounter in patient care.

177. D. These are also called "health care acquired."

178. B. Retrograde flow of urine commonly causes bladder infections. The urinary system is the primary site of nosocomial infections.

179. A. Be sure to wash hands before beginning the exam.

180. B. This question asks which item is not required for valid consent. A consent form is not always used.

181. B.

182. B.

183. A. Always observe standard precautions with every patient.

184. A. Handwashing is the number one method for preventing the spread of infection.

185. B. This protects the patient and the radiographer from injury.

186. C. Be sure to know what other departments to consult for relevant information.

187. D. This is a better answer than A, especially because alcohol is not always used.

188. A. Be sure to review the facts about sterile technique.

189. D. Portable machines go everywhere. Be certain that they are cleaned according to protocol.

190. B. This protects both the patient and the equipment from contamination.

191. D. Patient care is an integral part of the radiographer's responsibility.

192. C. Choice 2 is incorrect because this is beyond the radiographer's scope of practice. Choice 4 is incorrect because in a trauma situation, other health care workers need to be in the room and should be provided with lead protection.

193. D. This helps reduce cramping.

194. D. Some are nonionic, which rules out A and B. Contrast agents are not pure iodine, which rules out choice C.

195. B. Be aware of the possible complications when using these agents. Know all the details of these pharmaceuticals.

196. A. Although it does not occur often, recent exams involving iodinated contrast media should be brought to the radiologist's attention.

197. C. You can never assume there will be no reactions. Choice B is incorrect because other contrast examinations could include barium studies, which would not have a risk of reaction.

198. D.

199. D. Barium is a surgical contaminant.

200. D. As a professional, you need to know the continuing education requirements of your chosen field. Be sure to know your state's statutory requirements as well. Consult www.arrt.org.

CHAPTER 7

Answers to Challenge Test Number 3

1. D. Remnant radiation exits the body (choice A); gamma radiation is not produced in the x-ray tube (choice B). Choice C, nonionizing radiation, is incorrect because x-rays are ionizing radiation.

2. C. Choice A is incorrect because Compton produces scatter radiation. Choice B is incorrect because coherent scatter is produced at extremely low kVp levels. Choice D is incorrect because pair production occurs only at levels above 1.02 MeV.

3. A. Choice B is incorrect because coherent scatter occurs at extremely low kVp levels and does not produce a recoil electron. Choice C is incorrect because the photoelectric effect does not scatter the photon. Choice D is incorrect because pair production does not occur in diagnostic radio-graphy.

4. D. Choice A is incorrect because coulombs/kilogram is an SI unit. Choice B is incorrect because rem is the traditional unit of equivalent dose and effective dose. Choice C is incorrect because becquerel is the SI unit of activity.

5. B. Choice A is incorrect because coulombs/kilogram is the SI unit of in-air exposure. Choice C is incorrect because the curie is the traditional unit of activity. Choice D is in-correct because LET (linear energy transfer) is the amount of energy deposited per unit length of tissue irradiated.

6. A. Choice B is incorrect because the gray is the SI unit of absorbed dose. Choice C is incorrect because radiation weighting factor is multiplied by the absorbed dose to calculate equivalent dose. Choice D is incorrect because LET (linear energy transfer) is the amount of energy deposited per unit length of tissue irradiated.

7. D. Choice A is incorrect because rem is the traditional unit of equivalent dose and effective dose. Choice B is incorrect because the gray is the SI unit of absorbed dose. Choice C is incorrect because radiation weighting factor is multiplied by absorbed dose to calculate equivalent dose.

8. D. Choice A is incorrect because the becquerel is the SI unit of activity. Choice B is incorrect because the gray is the SI unit of absorbed dose. Choice C is incorrect because quality factor is multiplied by absorbed dose to calculate dose equivalency.

9. D. The rad is the unit of absorbed dose.

10. C. Linear energy transfer.

11. A.

12. D. Choice A is incorrect because contrast is produced by photoelectric effect, not Compton interaction.

13. B. Hence R = rads = rem for x-rays.

14. B. Genetic effects may express themselves in future generations as mutations.

15. D.

16. B. National Council on Ra-diation Protection and Mea-surements. Choice A, the International Commission on Radiological Protection, is incorrect. Choice C is incorrect, but the Nuclear Regulatory Commission does have enforcement power. Choice D is incorrect because the American Society of Radiologic Technologists is the professional organization for radiation science professionals.

17. C. Choices A and D are incorrect because there is no threshold dose regarding radiation protection. Choice B is incorrect because we do not assume a nonlinear response for radiation protection.

18. B. Choice A is incorrect because the inverse square law states that the intensity of radiation is inversely proportional to the square of the distance from the source of radiation. Choice C is incorrect because the reciprocity law states that mAs = mAs. Choice D is incorrect because Ohm's law states that voltage is equal to current times resistance in a circuit.

19. A. Indirect effect occurs when radiation strikes the cytoplasm. This causes the formation of free radicals and hydrogen peroxide, which damage the cell. Choice B is incorrect because the law of Bergonié and Tribondeau describes the radiosensitivity of cells. Choice C is incorrect because target theory explains that DNA is the master molecule of the cell. Choice D is incorrect because indirect effect causes about 95% of the cellular response.

20. D. Direct effect occurs when radiation directly hits the cellular nucleus. Indirect effect occurs when radiation strikes the cytoplasm of the cell.

21. C. Choice A is incorrect because 500 mrem per year is the absorbed dose equivalent limit for the general public. Choice B is incorrect because 5 rem per year is the absorbed dose equivalent limit for radiation workers.

22. C. The effective absorbed dose equivalent limit for radiographers is 5 rem per year. Choice A is incorrect because there are no quarterly absorbed dose equivalent limits. Choice B is wrong because 500 mrem per year is the absorbed dose equivalent limit for the general public. Choice D is incorrect because there are no monthly absorbed dose equivalent limits for radiographers.

23. D. Cumulative occupational exposure is calculated by multiplying the worker's age in years times 1 rem. Choice A is incorrect because the unit is incorrect.

24. C. The annual effective dose equivalent for the general public is 0.5 rem, or 500 mrem.

25. D. Choice A is incorrect because this term is no longer used. Choice B is incorrect because *ALARA* stands for *as low as reasonably achievable.*

26. D. Film badges are generally accurate down to the level of 10 mrem.

27. B. The exposure switch on a portable x-ray machine must be attached to a cord that is at least 6 feet long. This does NOT mean six feet is a safe distance. A lead apron must still be worn when performing mobile radiography.

28. B. Under no circumstances should the radiographer be exposed to the primary beam.

29. D. For proper radiation protection, x-ray tubes operating above 70 kVp must have total filtration of at least 2.5-mm aluminum equivalent. Lead is not used as a filter material.

30. B. Choice A is incorrect because gonadal shielding may obstruct the area of interest in some projections. Choice C is incorrect because male patients must also be shielded. Choice D is incorrect because the gonads must be protected outside of pregnancy as well.

31. D. The secondary protective barrier must overlap the primary protective barrier by at least $^{1}/2$ inch to prevent leakage after the building has settled.

32. A. The primary beam is never aimed at the control booth. The exposure switch in the x-ray control booth must have a cord short enough that the radiographer has to be behind the secondary protective barrier to operate the switch.

33. B. The exposure switch in the x-ray control booth must have a cord short enough that to operate the switch, the radiographer must be in the control booth, not simply behind the x-ray tube. The control booth is a secondary, not a primary protective barrier.

34. B. Waiting rooms and stairways are considered uncontrolled areas. They are shielded to keep exposure under 0.5 rem annually. Controlled areas are those occupied by persons who are trained in radiation safety and are wearing personnel monitoring devices. There is no specific area known as the off-limits area or the radiation area.

35. B. An uncontrolled area must be kept under 0.5 rem annually; this is the annual effective absorbed dose equivalent limit for infrequent exposure of the general public. Remember that 0.5 rem is equivalent to 500 mrem, not 5000 mrem.

36. A. Controlled areas are those occupied by persons who are trained in radiation safety and are wearing personnel monitoring devices. Uncontrolled areas are general public areas such as stairways and waiting rooms. There is no specific area known as the off-limits area or the radiation area.

37. D. Workload, measured in mA minutes per week, takes into account the volume and types of exams performed in the room. The use factor is the amount of time the beam is on and directed at a particular barrier. There is no specific shielding factor.

38. C. Workload, measured in mA minutes per week, takes into account the volume and types of exams performed in the room. Half-value layer is the thickness of absorbing material required to reduce the x-ray beam to half its original intensity. The amount of time the beam is on and directed at a particular barrier is called the use factor.

39. A. The amount of time the beam is on and directed at a particular barrier is called the use factor. Workload, measured in mA minutes per week, takes into account the volume and types of exams performed in the room. Occupancy is a determinant of barrier thickness that simply takes into account who occupies a given area. There is no specific shielding factor. Be sure to review the determinants of barrier thickness factors.

40. C. Leakage radiation from a diagnostic x-ray tube may not exceed 100 mR per hour, measured at 1 meter from the housing. This must be measured on a regular basis. Study tip: Be sure to read all choices carefully before choosing an answer. Choices A, C, and D are similar; they each contain the correct value of 100. However, only choice C uses both the correct value and the correct unit of measure for leakage radiation (mR per hour). If the units were expressed in R, the correct equivalent would be 0.1 R per hour.

41. B.

42. A.

43. D.

44. C.

45. A.

46. D. Choice A is incorrect because rectifiers change AC to DC. Choice B is incorrect because "generators" is an incomplete answer. Choice C is incorrect because timers determine the length of exposure.

47. C. Voltage is decreased but current is increased and sent to the filament during thermionic emission. Choice A is incorrect because a step-up transformer is not located in the high-voltage section. Choice B is incorrect even though mA going to the filament circuit is set at the autotransformer. Choice D is incorrect because a type of generator does not apply to this question.

48. C. The rectifier changes the incoming alternating current to direct current and sends it to the x-ray tube.

49. D. Be sure to review where the various components of the x-ray circuit are located and what function each one performs. It is not necessary to know the intricate functioning of these devices. Where they are and what they do will suffice.

50. D. This is the boiling off of electrons from the filament, which occurs when the rotor switch is activated.
51. C. Like charges repel, and this helps electrons leave the filament and travel to the anode.
52. D. More than 99% of the energy applied to the x-ray tube is converted to heat. The other interaction that produces x-rays is called characteristic.
53. B. Be aware that tubes are becoming outdated and are being replaced by solid-state components such as charge-coupled devices (CCDs).
54. C. Be sure to review the basic quality control standards listed in Chapter 3.
55. D. There is little tolerance for variability between exposures.
56. A. Although the collimator may be slightly "off," it still must be accurate within specified limits. This is for radiation protection purposes.
57. D. Be sure to review the basic quality control standards listed in Chapter 3.
58. A. An accurate timer should exhibit 120 dots for a 1-second exposure or 6 dots for a $1/20$-second exposure.
59. C. Because x-ray output never drops to zero with three-phase equipment, this test will display an arc. A $1/2$-second exposure will produce a half-circle, or a 180-degree arc.
60. A. Collimation must be accurate within 2% of the SID.
61. C. There can be a tolerance either way of 4 kVp.
62. C. Choice A is incorrect because the photocathode converts electron energy into light energy. Choice B is incorrect because the electron focusing lens helps restrict the electron beam toward the output phosphor. Choice D is incorrect because a Vidicon tube is used to send an image to the TV.
63. A. Tubes are becoming obsolete. Be aware that CCDs are the substitute technology. If asked this on the Registry exam, you will not have to choose between the two. The correct answer will be obvious.
64. B. The digital dosimeter has replaced many quality control test tools previously used.
65. C.
66. C.
67. C. In other words, 400 mA at $1/2$ second will produce the same density as 200 mA at 1 second; 200 mAs = 200 mAs.
68. The correct answer is C. If one uses 40 mAs and 90 kVp, an image with 4 times the density will be produced. If one uses 30 mAs and 92 kVp, the density will more than double. If one uses 15 mAs and 92 kVp, an image with less than double the density will be produced.
69. The correct answer is C. The inverse square law governs the relationship between distance and density.
70. C. Be familiar with the artifacts presented in Chapter 4.
71. B.
72. A. More radiation is required to create the image.
73. A. This results in lower patient dose.
74. A. Digital communication in medicine.
75. A. Digital communication in medicine.
76. A. Extremely high kVp is used with low mAs, resulting in too few x-ray photons making the image. This will cause noise or mottling of the image.
77. B.
78. B. This is mostly standard on modern x-ray generators.
79. C. Limiting the area being irradiated accomplishes both tasks.
80. B. Unwanted light or dark areas on an image.
81. D. H/D.
82. D.
83. A. According to Einstein, matter cannot travel as the speed of light.
84. D. 2% of the SID.
85. D.
86. C. Compton interaction produces scatter.
87. B. The average wavelength of the beam is shorter after filtration.
88. D.
89. D.
90. D.
91. D.
92. D. The central rays will still go through the grid, but the diverging rays will be absorbed in the lead strips.
93. C. As the diverging rays are more out of alignment with the angled lead strips, they will be absorbed by the grid. With lateral decentering, this will happen more on one side than the other.
94. B. Grid ratio is defined as the height of the lead strips divided by the distance between them. Choice A is incorrect because H & D refers to sensitometric curves. Choice C describes the reciprocity law. Choice D is incorrect because the 15% rule governs changes in technique involving kVp.
95. D. Using any SID out of range will result in grid cutoff.
96. A. Some believe these structures are imaged by scatter, but they are imaged by off-focus radiation.
97. D.
98. C. Tube, part, IR must be in parallel planes.
99. D.
100. B. mAs controls the flow of current through the x-ray circuit.
101. C. Beam restriction limits the occurrence of Compton interactions.
102. C. mAs has been doubled.
103. D. Be sure to review the Bucky factors.
104. A. Shorter wavelengths are more penetrating.
105. C. This is governed by the inverse square law.
106. D. There is more uniform penetration of the part, as well as an increase in the production of scatter.
107. D. There is a higher contrast because of photoelectric interactions.

108. D. The only factors listed that control recorded detail are SID and OID, and they are the same for each set of factors given.
109. A. Of all the factors listed, only kVp controls contrast. This set of factors has the lowest kVp and therefore exhibits the highest contrast.
110. C. Of all the factors listed, only SID and OID control magnification. This set of factors has the shortest SID.
111. A. Choice B would be correct if it included high kVp instead of low kVp. Choice C is incorrect because photoelectric interactions occur more often at lower kVp levels. Choice D is incorrect because Compton interactions occur at higher kVp levels.
112. D. This is why images at lower kVp tend to be more black and white.
113. B. Subject contrast is controlled by kVp and the atomic number of the part being radiographed. Choice A is true to a degree, but there is a better answer. Choice C is incorrect because recorded detail is a geometric function. Choice D is incorrect because characteristic radiation is produced at the anode.
114. B. Contrast increases because less scatter radiation is produced as a result of fewer Compton interactions. Choice A is incorrect because beam restriction reduces the number of Compton interactions, thereby increasing contrast. Choice C is incorrect because beam restriction reduces the number of Compton interactions, thereby shortening the scale of contrast.
115. D.
116. C.
117. B.
118. A.
119. B. Be sure to review these definitions. You are not likely to be asked more than one on the Registry exam, but you'll want to get it correct.
120. D.
121. C.
122. A.
123. D.
124. B. Review the various types of joints so you'll be able to handle any question you are asked about them.
125. D.
126. D.
127. A.
128. D
129. C. Be sure to review the major anatomy of the skull. Even though routine skull series are seldom performed, having been replaced by computed tomography, skull questions are still asked on the ARRT exam.
130. A.
131. B .
132. D.
133. B.
134. C.
135. B.
136. D.
137. D.
138. D.
139. D.
140. C.
141. D.
142. D. It is important to be able to "label" anatomy whether on drawings, on radiographs, or, as these questions illustrate, by using words.
143. C.
144. A.
145. B.
146. D.
147. D.
148. B.
149. C.
150. A.
151. A.
152. D. Be comfortable with answering questions regarding the alimentary canal and the urinary system. These types of questions are asked on the certification exam.

Study tips: For the following series of questions, be sure to know the exact centering point that you learned in positioning class and from Chapter 5 of this text. Also be aware that in some Registry exam questions you may be given ranges of angles from which to choose, making it easier to choose the correct answer. This may occur because not all positioning textbooks agree on certain angles.

153. D.
154. D.
155. B. This is difficult for a patient with an elbow injury.
156. A. Distinguish between PA and AP. Be sure to read carefully. Remember that the humerus and forearm must also be in the same plane.
157. D.
158. D.
159. D.
160. B.
161. A.
162. D.
163. A.
164. D.
165. C.
166. B.
167. C.
168. D.
169. D.
170. D.
171. B.
172. B
173. D.
174. C.

The preceding series of positioning questions has illustrated the level of knowledge you need going into the Registry exam. Be sure to review carefully and accurately. Don't panic. Just review some every day until you have mastered these facts.

175. D. Torts are a part of personal injury law.

176. C. Invasion of privacy involves violating confidentiality or improperly exposing the patient's body to viewing or radiation. Assault and battery involve threats and striking the patient.

177. D.

178. C.

179. B. *Respondeat superior* means "let the master answer." Gross negligence is a reckless disregard for life or limb. Slander is spoken defamation.

180. A. The heartbeat is regular but rapid.

181. C. Diastolic pressure is the blood pressure of the heart at rest.

182. D. Be sure to know the correct amount per unit time. Choice A would be damaging. The other choices would be inadequate. Read carefully.

183. B. The crash cart contains everything needed for a code blue, a defibrillator restores errant heartbeat, and the sp-hygmomanometer measures blood pressure.

184. C. The crash cart contains everything needed for a code blue, a defibrillator restores errant heartbeat, and the sphygmomanometer measures blood pressure.

185. D. Choice A is incorrect because hypovolemic shock is caused by a loss of fluids. Choice B is incorrect because septic shock follows massive infection. Choice C is incorrect because neurogenic shock causes blood to pool in peripheral vessels.

186. B. *Gastric* indicates that it flows into the stomach. Knowledge of medical terminology will greatly assist in ruling out some answers and carefully considering others.

187. D. You do not want urine to flow backward into the bladder, causing an infection.

188. A. Great care must be taken when performing a portable chest x-ray exam on a patient receiving mechanical ventilation.

189. D. Be sure to observe the F or C. You would not want to mix barium in water at 100 ° C.

190. A. Choice C does not make sense. Air is a gas, and iodine is not inert.

191. D.

192. A.

193. D. This can be caused by the mere suggestion of a reaction.

194. D. Literally, inflammation of a vein.

195. D. Contact is person to person, airborne is droplets and dust, and droplet is coughs and sneezes.

196. C. As explained in question 195.

197. A. As explained in question 195. Be sure to keep all of these straight.

198. B. Medical asepsis is not the complete removal, and gas sterilization is a way to sterilize equipment, not a patient care environment.

199. A.

200. D. Be sure to review the major medical terms you learned early in your program.

American Registry of Radiologic Technologists: *Radiography certification handbook and application materials,* St Paul, 2012, ARRT.

Bontrager K, Lampignano J: *Textbook of radiographic positioning and related anatomy,* ed 7, St Louis, 2009, Mosby.

Bushong S: *Radiologic science for technologists,* ed 9, St Louis, 2009, Mosby.

Callaway WJ: Graduate technologists and customer service, *Radiol Manage* 14:50, 1992.

Carter C, Vealé B: *Digital radiography and PACS,* St Louis, 2010, Mosby.

Ehrlich R, Daly J: *Patient care in radiography: with an introduction to medical imaging,* ed 7, St Louis, 2009, Mosby.

Eisenberg R, Johnson N: *Comprehensive radiographic pathology,* ed 5, St Louis, 2012, Mosby.

Fauber T: *Radiographic imaging and exposure,* ed 4, St Louis, 2013, Mosby.

Frank E, Long B, Smith B: *Merrill's atlas of radiographic positioning and procedures,* ed 12, St Louis, 2012, Mosby.

Gurley L, Callaway W: *Introduction to radiologic technology,* ed 7, St Louis, 2011, Mosby.

Jensen S, Peppers M: *Pharmacology and drug administration for imaging technologists,* ed 2, St Louis, 2006, Mosby.

Johnston J, Fauber T: *Essentials of radiographic physics and imaging,* St Louis, 2012, Mosby.

Mace J, Kowalczyk N: *Radiographic pathology for technologists,* ed 4, St Louis, 2009, Mosby.

National Council on Radiation Protection and Measurements: *Ionizing radiation exposure of the population of the United States,* NCRP Report No. 160, Bethesda, Md, 2009, NCRP.

National Council on Radiation Protection and Measurements: *Limitation of exposure to ionizing radiation,* NCRP Report No. 116, Bethesda, Md, 1993, NCRP.

National Council on Radiation Protection and Measurements: *Medical x-ray, electron beam and gamma-ray protection for energies up to MeV (equipment design, performance and use),* NCRP Report No. 102, Bethesda, Md, 1989, NCRP.

National Council on Radiation Protection and Measurements: *Quality assurance for diagnostic imaging,* NCRP Report No. 99, Bethesda, Md, 1988, NCRP.

National Council on Radiation Protection and Measurements: *Radiation protection for medical and allied health personnel,* NCRP Report No. 105, Bethesda, Md, 1989, NCRP.

Papp J: *Quality management in the imaging sciences,* ed 4, St Louis, 2011, Mosby.

Sherer M, Visconti P, Ritenour E: *Radiation protection in medical radiography,* ed 6, St Louis, 2011, Mosby.

Figures 2-1, 2-2, 3-2, 3-3, 3-4, 4-1, 4-2, 4-3, 4-4, 4-5 through 4-10—From Fauber TL: *Radiographic imaging & exposure*, ed 4, St Louis, 2012, Mosby.

Figure 3-1—From Bushong SC: *Radiologic science for technologists: physics, biology and protection*, ed 9, St Louis, 2008, Mosby.

Figures 3-5 and 7-15—From Malott JC, Fodor J III: *The art and science of medical radiography*, ed 7, St Louis, 1993, Mosby.

Figure 4-4—From *Mosby's radiographic instructional series: radiographic imaging*, St Louis, 1998, Mosby.

Figures 4-11 through 4-21 from Online Digital Imaging Academy, St. Paul, 2009, American Registry of Radiologic Technologists.

Figures 5-19 through 5-62 and 7-17 through 7-27—From Frank E: *Merrill's atlas of radiographic positions and radiologic procedures*, ed 12, St Louis, 2011, Mosby.

Figures 6-1 and 6-2—From Jensen S, Peppers M: *Pharmacology and drug administration for imaging technologists*, ed 2, St Louis, 2006, Mosby.

Figures 7-1 through 7-14—From Bontrager KL: *Textbook of radiographic positioning and related anatomy*, ed 7, St Louis, 2009, Mosby.

Please note:

The ARRT does not review, evaluate, or endorse publications. Permission to reproduce ARRT copyrighted materials within this publication should not be construed as an endorsement of the publication by the ARRT.